Happy Ending

by
Samuel A. Nigro, M.D.

Central Bureau, CCVA

Revised edition

$20.00
ISBN 1-887567-00-3

Published by

Central Bureau, CCVA
3835 Westminster Place
St. Louis, MO 63108

Dedicated to:

All those in Solidarity with Life, Liberty and the Peaceful Pursuit of Happiness.

Contents

FOR THESE *PROBLEMS* (AND RELATED ISSUES), GO TO THE CORRESPONDING *SACRAMENT* (NOTE: GRACE CAN ALSO APPLY TO EACH PROBLEM AS CAN OTHER SACRAMENTS AND VIRTUES

PROBLEM	***SACRAMENT***
Abortion	Baptism
Aggression	Holy Eucharist
Anxiety	Confession
Conflict	Matrimony
Death	Extreme Unction
Drugs/Alcohol	Confirmation
Employment	Holy Orders
Family	Matrimony
Future	Extreme Unction
Illness	Extreme Unction
Learning	Confirmation
Moods	Holy Eucharist
Peers	Confession
Pregnancy	Baptism
Religion	Holy Orders
Sexuality	Matrimony
Suicide	Baptism
Thoughts	Confirmation
Violence	Holy Eucharist
Withdrawal	Holy Orders
Work	Confession

Foreword

Samuel Nigro is a psychiatrist whose professional specialty is the family. Unlike the Hollywood cliché who is preoccupied more with his watch than his patients, Dr. Nigro is more than eager to work overtime in order to provide wise counsel, not only for his own patients, but for an expanded clientele of potential readers.

The title, *Happy Ending,* may conjure up images of fairy tales. Our cynical times no longer believes in either happy endings or fairy tales. But Dr. Nigro, who does believe in natural law, is realistic enough to understand how that can serve as a reliable basis for human happiness. Man has become alienated in the modern world: from himself, his nature, and his destiny. These essential parts have to be put back together again. Fragmentation is simply not natural. Spirit has fled, leaving us with mere matter to serve as a guiding star. Small wonder so many are lost.

For Dr. Nigro, nature is not as natural as it may look. It is really "charged with the grandeur of God." Hence, the main purpose of *Happy Ending* is to help people to see the spiritual through the material, to discern the harmony between science and religion, in short — to think and live sacramentally.

Happy Ending is Catholic in that it supports and reflects traditional Church teaching; it is catholic in that it incorporates what we have learned from science, history, life, and literature ("Sin is willful entropy."). It is a most unconventional tome, however, a veritable almanac (showing how *all men* should *act*). Though its conception is highly integrated, it is expressed in a highly unsystematic way. It is more a compendium of information than a piece of literature. At the same time, it represents a high regard, indeed, reverence, for the *word.* In fact, the words of another physician, Robert Southwell, could have served as an epigraph: "What thought can think, another thought can mend." Viktor Frankl has written about how unsound philosophies conveyed through misleading words and thoughts can be the root of a neurosis (Noögenesis or a noögenic neurosis). Dr. Nigro is most enthusiastic about reversing this trend. He employs the right words put in the right order to express the right thing. Confident about the healing potential of the word, he goes to considerable lengths in offering his readers verbal bromides, nourishing elixirs concocted of truth and thoughtful artistry. As a matter of fact, the bulk of the book is a compilation of epigrams.

Don Marquis spoke of the magical powers of the poet who can "stroke a platitude until it purrs like an epigram." Nigro wants us to see how matter shimmers with mysticism. Verily, as Whittaker Chambers has warned us, "Man without mysticism is a monster." A well-turned phrase, like philosophical insight, releases the spiritual component of each material event. It is precisely this spiritual component that enlarges our life and gives it wonder, direction, and purpose. A good psychiatrist wants to open doors for people (and not just the one that leads out of his office). He wants to free them from the claustrophobia of a one-dimensional existence. Even epigrams can open doors. Consider the following gem from the pen of Nathanial Hawthorne: "Happiness is a butterfly, which, when pursued, is always just beyond your grasp, but which, if you will sit down quietly, may alight upon you" (p. 230). Here, in an economy of words, we have a metaphor that explains why self-forgetfulness, rather than tenacity, is more likely to open the door to personal happiness.

Happy Ending is a cornucopia of intellectual and spiritual treats. It is engaging, enlightening, entertaining, instructive, and challenging all at once. Despite the seriousness of its subject matter, it is good fun, and, come to think of it, do we not enlarge our world when we forget our individual problems long enough to have some good, ol' fashioned fun?

Dr. Donald DeMarco
Kitchener, Ont.
July 12, 1995

PREFACE I:

THE GOOD NEWS IS TOO GOOD TO BE TRUE

After ignoring history and truth,
After lying, cheating, addicting, speeding,
After slandering and vilifying,
After violence and perversity.

After aborting, extorting, scalping, and killing,
After discriminating against, attacking, spying,
After delaying, wasting, stagnating,
After brutalizing, intimidating, blaming,

After fornicating, sodomizing, feminizing, masculinizing,
After raping and seducing,
After pornography and drugs,
After abandoning, ignoring, defeating, despiritualizing,

After cheating, dishonoring, debasing,
After reveling in animal passion,
After destroying and fouling,
After morbid boredom with created things,

After failed marriages,
After my children have become savages,
After decadence and barbarism,
After self-promoting "me, me, me,"
After stopping thinking, self-deceiving, and intellectual destruction,

After exploiting, fragmenting, dehumanizing, disintegrating and demoralizing others,
After sleepless nights without purpose,
After harried days without purpose,
After all has gone to hell,

Then I ask the perennial questions:

What are the final truths? What transcends to the highest perfection? What are the ultimate principles? What are the pressing things? The permanent things? What is? Do I know of my origins? Do I know my ultimate destiny? Have I rid myself of my sins?

And I finally ask:

Have I been to Confession?
Have I been to Communion?
Have I been to Church?
How is my relationship with God?
And what group has solidarity with the Ten Commandments?
And what group imitates Loving-Truth?
And what Church fights the tides of death and the evils of each age?
And therein I will find my true self as God made me,
And I will finally love myself, love God,
And I will find genuine Peace even on earth,
As a knowledgeable, praticing Roman Catholic.

And there is no reason to be sad when there is Joy—
the Catholic conclusion,

Because when with God, I am good no matter what!

PREFACE II:

HAPPY ENDING

"I'm tired of all the books, words and ideas and whatever — I want to know what's going on — I want to know how to live!" Thus spoke a young adult patient of mine.

The problem is in knowing "how to live" in a world where physical matter is prime. Scientific materialist emphasis on the physical world has resulted in an explosion of knowledge about the physical world such that religion seems to be a purely fanciful irrelevancy to the physical world. Before the knowledge explosion, the physical world was the mystery — and it was made understandable by religion. Now, the world is understood very well and religion seems unnecessary. But that is an illusion at best and massively wrong in the ultimate. Not only young adults are wanting "to know how to live," but it seems everyone is because they are engulfed in physical knowledge excluding religious understanding.

What this book is trying to do is to re-link the physical world to religious understanding by identifying the physical world counterparts to sacramental operations. A generation which only knows and even prefers physical facts needs to know significant spiritual analogues.

As a psychiatrist taking care of children, teenagers and adults of all ages for almost thirty years, "I want to know how to live" made me reflect on the secrets of life and whether they can ever be organized and given to everybody. Could a book be written not *about* life or about topics, but a book of living itself? Could a book be written which is a way of thinking and living regardless of what one believes. That is, be, believe, and act about everything as you want, but this is still the real way to live fully.

I next thought about myself as a psychiatrist who saw a lot, treated many, and read much and, who, finally, recognized how psychiatry and psychology have missed so much by denying the importance of religion...and how the mental health therapy field has not delivered well being for the people...and the case can be made that, by ignoring religion, matters have been made worse. And the idea occurred that somehow maybe what I learned, not only from my patients and family but from my readings could be organized and given to others to do with what they will. Everybody else can write *about* whatever. This book will accumulate *what is*. And it will be in people's well being emotionally, socially, culturally and spiritually.

The hubris of offering a book *of life* rather than *about life* must be apologized for, but I mean it just the same. I really believe that the material in this book contains the underlying themes and ways of thinking which are salutary for one's being regardless of what one knows, believes, or does. That is, it is "catholic." Or if you want, "Catholic" — meaning it is for everyone regardless. By reflecting on and living these messages, you can change your chemistry. You can change it for the better. In some instances, chemistry has gone haywire in our mental functioning and professional help will be needed, including medications. On the other hand, for most people, helpful messages will affect one's chemistry in a beneficial way just as extreme negative messages can influence the chemistry in our brains to develop and respond in negative ways that approach "evil." This book is to offer positive chemistry messages and a way of categorizing all messages sacramentally. It has been claimed that all life is sacramental, and if so, then all life is capable of being recognized as part of at least one of the sacraments. Once one begins to place all themes, messages, and activities into a sacramental mode, one becomes truly alive and lives life to the fullest. Doing such is merely not *about* life but IS life.

This book is divided into several parts beginning with a brief bewildering chapter condensing the interrelationships between sacraments and the physical world. The correlating charts are coherent but will be difficult because the ideas are new. The reader may find it beneficial to familiarize himself with the charts to some extent or to refer to them periodically as one goes through the remainder of the book. First is a chapter on the New Testament, the WORD, and words.

Next are chapters on each of the sacraments and grace. A body-soul/matter-spirit understanding of the sacraments is offered which is scientifically sound. With each sacrament and grace are offered many messages which can solve many problems and which can help one stay on a course of fulfilling Christian metamorphosis. These many messages have been allocated sacramentally...and present examples of how most of what you do can likewise be so allocated.

After the chapters on the sacraments, occurs a chapter of the most wonderful prayers for all purposes, followed by a brief chapter on virtues, gifts of the Holy Spirit, and sin. Next is a chapter on the Latin controversy with pro and con views presented and samples.

Then, three chapters on "Rapproachement. . . with" refer to Judaism, Islam and military service.

Finally, given is a brief chapter on anti-Catholicism is provided.

I hope the reader will learn to think sacramentally about everything and by living what is contained herein achieve a happy ending. Moreso, I hope the reader learns to understand all the spirituality in the physical world. Truly, the spiritual is more near than we usually realize.

It would be rude to not thank the man who edited, challenged, cajoled and laughed at my efforts. His task was one of Extreme Unction for me as well as Holy Orders, and I am deeply in his debt. He proved to me what I have always believed: That there is no where ever to be found a finer person than a good priest: in this instance Reverend John Miller, C.S.C. Thank you, Father Miller.

The extraordinary help of secretaries Norma Nero and Donna Mitchell was far beyond mere occupational effort encompassing Penance and Holy Eucharist...and if you read these chapters, you will know well what is meant.

Lillian Smith and Casey Koester provided the artwork as requested and I thank them for their patience and effort on behalf of my strange requests.

Finally, there are thousands of others whose sanctifying, civilizing, and sacramental messages should be added. But one has to stop somewhere. Nevertheless, I invite all to send to me their special messages which they believe should be incorporated into any future updating of this book.

Samuel A. Nigro, M.D.

Chapter 1:

BRIEF SACRAMENTAL OVERVIEW

Being a Catholic means following the personal live path to God by living within nature of the planet as sanctified by Jesus Christ. That is it in a nutshell. Anything other is extraneous and secondary.

It is a personal interaction between you and God. Again: Anything else is extraneous and secondary.

Yet, somehow, all extraneousness is related to by virtue of one's individual personhood — so all these extraneous aspects are not secondary when considered in the light of the path to travel to God. That is, there is a paradox in that our secondary and extraneous dimensions are all that we have in our personhood to achieve relating to God.

While the Church is in a sense also secondary and extraneous to our person relating to God, it nevertheless shows the way to God. By participating in our individual fullness as guided by the Church, we paradoxically embrace and participate in the total Church through the Mystical Body of Christ.

What people need to understand is that the way we do this individually is by the sacraments. We do not do this by promoting a political system, or an economic system, or a socialization phenomenon, or a military expansion, or any other ideology. Essentially, the sacraments keep personhood from being involved in any of these things to the degree that these things become primary. The sacraments set one above all of this. If the sacraments are followed, embraced and *lived*, one can somehow, not only participate still in any and all of these ideological aspects, but elevate them in a special way.

In this regard, Catholicism is the universal culture — it is the universal approach to all dimensions of life and can encompass them, thereby fulfilling the definition of Catholicity.

By the personal approach in this path to God, all is defined in personal terms whether it be evil or good. It has to do with one's own beingness as not involved in the earthly kingdom but seeking and following the trail to God in an extra-earth kingdom even though we are still on earth. We are enabled to achieve a personal holiness and thus achieve a personal resurrection, as one participates in the universe. But one must have the right messages reinforcing the right chemistry.

Through the Catholic Church the sacraments have been given which begin as rituals. These rituals are templates which start us and teach us much about how to follow the path to God. Each sacrament has its presence in the material of the universe. Once one grasps this fact, suddenly these rituals expand to encompass the world in an alarmingly exhaustive way. Suddenly soul and body are truly a total being embracing the physical world *and* the spiritual world. Thereby we suddenly become immune to the craziness of the world. We become beyond and above it because we recognize the first things and are more free therefore from the secondary ones. We realize that we are truly free.

Of course, this is what Jesus really brought us — *freedom.* Not "anything-goes" freedom, but genuine freedom, freedom which is the capacity to do good and the other transcendentals. Genuine liberty is the capacity to follow the trail of Jesus and fill one's life with the transcendentals *regardless* of where one is.

This is what the sacraments give us — ritually. It is very important for priests to see that these rituals are carried out. But even more important today, in a world filled with distractions of television, press and media, these rituals must be understood as something *to be lived* and not just undergone one or many times in one's life. The sacraments are to be lived.

When living the sacraments, one grows in personal *virtue*. The virtues enable personal growth and a personal relationship to God. Virtues actually are secondary living by-products of our interaction in natural law with the universe. Our beingness exudes virtue when we live our lives sacramentally — which means that we embrace the rituals with conscious awareness that the rituals are a sacramental way of participating in the physical universe. Thereby we will somehow extrude through life by a metamorphosis clearly given us by God. This confluence of our physical being with the spiritual is more and more difficult to imagine in today's world which almost completely emphasizes the physical to the exclusion of the spiritual. Whenever anyone comes to grasp the linkage with the physical and the spiritual, it must be far beyond the simplistic elaboration and foolishness offered in the press and media, as for example by astrology or New Age. Whatever others come up with will pale when compared to the profound depth offered by the Roman Catholic Church (read Dante).

While we live our lives in the city, country, social structures, church, employment states, educational experiences, political systems, and whatever else, we are enabled to be *free* of the negatives by virtue of the Catholicity of sacramental living, whether we realize it or not.

That is, we cannot be enslaved or injured by any of our cirumstances when we embrace the Church and live sacramentally. Our individual personhood, even if swamped by whatever is around us, cannot be negatively affected when we live the sacraments *personally*. The messages given in the book help promote such living. Actually, these messages *are* such living.

Physical/Spiritual Analogues

The contemporary emphasis on matter has tended to exclude the spiritual. This has been a tragedy in terms of outcome because essentially emphasis on the physical excludes free will and liberty. Science and matter result in a mechanistic philosophy negating free will unless the spirit can be found as a comprehensible, reasonable and automatic confluence with matter. What experience has been teaching us since the explosion of knowledge of matter during this century is that a mechanistic philosophy is no way to run the world.

Unless one can grasp the fundamental elements of physics as it describes matter and see in them the spiritual analogues, one will be doomed to follow a mechanistic approach to life which is unfree. Free will can only occur with the spiritual understanding of the physical world. There can be no genuine liberty without the concept of free will spiritually intoxicating people. This is only possible if one can see the transcendentals in all being. And this can only be accomplished if one can recognize sacramental living in our physical embracing of the universe.

The most fundamental description of basic physical components of matter have been appropriated from Stephen W. Hawking's *A Brief History of Time*. From that book, the most elemental understanding of the physical world is by eight constructs: event, spectrum, field, quantum, singularity, dimension, uncertainty, and force. Truly, if one does not understand something about those constructs, one does not really understand the physical world even though one knows an awful lot about the physical world. These eight elemental constructs in physics provide a structure analogous to what happens in the spiritual world. In a very real sense, that is what this book is all about: a scientifically consonant spiritual way of understanding the physical world and living therein sacramentally.

Stephen Hawking's eight constructs in physics are the following:

1. *Event* — a point in space-time of something that happens at a certain place in a certain time period.
2. *Spectrum* — the splitting of energy into position-time relationships.
3. *Field* — a matrix existing through space and time.
4. *Quantum* — the individual unit of receiving or giving energy.
5. *Singularity* — a point position at gravitational collapse wherein the space-time curve is infinite.
6. *Dimension* — Space coordinates in time.
7. *Uncertainty* — accuracy of position is inversely related to the accuracy of movement.
8. *Force* — that which affects the matter of particles.

This list is duplicated on the Sacramentalization Of The World Chart (p. 7) in the center under *BODY* as the third *PHYSICAL* column. Reading down this third column of body and physical constructs, physical existence is recognized to be a series of events by spectra in a field of quanta tending to collapse to a singularity in dimensions with uncertainty and force.

What can be recognized is that each physical construct has its counterpart in the psychological realm under the *MIND* which is the column immediately to the left of these physical constructs, and that each physical construct has its transcendental analogues as attributes of the *SOUL* in the column immediately to the right of the physical constructs. In addition, each physical construct has its analogue in the spiritual realm in the far columns of SACRAMENTS and GRACE as well as in the INCARNATING ACTS manifest by virtues as analogues to the physical constructs also.

That is, all physical constructs are spiritual in column one by Baptism, Penance, Communion, Confirmation, Extreme Unction, Holy Orders, Matrimony, and grace. This results in the permutations of the transcendental outcomes on the soul in column 4 resulting in dignity, unity, integrity, identity, spirituality, life, liberty, and the pursuit of happiness. The actual activities produced are listed in column 5, the incarnating acts of the virtues of faith, hope, charity, prudence, justice, fortitude, temperance and holiness.

In a world dominated by physical emphasis, these analogues emphasize the spiritual presence hidden and unrecognized unless listed, reflected upon, and practiced. One cannot alter or deny the laws of physics but properly understood, the physical universe can be spiritual and sacramental.

Roman Catholic Humanbeingness

The Roman Catholic Humanbeingness Chart (p.8-10) is actually natural law in action. It is merely a further elaboration of the first chart already reviewed.

This is more technical, but if one wants to understand the spiritual components of a physical world which is absolutely essential when one is being told that the physical is all there is, then reflection is necessary.

On the Humanbeingness Chart, the first column is that of statimuum (from the Latin "statim" meaning "immediately," i.e. the opposite of "continuum." The statimuum is wherein all is in all, the width and breadth of it personally experienced in total universe in one never ending moment — a forever all momentary compression of eternal immediacy — a scientific way of saying "heaven"):

> There is a very profound truth about the true excitement and inexhaustible poetry of life. The truth is not so much that eternity is full of souls as that one soul can fill eternity.
>
> G.K. Chesterton

Statimuum — that is, if there are "black holes" in the universe in which matter compresses to an incredible nothing, there must also exist a spiritual expansion encompassing all — a "white totality." Not a space-time continuum, but a spiritual STATIMUUM — the never-ending estay of Love and Truth surfeited eternally and infinitely — only feebly adumbrated by the best personal feelings ever experienced.

Back to the chart, the statimuum column links the sacraments with the psychological counterparts. That is, the psychologically and spiritual coincide in the statimuum as follows: in Baptism by relating to *living things are precious*; by Penance daily through *selectively ignoring* that which is negative; by Holy Eucharist through *subdued spontaneous charity but being true to one's self*; by Confirmation through *emotional self-control and affect assistance*; by Extreme Unction through *detached warmth and gentleness*; by Holy Orders through *non-reactive listening*; by Matrimony with *person-entered candidness*; and by grace as *relating with holiness* to all around.

The second column under the Roman Catholic Humanbeingness Chart is that of continuum — the space-time continuum. To continue the analogical description: every day has us participating in a *continuum physically*: in an *event*, with our energy split by *spectrums*, in a *field* of interaction, with a *quantum* of receiving or giving energy, near a *singularity* approaching infinity (because physical death is always near), within the *dimensions* of our existence, in an *uncertainty* of who and where we are, and by *force* which affects other materials and entities. This is a description of our body's interaction in the physical world at every moment of life.

Under the humanness column, it should be evident that each human being maintains *dignity* with each event, *unity* by a spectrum of energy, *integrity* throughout the fields of existence, *identity* in the giving and receiving of energy by quanta, *spirituality* by approaching singularity, *life* within all dimensions, *liberty* associated with its uncertainty, and maintain a *pursuit of happiness* with the forces within one's grasp.

Finally, the activity column reveals virtuous outcomes analogous to the physical world embraced according to right reason and spirit.

Summary

That is, what each person has through Catholicism and sacraments is a different understanding and level of existence for birth, development, suffering and death. Through the impact of Jesus and His Church (and Mary and Joseph and the saints too, but they are secondary helpers and in a real sense unnecessary but historically important in at least being reminders, models and intercessors), the world is changed because our chemistry has changed into a different level of totally profound grasp.

This is an extremely *personal* experience which of course involves us in the universe wherever we are and with whomever we have come into contact.

By sacramental living, a different life is being lived. By virtuous dealing with all and remaining true to natural law with all, we literally spiritually escape from all that surrounds us, but we engage *for the better* all that is around us enabling a transition as experienced on the earth as in another presence because by being this way, we are "not of this world," even though we engage this world. Finally, such living will enable us to undergo a transition through our efforts but still absolutely made possible by Jesus showing us the way and opening the way as a free gift to all. The way was opened and the method was only made known and paid for by Jesus whose example from birth, development, suffering, and death was a realistic and graphic exposition of what we are undergoing.

Thus, the sacraments understood, embraced, and *lived* make us free! Not of this world! And ready at any time to make the transition joyfully (at all times) into the next.

Somehow, hopefully realized will be that the sacraments of the Church offer the supernatural. The sacraments give grace. They enable thinking in the finest sense. The sacraments give Loving Truth. The sacraments give the very life of God. . .here on earth. . .and possibly forever. And the sacraments should be lived day in and day out.

The myriad messages offered in this book are consistent with the charts. Almost all human activities can be allocated sacramentally according to the psychology of the activity itself. Living one's life with this interaction is to *live* in a physical world in a spiritual way. Deeper reflection and meditation on each message will enable one to spiritualize the physical world. Indeed, one will be linked into the physical world in a way that brings it to a higher, different level and into a metamorphosis that we cannot fully understand but still can aesthetically sense. Once one begins to do this, almost all messages and activities can be placed in a sacramental category. Thereby the world of thinking changes. As you read and hear about anything and everything, keep it in sacramental and transcendental perspective and then think and live this way. This is the way really to live. It places one beyond the physical senses. It gives one a self-knowledge and a divine intuition.

The summary chart on the page eight outlines *ROMAN CATHOLIC HUMANBEINGNESS* which is "Natural Law in Action." Four columns are presented with the items in each column coinciding at the same level with items in other columns.

The first column is STATIMUUM. Therein, the *forms* of things in the universe are engaged by the *soul* in terms of *appetite*, i.e., desirables (that which attracts) or aversives (that which repels). The first item is *Baptism*, the pattern of which is "living things are precious."

CHART: THE SACRAMENTALIZATION OF THE WORLD

SACRAMENTS and GRACE	combine *MIND*,	*BODY*, and	*SOUL* to	*INCARNATING ACTS*
Spiritual	*Psychological*	*Physical**	*Transcendental*	*Virtues*
Baptism	Living things are precious	Event	Dignity	Faith
Penance	Selective ignoring	Spectrum	Unity	Hope
Holy Eucharist	Subdued spontaneity nonself excluded	Field	Integrity	Charity
Confirmation	Affect assistance	Quantum	Identity	Prudence
Extreme Unction	Detached warmth and gentleness	Singularity	Spirituality	Justice
Holy Orders	Noncreative listening	Dimension	Life	Fortitude
Matrimony	Person entered Candidness	Uncertainty	Liberty	Temperance
Grace	Allegiance to mankind through Jesus and his church	Force	Pursuit of Happiness	Holiness

A sacrament is an outward sign instituted by Christ to give grace. It involves three things: an outward or visible sign, the institution of that sign by Christ, and the giving of grace through the use of that sign. Each sacrament is based upon Scripture and has its origin traced back to its early use by the first members of the church instituted by Christ from the very beginning. Sacraments are the ancient secret formulae which allow space-time creatures to transform into eternity.

* From a *Brief History of Time* by Stephen W. Hawking

ROMAN CATHOLIC HUMANBEINGNESS

[Natural Law in Action]

STATIMUUM* [Form] [Soul] [Appetite]	CONTINUUM [Matter] [Body] [Senses]	HUMANNESS [Intellect] [Truth] [Senses]	ACTIVITY [Will] [Loving-Beauty & Goodness] [Appetite]
Baptism *Living things are precious.*	Event A point in space-time of something that happens at a certain place and a certain time.	Dignity	Faith—assent to God
Penance *Selective Ignoring*	Spectrum The splitting of energy into position-time relationships.	Unity	Hope—Trust in ultimate positivity and asension
Holy Communion *Subdued spontaneity, non-self excluded.*	Field A matrix existing through space and time.	Integrity	Charity—Conscious commitment to perfection
Confirmation *Affect assistance*	Quantum The indivisible unit of receiving or giving energy.	Identity	Prudence—Pratical reason seeing and reognizing the will of God in all things and aware of the interdependence of all virtues in life.
Extreme Unction *Detached warmth and gentleness*	Singularity A point position at gravitational collapse wherein the space-time curvature is infinite.	Spirituality	Justice—Regard for and giving to all that is due them.
Holy Orders *Non-reactive listening*	Dimension Space coordinates and time	Life [Father]	Fortitude—Strong, firm, assured practice of all virtues in pursuit of Good.
Matrimony *Person-entered candidness*	Uncertainty Accuracy of position is inversely related to the accuracy of movement	Liberty [Son]	Temperance—Moderation and self-control
Grace *Relationship*	Force That which effects matter particles.	Pursuit of Happiness [Holy Spirit]	Holiness—Dedicated and Consecrated to God's service.

*from the Latin "statim" meaning "immediately" — the opposite of "continuum" — statimuum — wherein all is in all, the width and breadth of it personally experienced in total universe in one never ending moment — a forever all momentary compression of eternal immediacy — a scientific way of saying "heaven"

The second column is CONTINUUM which is the temporal-spatial world wherein the *matter* of objects is perceived by the person's *body* through the *senses.* The first item is *event* and is defined from Stephen W. Hawking's book "A Brief History of Time" (as are all the items listed under the CONTINUUM column).

The third column is HUMANNESS which is composed of those transcendental principles by which the intellect grasps *truth* through the *senses*. The first item in the HUMANNESS column is that of *dignity*.

The fourth column is ACTIVITY in which the free *will* seeks *loving* through its orientation towards the appetites (desirables or aversives). The first item under the ACTIVITY column is that of *faith*, which is the assent to God.

The horizontal linkage of each item in the four columns requires reflection:

Baptism patterns the form of "preciousness of life" just as *event* emphasizes a space-time point of existence. For the human, this means the intrinsic *dignity* of that point of human life. The awareness of this results in not only an assent *(faith)* to the individual but seeks the higher good through recognizing God as the basis for this Being.

The second item is *Penance* wherein negative occurences are to be "selectively ignored" and split to insignificance. This coincides in the physical-temporal world with *spectrum* wherein energies are split. For the human, the principle of *unity* is forthcoming, accompanied by *hope* in that the negativity will be selectively ignored and positivity will create ascension.

The third level linkage is *Holy Eucharist* (patterning of "spontaneity and genuineness") which coincides in the physical world with *field*, i.e., a matrix of space and time. The resulting human principle is that of *integrity* wherein *charity* results by the conscious suffering commitment to personal perfection, spontaneously and genuinely pervading the universe.

The fourth level is that of C*onfirmation*, a pattern of "assisting emotions" as coinciding with *quantum*, i.e., energy units being given and received in the physical world. The resulting human principle is *identity* leading to the activity of *prudence* wherein one's own identity is willed to energize all interdependently as well as in concert with God.

The fifth level items begin with *Extreme Unction* patterned by "detached warmth and gentleness." It coincides with the physical *singularity* at which point infinity is approached at gravitational collapse. The humanness principle here is *spirituality* enabling the activity of *justice* to be forthcoming because at infinity all is given which is due.

The next items begin with *Holy Orders* wherein the universe is "non-reactively listened" to in the *dimensions* of poverty, chastity, obedience and timelessness (coinciding with the physical *dimensions* of space coordinates and time), evoking and emoting the human principle of *life* (personified by the Father) activated by *fortitude*, i.e., the courageous practice of virtues in pursuit of good while confronting adversity.

The seventh level is that of *Matrimony* wherein "person-conscious centered" open relatingness occurs coinciding with *uncertainty* in the physical world meaning that all accuracies are not known. The human principle resultant is that of *liberty* (personified by the Son) resulting in the activity of *temperance* wherein moderation and self-control results enabling two to become one.

The final level of items begin with *grace*, the "strings" between human particles manifest in the physical world by *force* affecting matter particles. The human principle resulting is that of *pursuit of happiness* (personified by the Holy Spirit). The activity resultant is that of *holiness* by dedication to the service of God.

In summary, Natural Law in action is Roman Catholic humanbeingness. The spiritual world of the Statimuum has counterparts observable in the physical world of the space-time continuum. The fundamental principles of humanness have counterparts in the world of activity and choice. By full participation in the physical world at the level of humanness, one participates in the Statimuum. By such, you are Roman Catholic. You will ascend. Joy will be yours. There is a happy ending.

CHAPTER 2:

THE GOOD NEWS — THE NEW TESTAMENT — THE WORD (and words)

Presaging Christ, Socrates discerned: "Be of good cheer and know this of a truth-that no evil can happen to a good man either in life or after death." Socrates went on to say that the good man is one doing things with right reason and virtue. Add the sacraments and he would have had Roman Catholicism. All this is a simple way of saying that only by adhering directly or indirectly to the principles of the Roman Catholic church can no evil happen and can people be saved. This is because the church stands for the supernatural and for the best of the natural. The church and her principles from Christ stand the test of time as they adhere to Jesus and the Apostles. This is the Good News. And it is an old message written down as the New Testament by the church itself.

Even so, Good News language seemingly fails to clarify "What is God?" Indeed language is inadequate for humans to grasp God as fish cannot communicate to each other: What are people? Belief is not the problem, but simple stories, puzzling parables, and inadequate words constitute communication deficiencies which account for disbelief. Humans only have the language of each epoch and that language often does not ring true to those following or preceding (can we understand two thousand year old words? could people of those centuries understand our describing today?)

So how then can God inform us without massively overwhelming us?

Using one's wildest imagination, how would God come to us? And then how would God come to us in a way which would enable the existence of human freedom which is necessary for us to be in the image and likeness of God?

Paradise?

First, would God give us everything? Would God give humans a totally fulfilled paradise as inadequately described by the story of the Garden of Eden? Imagine that Garden! Imagine God giving man all Paradise, and a Paradise to be paradise *must* include freedom. As in Genesis, freedom in such a paradise could be present by one simple free choice about a specific act of taking or avoiding a forbidden fruit amidst all the startling cornucopia of good. According to ancient human tradition known as Divine Scripture, we know this is exactly what was provided to mankind in the beginning, and that we humans failed that simple freedom. God giving "all" with freedom present by one simple choice was not enough. Humans still did not grasp God as total Goodness and disobeyed the simple single prohibition offering free choice. Given paradise minus one small choice, humans chose the one wrong thing! Clearly giving humans almost everything did not work. This ancient biblical description seems simple and it is because of its age, but certainly a scientific story could not be forthcoming 2,000 years ago (the language problem alluded to earlier?). But it is not an irrational explanation and it clearly conveys a massively possible message that "all was given but lost." The creature God created has a strong propensity to choose wrongly even when life is easy because he is surrounded by everything positive. . . .Tell me about it!

Terror?

So what next? How about terror? Would God come to us with fear and violence as graphically described in the Old Testament? That obviously was done (Sodom and Gomorrah, for examples), but just as in the Garden of Eden, humans could neither understand nor identify God's arrival in fear and violence. Humans are slow learners and fast forgetters. Nay, humans did not persistently grasp God in massive violence but in fact imitated the violence in massive arrogance. Thusly, after Paradise, terror did not work either, and God laughed joyfully at the free but weird creature He created whom He could no longer bribe and could no longer scare.

The cosmos?

If not by All Goodness or by Abject Fearsomeness, how else would God come to us and still give us choice (Freedom is necessary!)? Something spectacular would certainly do it. . .something similar to a laser light show panorama in contemporary entertainment but magnified almost infinitely! But this method of presentation of God would deprive humans of freedom by the overwhelming awesomeness of it all if it were continuous. But even then, it is possible that humans would develop tolerance to the grandeur and gradually pay it little mind. And if the Grand Spectacular were not continuous, written or oral history from the actual viewers would probably fail to convey it anyway to those who had not seen it. A growing number of skeptics would just not be convinced. However, if the Grand Spectacular were continuous and tolerance did not develop, such a dazzling cosmic splendor would deprive humans of that very freedom which is essential for humans to return to God by being able to *choose* Loving-Truth. That is, there is no real choice, no real freedom, in facing such an awesome cosmic spectacular, so this splendorous percept does not seem reasonable (unless it is the Universe itself? — that is, the universe itself could be the ongoing Grand Spectacular to which we indeed *have* developed tolerance??).

The Word **(and words)!**

When one deeply reflects on how God would come to us and leave our freedom intact, one is left with the reasonableness of what the Good News says actually did happen: God communicated with us and joined us by sending a man who rose from the dead after giving witness to a bizarre, out-of-this-world, never-contemporary Loving-Truth, and the Man He sent to us is somehow mystically God Himself. What happened is not unreasonable: The appearance of Jesus Christ, the God-Man, entering the poorest of the poor, establishing genuine freedom, espousing profound love, witnessing precise truth, fulfilling hundreds of ancient prophecies, performing miracles, all as *one-of-us*, demonstrating human emotions, participating in a terrible death by crucifixion, and then opening the awareness and possibility of existential infinity by rising from the dead, opening the doors to dimensions of existence whose boundaries are truly spiritual and immeasurable, but more real than the events, spectra, fields, quanta, singularities, dimensions, uncertainties, and forces of the spirituality with which our physicists struggle to define the space-time universe.

After Paradise and Terror failed successively and the cosmos taken for granted, it is perfectly reasonable for God to try something else — like becoming human Himself. This Christianity clarifies: *that the Divine Spectacular is provided in a human manner with freedom intrinsic to choosing belief or unbelief.* The awesomeness is calibrated with startling vividness but humanized with the vacuity of choice — a rational balance between the overpowering and the deliberating. The divine is offered in a human way!

If one believes that there is a God, then it is difficult to believe that an effort would not be made to communicate and to have a relationship with His creatures. In such regards, there is nothing unreasonable about Jesus Christ and his Roman Catholic Church which rigidly maintains trust and allegiance to the Loving-Truth as Jesus Christ presented it: a Loving-Truth which is the Body of Christ, which is human and divine, which is matter and spirit, which is physics and theology. This is the Good News: the Gospels and Tradition. The church tells the Good News, not what you *want* to hear. Lovingly, the true church will tell you God's messages which need to be heard. . . The Word of God.

The first source of all "heard" (word) knowledge is the New Testament. Today in addition to having the Bible as a traditional book for a household, a set of audio cassette tapes of the New Testament is highly recommended. No young adults should claim they are Catholic (or Christian) without having *read* or *heard* the New Testament *at least once*! Audio cassettes nicely fill this function. Youths must be challenged to *listen* to the New Testament from start to finish if they proclaim themselves to be believers in one God.

Two thousand years ago, our world was filled with uncivilized pagan savagery and disgust. There was no Pollyannish, happy, innocent, idyllic life (a commonly held myth resulting from surmising that the past must have been better than the present since our present world seems so negative). Actually, two thousand years ago and before was a nightmare of primitiveness. Anthropologists to the contrary, life without missionaries was pretty grim.

Pre-Christ life, like life without Christ now, was, with few exceptions, incapable of sustained ascendancy in thought, in search for truth, in advancement of knowledge, and in fulfilling relationships.

However, like a bolt of lightning, love and truth (at times painful, unwanted, and unpleasant) appeared on the scene, offering not a Revolution but a Lovelution — a gift which has lasted over two thousand years. To listen to the New Testament is to hear what took place and realize that what happened was from out of this world! Here were ideas never heard before. Imagine being there and experiencing New Testament history as it happened. compare it to what was common in other primitive societies. Perhaps it will become understandable how startling is the nature of the New Testament message.

The apostles forged Christ's message into really *new* ideas — forever new! Regardless of young people's proclaiming "newness," everything else has been tried and found wanting — but each generation appears to have to try the old ideas again and again. Thankfully, a few souls do discover and apply the new ideas of the New Testament. . .and live as happily as one can on this earth. The rest wallow in the pseudo-new — and wonder why it does not work.

Sadly, most of us take the Good News for granted when in fact the Word is needed as much now as in the days of the apostles.

All should listen to the New Testament as if hearing secret documents containing the secrets of life. . .because that is what is being heard. New Testament characters were not whimpering around saying "we love everybody." They *lovingly told the truth* (with words!), enabling themselves and others that followed to be free. They challenged. They enlightened mankind as to the issues of right from wrong. Jesus, the God-man, was killed for telling the truth and His followers were persecuted and killed also. Today is not different. Pay heed to what is presently attempted to discredit and hurt the Roman Catholic Church as it proclaims Jesus' loving messages (words) of truth — the Good News as given to the world by the Roman Catholic church.

OTHER WORDS IN EXISTENCE — ANGELS

St. Paul says "If I speak in the tongues of mortals and of angels. . ." (1 Corinthians 13). To that, I say: Interesting that he groups mortals and angels together! And more interesting is that he implies that he indeed can "speak in the tongues of mortals and of angels!"

Jesus is the WORD — an apt description with implications not fully developed especially in terms of God's other creation in His image: angels.

This hypothesis is put forward: words create (temporally, not in the absolute) and coincide with the angelic hierarchy (not all words. . .but most do!).

Think about it: Every word conjures up an image. . .a quasi-spiritual accompaniment. Words, phrases, and language have metaphysical dimensions and metaphysical stature of sorts. When Ralph Waldo Emerson writes that "Nature itself is the symbol of spirit" and "the whole of nature is a metaphor of the human mind," he is getting close. He, as others, stops too soon. Nature can only be described, symbolized, named, defined, and imagined by *words*. The same goes for intuition and thinking. With words are the sense of spirit, the sacred, and secrecy. Words transcend as they corrupt. Are they therefore wrongly thought of as being angels or demons?

Words are the nearest things existing which approach that which we understand angels to be. That is, if angels are created beings without *res* (matter) but with *ens* (an existence) and the other transcendentals of *aliquid* ("definition" or identity/form/essence), *verum* (truth), *unum* (oneness), *bonum* (good) and *bella* (beauty), then angels can be seen analogically as words! After all, words are limited to conscious-of-consciousness capable creatures (thus far, such creatures appear limited to human beings alone by mankind's direct experience).

Furthermore, words can be hierarchically categorized. The existence of words and the temporal semi-material order for mankind gives evidence (by the very non-materiality of words) to more spiritual and less material fully existent comparable phenomena (angels).

As the WORD traditionally is identified as the ultimate spiritual entity of Jesus the Christ, Son of God and God Himself, so too can *each word* be postulated as having a spirit angelic counterpart whose existence needs acknowledgement, whose power needs invoking, and whose aid needs be given thanks. Each word is or has an angel. . . No one knows which it is or if it is even both or not at all. Regardless, how could we name all the angels without using the words we have? Needless to write, only the proper use of each word would allow its full angelic impact.

In this regard, angels indeed are everywhere and we use them everyday by words leading us to the WORD.

Analogies

It is interesting to reflect on descriptions of angels in the past in the light of this hypothesis: that they are somehow identifiable with words.

The letters of St Paul and St. Peter and describe the presence of angels and the Old Testament confirms that angels were "ministers and servants of the Lord."

John Henry Newman has described angels as "the agency of the thousands and the ten thousands of His unseen servants." To identify angels as words while reading St. Thomas on "The Angels" is to have at least a glimmer of insight. . .just perhaps. . . And Leon J. Podles has written:

> Angels present an interesting philosophical question to Aquinas — If matter is the principle of individuation in the species, each angel is a species. That is, angels differ among themselves as much as an elephant differs from an alligator.

But cannot the same be said about words?

Podles also states:

> All actions in the material world are accomplished through the agency of angels, who conduct the divine light to the world through their hierarchies as the ecclesiastical hierarchies conduct grace throughout the church. . . .Perhaps angels are the channels of invisible communication among men, the hidden messengers that allow us to see briefly into the mind of another person.

And about preternatural events that defy rational explanation, Podles says: "They have the mark of personality." It is difficult to deny "words" as analogous to all the above.

Dante calls angels the "birds of God." And one cannot help but think of a dictionary when he writes:

> . . .and all around that enter, wings outstretched
> I saw more than a thousand festive angels,
> each one distinct in brilliance and in art.

Dante has Satan's hideous body frozen upside down in ice flailing his wings thereby cementing himself more frozen, but cold inarticulate breezes waft from him permeating the universe as demonic lies, the unspeakable, and deforming sounds of corrupted language.

One thinks of John Milton's:

> The mind is its own place, and in itself
> can make Heav'n of Hell, and Hell of Heav'n.

And it does all this with words — angelic or demonic! As Milton also writes:

> To visit oft the dwellings of just men
> Delighted, and with frequent intercourse
> Thither will send his winged messengers
> On errands of cupernal grace.

Furthermore, Milton's other word for the study of angels was "pneumatology"!

Marion Montgomery has written:

> Dr. Johnson remarks of *Paradise Lost*. . .that spirit allows no image, and most especially imagery is disallowed to that perfect intellectual creature, the angel. . . [A]ccording to the limits of man's nature, [man] is inescapably imperfect as maker because [he is] a fallen and so imperfect intellectual creature. Further, he is burdened by a discursive intellect dependent upon the orders of nature for initial understanding of being itself. As incarnate soul, that nature sets him quite apart from that pure spiritual being peculiar to angelic natures, in envy of which we have sentimentalized that angelic nature as if our own.

One can live with that — and even think of words as angels, because such a construct may be the best and nearest way to understand angels.

Paul Claudel has written "The Hymn of the Holy Angels" and one part of it is the following:

> God the Father — God who knows
> all His nestlings by their names —
> has gathered in his mansion, sealed
> with seven seals, these winged seeds
> in all their myriad multitudes,
> different each from each in kind,
> being, from Angels to the Seraphim,
> the types and prophecies of all
> Creation and, within the Eternal
> Zion, Preface to the Holy Mass.

Can this not apply to words as angels?

And remember St. Hildegard's reflections on God's impact: "Mine is the blast of the thundered word by which all things are made." Indeed, if the Word was made flesh, cannot words be made spirits?

Psalm 91:12 says: "For you, he has commanded angels to guard you in all your ways." Pray tell, how except by words. And the Psalms seem filled with such imagery: "Oh voice of mercy! Oh words that give to our hearing the joy of salvation!" and "abyss calleth an abyss" and "the voice of power". . . Psalm 85:11-12 proposes: "Mercy and truth will meet; justice and peace will kiss. Truth will spring from the earth; justice will look down from Heaven." One can begin to sense the spirit coinciding with words. Psalm 94:10 states: "Yahweh, the teacher of mankind who knows exactly how we think, how our thoughts are a puff of wind."

And Proverbs 9:1 says: "Wisdom hath built herself a house, she hath hewn out her seven pillars." Is wisdom an angel?

Words worked their wonders and misdeeds for the Romans too who called angels *boni et mali Genii*.

Thomas Decker writes: "We are never like angels 'til our passion dies." Can such not apply to our *good* words in contrast to the passionate demonic ones?

Please think of *words* as others have written about angels:

'Tis only when they spring to Heaven that angels
Reveal themselves to you.

Robert Browning

The angels are dispensers and administrators of a Divine beneficence toward us; they do regard our safety, undertake our defense, direct our ways, and exercise a constant solicitude that no evil befall us.

John Calvin

Make yourself familiar with the angels, and behold them frequently in spirit; for without being seen, they are present with you.

St. Francis de Sales

An angel is a spiritual creature created by God without a body, for the service of Christendom and the church.

Martin Luther

In this dim world of clouding cares
we rarely know, till 'wildered eyes
See white wings lessening up the skies,
The angels with us unawares.

Gerald Massey

The angels may have wider spheres of action, they have nobler forms of duties; but right with them and with us is one and the same thing.

Chapin

Words are the only things that live forever.

G.K. Chesterton

St. Bernard translates Isaiah 11:2-3 as follows:

And the Spirit of the Lord shall rest upon Him: The spirit of wisdom and of understanding, the spirit of counsel and of fortitude, the spirit of knowledge and of piety, and he shall be filled with the spirit of the fear of the Lord.

This fits well when St. Bernard writes: "Say the word and receive the Word."

About angels, Hebrews 1:14 says: "Are they not all ministering spirits, sent to serve for the sake of those who are to inherit salvation?" What else but words!

Without awareness of this hypothesis linking angels and words, in a personal communication to me, Father Fred Barnett of the Motherhood Shrine in Laurie, Missouri, described his vocal cords as "angel wings" when he viewed them as part of a medical examination. His description did not surprise the physicians and others involved in laryngeal studies and treatments, because vocal cords have been

ANGELS AS THE WORD SPECTRUM

Each word has (is?) an angel?

(Latin, Scripture & Tradition)

Seraphim
- Transcendentals!
- Executive-Leadership

Cherubim
- Wisdom-filled
- Operating Knowledge
- Faith/Events
- Legislative
- Operating Words

Thrones
- Free Judgments
- Interrelating
- Hope/Spectrum
- Judiciary
- Judgmental Words

(Latin and cross-cultural words)

Dominions
- Reason and creation
- Perfection in Space/Time
- Theology
- Charity/Field

Virtues
- Operational Order
- Spatial Identities
- Law
- Prudence/Quanta

Powers
- Protective Function
- Spiritual Infinity-Closeness
- Medicine and Safety
- Justice/Singularities

(Cultural words)

Principalities
- Groups of groups and community time-based coherence
- Community life-nations/cities/political-social
- Fortitude/Dimensions

(Sub-Cultural Family Words)

Archangels
- Groups of individuals linked and co-existing in moment and position
- Family and extended family groupings
- Temperance/Uncertainties

(Daily Living Words)

Angels
- Individual guardians of individual men
- Pursuit of Happiness
- Holiness/Force
- Each person has a guardian angel carrying the person's name

---

("Fallen" Angels)

Demons
- Anti-Words: hateful, violent, manipulations and suggestions to sin
- Lies
- Astrology and Television/Movies and the language of the foul and demeaning
- Fools with long words and large vocabularies that do not coincide with transcendental existence

called "angel wings" almost since the beginning of the use of vocal cord observation instruments! This is truly an unanticipated, astonishing coincidence.

The reader is encouraged to review the following summaries: "Angels as the Word Spectrum" (page 19), "The Hierarchy of Angels", and "The Universe, Angels, and Words in Action (page 22)." Then page through a dictionary reflecting on the angelic counterparts to words.

THE HIERARCHY OF ANGELS

A hierarchy exists consistent with God's governing all created being and establishing order in the universe. This hierarchy has been known for thousands of years in the generic sense as "angels." An ancient secret is that to function effectively in the universe an elementary knowledge of the hierarchies of angels is important especially if one wants to exert maximum influence on the governing spirits existent. Without a doubt, angelic influences are more real than any of the emotional, flashing, flickering light charlatans in television, movies and light shows.

The following three categories of angels constitute the first hierarchy according to the description by St. Thomas. Essentially, they constitute the balance of powers available to us in a higher level of the universe and society: Executive, Legislative and Judiciary.

Seraphim are those angels nearest to God in perfect contemplation of the intelligible transcendental essences within God. Love of genuine Form, Truth, Oneness, Good and Beauty ending in God are what these angels embrace. Whatever little Seraphim have to do with humans is limited to the highest executive levels of mankind. Therefore, one should only appeal to Seraphim in regards to one's leaders and rulers and a quest for total Transcendental Love.

Cherubim are those angels which contemplate divine goodness via wisdom with operating knowledge of God's confluence with the universe. Whatever Cherubim have to do with humans has to do with the legislative implementing operational aspects of the universe. The events of these angels are natural operations. If witnessing to Transcendental confluence is desired, more faith can be placed in Cherubim.

Thrones are those angels which contemplate dispositions of divine judgments in terms of the outcomes of events in a free universe. Whatever Thrones have to do with humans is linked to judiciary dimensions existent, and these angels should be invoked for judicial matters. Thrones are a good example of how angels are split energy forms intellectually required by and for the unity of the universe. If all creation is balanced by a spectrum of unrecognizable interrelating, more hope can be placed in Thrones.

The next three categories of angels constitute the second hierarchy in St. Thomas' description and have to do essentially with the learned professions: Theology, Law and Medicine (safekeeping).

Dominions (or Dominations) are those angels who know the reason of things in universal ordering of created life. Whatever Dominions have to do with humans has to do therefore with the highest level of thinking at a theological level. In such regards, Dominions reveal that angels are the creatures spanning space and time linking perfection. All being in a field of spontaneous total rationality will have more charity by considering the Dominions.

Virtues are those angels involved in the operational effectuation of universal ordering. Whatever Virtues have to do with humans, they are involved in legal aspects and laws — all laws. In such regards, Virtues reveal that angels are quanta affirming spatial identities. In considering the giving and taking of ordered energy, more prudence comes from considering the Virtues.

Powers are those angels involved in the protection from evil influences and confusion. Their involvement with humans has to do with medicine, military, and safety services for general functioning. As such, Powers reveal that angels are singularities in and at spiritual infinity. If good and beauty are to be maintained, then more justice will come from considering the Powers.

The last three categories of angels constitute the third hierarchy of and have to do with the general functioning of mankind: Nation/Cities, Family Groupings and Individuals.

Principalities are those angels concerned with the course and general good of human grouping of groups such as the general good of nations and cities. Whatever Principalities have to do with humans is related to community life in the broad sense. In such regards, Principalities reveal that angels are dimensions of life required for a coordinated time-bound, coherent universe. If good is to be personal in such existence, more fortitude will come from considering the Principalities.

Archangels are those angels concerned with individuals in groups of linked relationship. Whatever Archangels have to do with humans is ordinarily related to a family-like situation. Archangels reveal angels to be uncertainties in the freedom between movement and position. If self-control and motion are sought to coexist, more temperance will come from considering the Archangels.

Angels are those specific angels (in contrast to the generic term "angel") who are concerned as individual guardians of individual men (male and female). Whatever Angels have to do with mankind, it is at the individual personhood level from the moment of conception to the end of one's life at least. In this regard, Angels are forces of the pursuit of happiness. If God is a belief, more holiness will come from considering the Angels.

THE UNIVERSE, ANGELS, AND WORDS IN ACTION

If one does not study thoughtfully and pray for angelic help at the appropriate levels as described, one ends up with fortune tellers, astrologers, enneagrams, New Age feel good fantasies, and other ineffective approaches that get one nowhere. One must pray to the right category of angels as they are linked to the universe to be effective in using their forces. And it helps to know the right words using and praying with them as if angels. . .because they probably are.

Area of concern	*Angels to Whom to Pray for Aid*	*Corresponding Words*
Leadership-Executive-Transcendentals	Seraphim	Latin, Scripture & Tradition
Legislative-Operational-Wisdom-Faith/Events	Cherubim	Latin, Scripture & Tradition
Judiciary-Free Judgment-Interrelating-Hope/Spectrum	Thrones	Latin, Scripture & Tradition
Theology-Reason and all Creation-Perfection as Spectrum-Charity/Field	Dominions	Latin & cross-cultural Words
Law-Ordering-Operational Order-Spatial Identities -Prudence/Quanta	Virtues	Latin & cross-cultural Words
Medicine and Safekeeping-Protective Functioning-Spatial Infinity Closeness-Justice/Singularities	Powers	Latin & cross-cultural Words
Nations, States, Cities-Community Time-Bound/Coherence in Political Social Realm-Fortitude/Dimensions	Principalities	Cultural Words
Family Groups-Groups of Individuals linked in Motion and Position-Temperance/Uncertainties	Archangels	Subcultural Family Words
Self-Individual Guardians-Genuine Pursuit of of Happiness-Holiness/Force	Guardian Angels	Daily Living Words
Evil	Demons (always present when called — one does not pray to them)	Anti-words: sins, lies, misused words, hateful and violent words, manipulations and suggestions to sin

While the hypothesis that words are angels is tenable, the concept that each word spiritually coincides with an angel is actually comforting. Suddenly there are angels everywhere whizzing about. . .and words are realized as more powerful, more meaningful and more requiring of respect and deliberative use than ever before. If Jesus is the Word, angels are indeed not only as Dante wrote "birds of God" but are "words of God" too. Therefore, words must be used carefully and respectfully. . . They are more powerful than heretofore realized. They can be angelic or demonic. Can it be that angels have been literally right under our noses the whole time? And since Jesus is the Incarnate Word, are not all words potentially incarnating because they are of spirit too?

When humans speak, is there not a spiritual aspect? And do not words have great energetic significance? Whenever a word is used, can it be that we, like, "speak in the tongues of mortals and of angels?"

To all that must be added the Hebrew tradition, told to me by Mary Kay Kantz, that the word for "creating" is the same as for "speaking"; and in Genesis, therefore, when "God said. . .and there was. . .God said. . .and there was. . .God said. . ." and things happened! God named and created at the same time! God created the universe by speaking it and it was there! Why not? When God speaks, something must happen. It follows that if God created angels, he spoke and words became real beings. Can all the words be our words? What else is there that has spirit which can fit?

And, is it not true then that *all creation* (of old and new beings alike) IS God speaking? If this is tenable, how can the universe ever be despiritualized again? If you listen, will you not see? THE WORD by the words?

Does not such an understanding respiritualize all the universe? Can it be that when we speak, we send forth angels. . .but no doubt one must ordinarily be concentrating on doing just that. And when we hear what comes from radio, television, movies and other communication technologies, do we not need to recognize demons when angels are not forthcoming?

Now do you know why it is important to use words transcendentally and thinking of the angels? Try it! When you use words, are you sending angels about. . .or demons?

Once realized, words aquire new meaning and new power. Should we not say: Beware! Angels are at work!

The reader is encouraged to read the sacramental categories of spirit words in the following chapters thinking of angels all the time.

CHAPTER 3:

BAPTISM

In the physical order, an *event* is a point in space time of something that happens at a certain place and a certain time. Your human beingness is an event.

In the spiritual order, *Baptism* is an *event* of your intrinsic *dignity* of respect for life conveying an ascent of *faith* that "living things are precious" and that one came from God with nothing and will return to God with all.

"Truly, I say to you, today you will be with me in Paradise."

Baptism makes you an event — a point of dignity and faith by respecting life.

Live Baptism — a rebirth to existence in the world of spirit.

To cleanse one's soul and to become alive.
To enter the realm of God and
to participate in the Incarnation.

In physics, an *event* is a point in space-time of something that happens at a certain place and a certain time. So is Baptism.

Baptism is a Sacrament which cleanses us from original sin, makes us Christians, children of God, and Heirs of Heaven. Baptism is an *event*.

Baptism patterns the form of "preciousness of life" just as *event* emphasizes a space-time point of existence. For the human, this means the intrinsic *dignity* of that point of human life. The awareness of this results in not only an assent *(faith)* to the individual but seeks the higher good through recognizing God as the basis for Being.

Living things are precious. . .

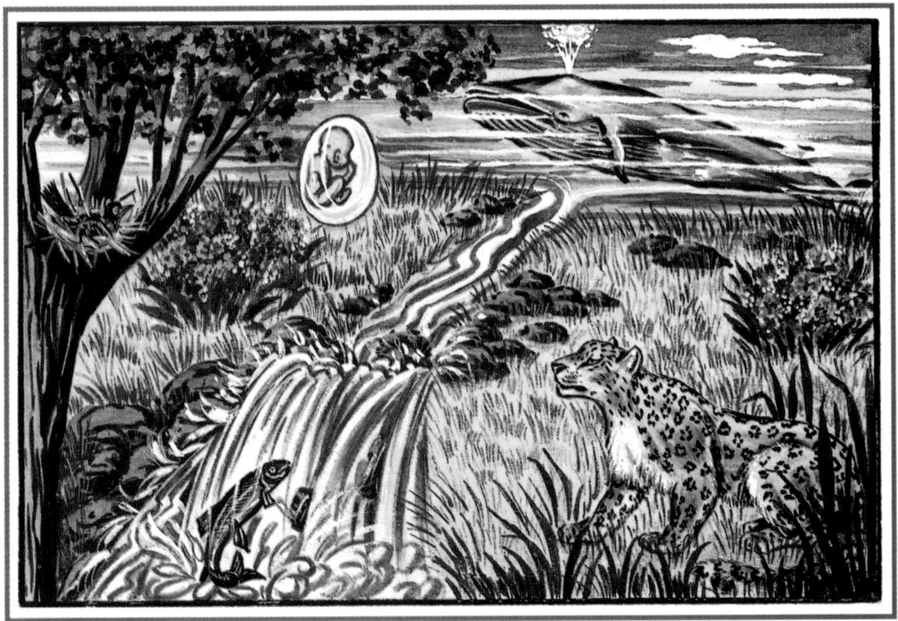

. . . The First Law of the Universe. In a cosmically short, humanly long 600 million years, matter has organized itself into living things. In this process, no species has been able to foresee the next step forward in the mental direction of evolution. Therefore, activities that hurt any living thing should be consistent with evolving life and respect the dominant species existant. For acting counter to this protean law spoils water, soils air, ruins land, kills living things, and may postpone the next higher level of evolution, which hopefully will have supra-human Men living peacefully together in a fuller Humanity that our minds cannot foresee. Choose Life, hurt less, and kill little.

LIVING THINGS ARE PRECIOUS

Life and personal development are often said to "unfold." This is not so. Actions may be considered brief "unfoldings" of that within oneself, but development is the opposite.

Life and personal development are a series of foldings back on ourselves by influences from one's surroundings. From macromolecules to cerebra, from data to wisdom, from numbness to rage, from passivity to activity, from isolation to stimulation, from mental disruption to mental defenses, and from baptism to spiritual ascendancy, all life events impact on humans by an internal folding back on that which we are, resulting in that which we have become.

Life and personal development are anti-entropic processes of organization and complexification in a spiritual direction by the interaction of great numbers.

* * * * *

Everything that happens to you is a gift.

St. Ignatius of Loyola

I like God's finest whispers.

11 Year Old Down's Syndrome Girl's
Tapped Out First Line on a computer

A person is the actual unique reality of a spiritual being, an individual whole existing independently and not interchangeable with any other.

Max Muller

Don't tell me how you work. Tell me how much you get done.

James Ling

Try to want less and less so you will thank more and more.

Brother David

Victims have no fun.

Samuel A. Nigro

What we wish, that we readily believe.

Demosthenes

The mere fact that we ignore something does not make it cease to be.

Donald DeMarco

And the mere fact that we think we believe something does not make it be.

It is possible that blondes also prefer gentlemen.

Mamie Van Doren

The best of all things is to learn. Money can be lost or stolen, health and strength may fail, but what you have committed to your mind is yours forever.

Louis L'Amour

All evolution which has increased our power was an adaptation to the as-yet unknown. A planned evolution would be the end of evolution itself. Moral evolution in particular cannot and does not move in the direction that man wishes. And if it did follow human direction, it would soon cease to preserve what it has created.

Friedrich Hayek

If evolution is as real as scientists say, then there must be a free flow of life. No man could have conceived, implemented and orchestrated life to this level. To assume, then, to take over the genetic code is to destroy evolution.

Samuel A. Nigro

Justification comes through Baptism, is received by Faith, consists in God's inward presence, and lives in Obedience.

John Henry Newman

Very often a change of self is needed more than a change of scene.

A.C. Benson

When one is out of touch with oneself, one cannot touch others.

Ann Morrow Lindbergh

One example of friendship remains with me as vividly as the moment I first heard of it as a boy. In his first season with the Brooklyn Dodgers, Jackie Robinson, the first black man to play Major League Baseball, faced venom nearly everywhere he traveled — fastballs at his head, spikings on the bases, brutal epithets from the opposing dugouts and from the crowds. During one game in Boston, the taunts and racial slurs seemed to reach a peak. In the midst of this, another Dodger, a Southern white named Pee Wee Reese, called timeout. He walked from his position at shortstop toward Robinson at second base, put his arm around Robinson's shoulder, and stood there with him for what seemed like a long time. The gesture spoke more eloquently than the words: "This man is my friend."

Willie Norris

We need to teach our children that they can't cheat. There is no way to pull it off; you can't lie to life. You may deceive your teacher about what you know, but you can't deceive life. What you haven't learned leaves a hole that nothing but that learning can fill and no amount of covering over can disguise.

Reverend Edward R. Sims

Next to knowing when to seize an opportunity, the most important thing in life is to know when to forego an advantage.

Benjamin Disraeli

A CATHOLIC NATURAL LAW MANIFESTO FOR LIFE AND SEXUALITY

Awareness of the environment has demonstrated the interdependence of all creatures. Indeed, environmental concerns collide with John Stuart Mill's promotion that "liberty" may allow whatever does not affect others. Experience with the environment has demonstrated that *all* affairs may deserve consideration as affecting others. In ways subtle and obscure, others *are* affected by what only *seems* not to be affecting them. Thus, even "liberty" must be consonant with nature because when nature is thwarted, all may be affected.

The growing awareness of mankind's interdependency with nature coincides with global concerns for the planet. Respect for planetary processes must include the geosphere, the atmosphere, the hydrosphere, the biosphere, and the behavior-sphere of the animal kingdom.

Furthermore, respect for behavioral patterns intrinsic to the animal kingdom must include mankind as a part of that kingdom at least as a creature natural (and more) to the planet. Therefore, to respect the planet is necessarily to reinforce mankind's behavior in all aspects as *part of* nature. Respect for gender, mating, conception, gestation, development, behavior (including sexuality and violence), and habitat (nests, dens, homes, activity locales, et.) of animals must include comparable consideration for mankind. *To be consistent with the planet human sexuality and violence must also be in concert with natural processes.*

Also, fundamental social units exist in the animal kingdom which are generally species specific for male/female procreative and unitive togetherness. For humans the *family* is overwhelmingly the social unit, and it deserves as much respect and consideration as other social units in the rest of the animal kingdom.

In addition, nonprocreative, nonunitive, body-focusing behaviors are maladaptive, overwhelmingly absent, and if exaggerated are generally incompatible with healthy species maintenance. Examples of these behaviors are anal sex, oral sex, masturbation, and procreative/unitive miscuing. None of these regularly occur in the animal kingdom. Deviations such as these almost always create risk for survival. For humans, the AIDS epidemic is proof that even private consensual sexual behavior can have negative environmental impact affecting others. It is difficult to think of any behavioral disruption for any creature's procreative gender processes which do not thwart nature and which do not have a negative impact on all.

If planetary processes are of import, then to be environmentally sound, in concert with the planet and in synchrony with nature, human sexuality must also conform. If ecology has discovered that *all affects all*, even sexual behavior is never totally private.

Therefore, for *human* life and sexuality to be ecologically sound as a planetary process, the following principles are set forth as derived from the animal kingdom of which humans are a part.

1. Respect for nature includes the natural processes which have defined us thus far. Nature can *never* be supplanted by any man for any reason. We have come from nature's God out of nothing, and, saved and serving "environmentally," we shall return to nature's God with everything. Nature must be profoundly respected but not adored (For believers: Thou shalt not have strange gods before Me).

2. Natural processes can be studied and modified within limits of absolute respect for, relative subservience to, and unique individual fulfilling membership in nature. Therefore, natural processes should never be controlled by an independent self-proclaimed *controller* of nature. Natural processes should be cleanly respected without abuse (For believers: Thou shalt not take the name of (and nature from) the Lord thy God in vain.
3. Natural biological diversity is healthy and incompatible with any species controlling its own gene pool except within the safety of the randomness of natural consciousness which it has developed. Therefore, creation, total and individual, requires a ritualized respect (For believers: Remember, thou shalt keep holy the Sabbath Day. . .of respectful remembrance of all Being).
4. Every creature has the right to its social unit, environmentally identifiable in the animal kingdom which must be maintained and respected. The fundamental social unit of sexual behavior for mankind is a procreative/unitive and male/female complementary duality which creates a *family* defined as a head of a household living with one or more related individuals in a process of shared responsibility, mutual growth, reciprocal commitment and self-sacrificing performance. This is "marriage": A conscious promise between a man and a woman to live as one quadruped creature in conformity with the planet. (For believers: Honor thy father and thy mother — and thy family).
5. I*ndiscriminate* killing is not found in nature and violence is limited to survival. Consistent with this is the rearing of offspring in nature as a unitive (protective-caring) function predominantly female but also often with male support. Therefore, living things are precious and violence is to be avoided including that against one's offspring (For believers: Thou shalt not kill).
6. Extraprocreative and extraunitive sex is anti-environmental. Adult females will only accept sexuality of a male in a procreative/ unitive marital oneness as is overwhelmingly consistent with femaleness in nature. (For believers: Thou shalt not commit adultery).
7. It is environmentally sound that everyone has a right to his own personal and private property which includes his or her sexuality. Misleading stimulative behavior will be avoided because it is ordinarily not found in a healthy planetary process. Mature adults will seek sexual behavior by giving clear, unambiguous messages of receptivity or rejection. Sexual receptivity messages are environmentally personal and make clear the existence of individual, private ownership of at least some aspect of an individual's own space. (For believers: Thou shalt not steal — even sexuality from oneself or from another).
8. In nature, adults seek sexual release but always defer to partners as overwhelmingly consistent with gender defined by nature. To live with other creatures in confluence with the realities of maleness and female-

ness is *truth* in nature (For believers: Thou shalt not bear false witness (unnatural sex) against thy neighbor. . .or anyone else).

9. To be environmentally sound, adult maturity is always present and no *pre-adults* are disturbed by *adult* sexual behavior. All relationships are to be kept holy, uplifting, and honorable (For believers: Thou shalt not covet thy neighbor's wife — or the personhood of anyone else including the immature).
10. Sexual behavior is procreative and/or unitive and never recreational. Sexual behavior has a pattern and purpose in nature. Trivialization of sexuality into a "product" is pollution. Material objects should not run one's life (For believers: Thou shalt not covet thy neighbor's goods).

In the final analysis, if the state or the nation has a compelling interest in the health and safety of the planet, a concept of "liberty" cannot be entertained which allows human behavior to be *inconsistent* with nature. Thus, there is no privacy (except in social manners) because the ecosystem includes most all of what we do including sexuality. Dysphoria and dysfunction are the incontrovertible result of allowing privacy to rule.

If the environment is to be respected, reason must be followed. If individuals of a species are to be cleanly protected, feelings and reason must conform. If reproductive diversity is promoted, gene integrity must be fulfilled and maintained. If trees are to be respected, then so must social units of the animal kingdom including the human family. If condor embryos are to be nurtured, so must human embryos. If the rain forest is to be respected, then so must mating behavior. If the ocean is to be kept clean, then pregnancies must be allowed to proceed. If a sound environment is of concern, then truth and good must define personal liberty. If nature defines gender patterns, humans must comply. If the atmosphere is to be clean, then so too must human behavior, and both must be in conformity with the planet. Nature does not forget its reasons nor does it forgive abuses.

This manifesto conforms humanity to the planet with God or evolution or both. Regardless, nature decrees a fantastic future if ecologically sound principles about human sexuality, among other things, are followed. And when these ecological principles are thwarted, everyone is affected.

By these principles, the Roman Catholic church conforms to the planet as the soul of nature. Actually, the church's teaching such principles provides the substance for humans as individuals or groups to be environmentally sound, to be in concert with the planet, and to be able to develop further in a way almost unbelievable.

Samuel A. Nigro

Life is a card game in which everyone is dealt a hand that he must accept. His success will depend on his playing it as well as it can be played. A very large proportion of failures in life occur because men refuse to do this and instead insist on playing the hand that they think they should have been dealt.

Lord David Cecil

After a while you learn the subtle difference between
holding a hand and chaining a soul,
And you learn that love doesn't mean learning and company
doesn't mean security,
And you begin to learn that kisses aren't contracts and
presents aren't promises,
And you begin to accept your defeats with your head up and
your eyes open, with the grace of an adult, not the
grief of a child,
And you learn to build all your roads on today because
tomorrow's ground is too uncertain for plans.
After a while you learn that even sunshine burns if you get too much. So
plant your own garden and decorate your own soul, instead of waiting for
someone to bring you flowers. And you learn that you really can endure
. . .That you really are strong,
And you really do have worth.

Anonymous

To be fully alive involves the renunciation of one's past and one's future. . .to do otherwise is to kill the present.

Anthony de Mello

Laziness may appear attractive, but work gives satisfaction.

Anne Frank

If you cannot do it right, don't do it at all.

Evelyn Nigro

If you *must* beat a child, use a string.

Anonymous

There is no such thing in anyone's life as an unimportant day.

Alexander Wollott

The more I want to get something done, the less I call it work.

Richard Bach

A winner never quits. A quitter never wins.

Anonymous

To be or not to be, that is the question.

William Shakespeare

The answer is, "To be. Always: TO BE."

Samuel A. Nigro

You knit me in my mother's womb. . . Wonderful are your works.

Psalm 139:13-14

Trifles make perfection — and perfection is no trifle.

Michelangelo Buonarroti

The thing that impresses me most about America is the way parents obey their children.

Duke of Windsor

It's a chance to do something patriotic for your country without killing anybody.

George Raveling (Asst. U.S. Olympic Coach)

Every evening I turn my worries over to God. He's going to be up all night anyway.

Mary C. Crowley

The art of living sucessfully consists of being able to hold two opposite ideas in tension at the same time: First, to make long-term plans as if we were going to live forever; and second, to conduct ourselves daily as if we were going to die tomorrow.

Sydney J. Harris

The difference between capitalism and communism is that capitalism offers a larger share of the doughnut and communism offers a larger share of the hole.

Al Bernstein

The most important thing a father can do for his children is to love their mother.

The Reverend Theodore Hesburgh

We're equipped three ways to have all the answers — we've got an encylopedia, a home computer, and a teenager.

Laurene J. Peters

Man without mysticism is a monster.

Whitaker Chambers

. . .The strict rationalist who denies the acceptability of all beliefs based on anything but experience and reasoning, tends to become a barbarian.

Friedrich Hayek

Human progress is slow and difficult precisely because imagination alone is not enough. Some beautiful dreams, when implemented, turn out to be hideous nightmares. . . . Whatever is desired must not be so strong that it tries to impose itself all by itself, without due regard for the knowledge and love that are needed to render justice to the relevant existing realities.

Donald DeMarco

If you could build a small package, something small enough to carry in your coat pocket, a machine which would instantly start and stop, in which you could instantly reverse yourslf or go forward, which would require no batteries or other energy sources, and which would provide you with full information on an entire civilization, what would you have? A book.

Isaac Asimov

Baptism is a Sacrament which cleanses us from original sin, makes us Christians, children of God, and heirs of heaven.

Baltimore Catechism

Civilization took *the pill*, got sick, and died.

Anonymous

Nothing happens unless first a dream.

Carl Sandburg

Evolution appears to be a process of organization and complexification in a mental-spiritual direction by the interaction of great numbers of matter. If evolution is true, then humanity (as sanctified or energized) has enveloped all evolutionary energy, not as a species, but as individuals, each on a personal basis. Such has been so since ensoulment. Evolution then, if it is true, is now uniquely personal, with each individual freely choosing to evolve (ascend) or not to evolve further, depending upon the developmental axis personally chosen. The psychosocial axes available lead, as evolution demands (if evolution is true), to a spectrum of outcomes varying from annihilation to stagnation to transition to Beatific Assimilation. The most efficient path to evolving personally into the next ultimate level of existence is the Catholic Species of Loving Truth of the Roman Catholic Phylum of Life (Father), Liberty (Son), and the Pursuit of Happiness (Holy Spirit).

Samuel A. Nigro

Allowing for error, good is obtained by reception and mastery of the forces of nature, and through voluntary association of individuals in equal free choice.

Isabel Paterson

Alexander the Great, at the acme of his power, asked Diogenes: "Is there anything I can do for you?" And Diogenes replied: "You can stand aside from between me and the sunlight."

Name Lost

No edict or law can impart to an individual a faculty denied him by nature.

Isabel Paterson

And no edict or law an deprive an individual of a faculty given to him by nature without due process.

Government then is solely an instrument or mechanism of appropriation, prohibition, compulsion and extinction; in the nature of things it can be nothing, and can operate to no other end.

Isabel Paterson

Any woman who is pregnant and does not want to be has not been choosing properly. Of all the birth control choices and of all the choices for behavior, and she still finds herself pregnant, it is obvious she cannot make choices already and has forfeited her chance for any more choices.

Samuel A. Nigro

Let the children be, do not keep them back from me; the Kingdom of Heaven belongs to such as these.

Matthew 19:14

The youth of the nation are being destroyed. Without mountains of shoes. Without piles of clothes. Without gunfire. Without ovens. But we are smotheringly buried alive under heaps of clean carnage by abortion.

Samuel A. Nigro

Pregnancy is nine months. Childraising is nineteen years. Abortion is forever.

Name Lost

New human life is a gift not a product, and should be invoked only in an atmosphere of conjugal love in which husband and wife renounce power and control both over each other as well as over their progeny.

Donald DeMarco

Go, therefore, teach ye all nations, baptizing them in the name of the Father, and of the Son, and of the Holy Spirit.

Matthew 28:19

All power is given to me in heaven and in earth. Going, therefore, teach ye all nations, baptizing them in the name of the Father, and of the Son, and of the Holy Spirit. Teaching them to observe all things whatsoever I have commanded you: and behold I am with you all days, even to the consummation of the world.

Matthew 28:18-20

For had ye believed Moses, ye would have believed me. For he wrote of me. But if ye believe not his writings, how shall ye believe my words?

John 5:46-47

Therefore, everyone who acknowledges me before men, I also will acknowledge him before my Father in heaven. But whoever disowns men before me, I in turn will disown him before my Father in heaven.

Matthew 19:32-33

I and my father are one.

John 10:30

I am the Way, the Truth, and the Life. No one comes to the Father except through Me.

John 14:6

We see things and people not as they are but as we are.

Anthony de Mello

The missing link is God.

Samuel A. Nigro

Truly thou art the Son of God.

Matthew 14:33

If you abide in my word, you shall be my disciples. Indeed, you shall know the truth and the truth shall set you free.

John 8:31-32

A condition of complete simplicity (costing not less than everything).

T.S. Eliot on Christianity

Premature sexual information and excitement for children interfere with the most important thing a child can do: Play — play at things which are in the realm of childhood rather than adulthood.

Anonymous

A man who does not know what happened before his birth will always remain a child.

Cicero

In the 15-20 billion years of the universe, we each get our finite moments, so make the best of them and you can embrace it all! The billions of years have been done without the know-it-all's too. So, don't you think you should have your kids and/or do something decent during the time you have? And after looking at the billions of years, is it not obvious that humans, regardless of any observations to the contrary, are more alike than different. Live your life fully for all there is, and all will be yours.

Samuel A. Nigro

When God created us, he did not intend for us to die; he made us like Himself. It was the Devil's jealousy that brought death into the world and those who belong to the Devil are the ones who will die.

Wisdom 2:23-24

The secret of contentment is the realization that life is a gift, not a right.

Anonymous

Now we have received not the spirit of the world, but the spirit that is from God, that we may know the things that have been given us by God. These things we also speak, not in words taught by human wisdom, but in the learning of the Spirit combining spiritual with spiritual.

1 Corinthians 2:12-13

For you were buried together with him in Baptism, and in Him also rose again through faith and the working of God who raised him from the dead.

Colossians 2:12

But when the goodness and kindness of God our Savior appeared, then not by reason of good works that we did ourselves, but according to his mercy, he saved us through the bath of regeneration and renewal by the Holy Spirit; whom he has abundantly poured out upon us through Jesus Christ our Savior, in order that, justified by his grace, we may be heirs in the hope of life everlasting.

Titus 3:4-7

Amen, amen, I say to thee, unless a man be born again of water and the Spirit, he cannot enter into the Kingdom of God.

John 3:5

Do you not know that all we who have been baptized into Christ Jesus have been baptized into his death? For we were buried with him by means of Baptizing into death, in order that, just as Christ has risen from the dead through the glory of the Father, so we also may walk in the newness of life.

Romans 6:3-4

Every human being has been brought into the world according to the will of God. And God created us in such a way that every human being can either save his own soul or destroy it. Man's task in life is to save his soul. In order to save our souls, we must live according to the ways of God, and in order to live according to the ways of God, we must renounce the sensual pleasures of life; we must labor, suffer and be kind and humble.

Leo Tolstoy

Do not make yourself low; people will tread on your head.

Yiddish proverb

He who draws the image of man draws the image of God.

G.K. Chesterton

God wants you to be a saint.

Mother Angelica

The very idea of freedom presupposes some objective moral law which overeaches rulers and ruled alike. Subjectivism about values is eternally incompatible with democracy. We and our rulers are of one kind only so long as we are subject to one law. But if there is no Law of Nature, the ethos of any society is the creation of its rulers, educators and conditioners; and every creator stands above and outside his own creation.

C.S. Lewis

However far you traced the story back, you would never find the laws of Nature causing anything. The dazzlingly obvious conclusion. . .: In the whole history of the universe, the laws of Nature have never produced a single event. They are the pattern to which every event must conform, provided only that it can be induced to happen.

C.S. Lewis

Start off everyday with a smile and get it over with.

W.C. Fields

Read nature; nature is a friend of truth.

Edward Young

You must love all that God has created, both in his entire world and each single tiny sand grain of it. Love each tiny leaf, each beam of sunshine. You must love the animals, love every plant. If you love all things, you will also attain the divine mystery that is in all things. For then your ability to perceive the truth will grow everyday, and your mind will open itself to all-embracing love.

Fyodor Dostoyevsky

Do thyself no harm.

Acts 16:28

I deplore the horrible crime of child murder. . . We want prevention, not merely punishment. We must reach the root of the evil. . . It is practiced by those whose inmost souls revolt from the dreadful deed. . . No matter what the motive, love of ease, or a desire to save from suffering the unborn innocent, the woman is awfully guilty who commits the deed. . . But oh! thrice guilty is he who drove her to the desperation which impelled her to the crime.

Susan B. Anthony

Nothing is perfect unless it is personal.

G.K. Chesterton

If frogs believed in humans, they would no doubt, if they could, try to communicate with us. If we humans believe in angels, we would be fools not to pray for their intercession and their power! Are we humans arrogant frogs refusing to believe that there is more to the universe than our own immediate sensations? Or do we humans have enough understanding to recognize that there is more to life than what subhuman creatures and we ourselves perceive? So, pray to your Guardian Angel. Pray intently — you will be pleasantly surprised.

Samuel A. Nigro

Only those who persist, succeed.

Name Lost

Has any one supposed it lucky to be born? I hasten to inform him or her it is just as lucky to die, and I know it.

Walt Whitman

I cannot prove to you that God exists, but my work has proven empirically that the pattern of God exists in every man and that this pattern in the individual has at its disposal the greatest transforming energies of which life is capable. Find this pattern in your own individual self and life is transformed.

Carl Jung

Women give form. Men give matter.

Name Lost

My fetal life meant a lot to me. . .it still does. . .you never lose your dependency on it.

Samuel A. Nigro

The best way that a man could test his readiness to encounter the common variety of mankind would be to climb down a chimney into any house at random, and get on as well as possible with the people inside. And that is essentially what each one of us did on the day he was born.

G.K. Chesterton

It is almost a matter of religion that every infant is a terrible infant. Every child is, both in the most superficial and in the most solemn sense, a holy terror.

G.K. Chesterton

No Catholic thinks he is a good Catholic; or he would by that thought become a bad Catholic.

G.K. Chesterton

Well, on the day I was born, God was sick. . .

Ce'sar Vallejo

Another example of simplistic (I feel this way so it is this way) Gnosticism.

Samuel A. Nigro

Getting born is a very important decision. Who made yours? Indeed, what did your fetal life mean to you?

Samuel A. Nigro

God is an early Riser.

John Donne

They should not hear a word from me
Of selfishness or scorn
If only I could find the door
If I were only born.

G.K. Chesterton

A woman who does not control her body has no right to kill the child that results.

Anonymous

To watch or pay to watch pornography? That's like paying to watch an abortion.

A virtuous college student

The care of human life and happiness, and not their destruction, is the first and only object of good government.

Thomas Jefferson

Prevention is not only not better than cure, prevention is even worse than disease.

G.K. Chesterton

While all men are created equal, they differ greatly in the sequel.

Fisher Ames

Human life itself is an adventure as risky as hitting the policeman.

G.K. Chesterton

It seems to me as clear as daylight that abortion would be a crime.

Gandhi

Life is unfair. And it's not fair that life is unfair.

Edward Abbey

Shall I tell you the secret of the whole world? It is that we have only known the back of our world.

Gabriel Syme, The Man Who Was Thursday

The only reason you have any rights at all is because the women in your family, for hundreds of years, did not violate the right to life of their unborn children, and that includes you.

Samuel A. Nigro

Man is never the better for having a fine gown.

Baruch Spinoza

I praise you for the wonder of my being.

Psalm 139

She taught me the most valuable lesson of my life; no matter how bad the pain is, it's never so bad that suicide is the only answer. It's never so bad that the only escape is a false one. Suicide doesn't end pain. It only lays it on the broken shoulders of the survivors.

Anne Grace Scheinin, describing the
suffering caused by her mother's suicide

Even if one does not believe in God, suicide is not legitimate. . . Only in the courageous facing of things as they are is authenticity realized, is one's destiny fulfilled. . . Murder and suicide are one in the same thing. . . From the moment life is recognized as good, it becomes good for all.

Albert Camus

I have set before you life and death; choose life.

Deuteronomy 30:19

Before I formed you in the womb, I knew you, and before you were born I consecrated you.

Jeremiah 1:5

What the universal church holds, not as instituted (invented) by councils but as something always held, is most correctly believed to have been handed down by apostolic authority. Since others respond for children, so that the celebration of the Sacrament may be complete for them, it is certainly availing to them for their consecration, because they themselves are not able to respond.

St. Augustine, A.D. 400 on Baptism

You were a thumbsucker, and it took a long time to wean away. You never put down your blue-and-white blanket either. After I washed the blanket, you would stand sucking your thumb, holding onto it while it was drying on the clothes line.

The mother of Edward A. Malloy, C.S.C., President of University of Notre Dame, telling how he was at the age of 4

Every woman knows that if she were free, she would never bear an unwished-for child, nor think of murdering one before its birth.

Victoria Woodhull

Freedom is obedience to love while slavery is obedience to purposelessness.

Name Lost

Unable to compete in the field of Total Humanity, some exhaust themselves in an ignoble battle on behalf of something less, such as femaleness, blackness, hedonism, or some religion that restricts Love.

Anonymous

Therefore, if any one is in Christ, he is a new creation; the old has passed away, behold, the new has come.

II Corinthians 5:17

Perfection begins by getting up early and on time.

Cardinal John Henry Newman

No one ever really owes anybody anything unless it is something of monetary value specifically borrowed.

Michael D. Nigro

You were a human being when you were a fetus.

Anonymous

Cursed is the man who trusts in human beings, who seeks his struggle in flesh, whose heart turns away from the Lord. . . Blessed is the man who trusts in the Lord, whose hope is the Lord.

Jeremiah 17:5-8

At the creation of the world, God moved the heavens with motions identical to the ones with which they actually move. Therefore He then imparted to them *impetuses* by which they continue to move uniformly.

Jean Buridan in the early 14th century

At some time, each human being, to be genuinely human, must ask: "What am I going to do to save the world?"

Anonymous

There is not one class of human beings that has dignity and another that does not. Classifying human beings in such a manner would represent the most invidious form of prejudice imaginable.

Donald DeMarco

There is nothing sweeter than love, nothing stronger, nothing higher, nothing wider, nothing fuller, nothing better in heaven or earth; for his love is born of God and only in God, above all that He has created, can it find rest.

Thomas a Kempis

In Genesis' first three chapters, the fatal flaw of Earth's children is revealed. It is the authority problem.

Nancy M. Cross

Obedience is a blessing and disobedience a curse. Submission to the plan looks like bliss, and rebellion against the plan looks like hell. If the creature in his freedom chooses not to heed his creator, then the creature must live with all the authority problem brings upon him.

Nancy M. Cross

An abortion kills the life of a baby after it has begun.

Planned Parenthood in 1963

The concept that the fetus is a patient, an individual whose disorders are a proper subject for medical therapy, has been established.

Medical and Health Annual of the Encylopedia Britannica in 1963

The father's blessings establish the houses of his children, but the mother's curse rooteth up the foundation.

Sirach 3:9

Man is a statue of God walking about the garden.

G.K. Chesterton

If I knew then what I know now, you never would have died.

Linda Allison-Lewis, the beginning of her prayer for healing to the child she aborted ten years before.

The Biblical subordination of women to men is the psychosocial manifestation of an existential truth evident in all creatures which have gender differences. The truth is that the female of almost all species, by virtue of transcendental projection of identity, oneness, and beauty, is absolutely necessary to bring out the best of both males and females of the species. The existential, biological priority (and superiority?) of the female is (for every action, there is a reaction) reacted to and complemented by a psychosocial subordination to the male in almost all species. This is how Nature IS. . .of which Mankind is a part.

Samuel A. Nigro

I baptize thee in the name of the Father, and of the Son, and of the Holy Spirit.

Form of Baptism

What every thinking person longs to avoid being: a product of his times.

Maggie Gallagher

Choice is the opiate of the liberal.

Maggie Gallagher

To say that in order to be equal with men it must be possible for a pregnant woman to become unpregnant at will is to say that being a woman precludes her from being a fully functioning person. . . Of all the things which are done to women to fit them into a society dominated by men, abortion is the most violent invasion of their physical and psychic integrity. . . It is a deeper and more destructive assault than rape, the culminating act of womb-envy and woman-hatred. . .

Daphne DeJong

The simplest solution to the problem of unwanted children is to *want* them.

Joan Andrews

A woman who deliberately destroys a fetus is answerable for murder. And any fine distinction as to its being completely formed or unformed is not admissible among us.

St. Basil the Great, Circa 350 A.D.

Christian is my name and Catholic is my surname. The former qualifies, the latter manifests me for what I am. And, if I initially must explain the word "Catholic" and translate it from the Greek into the Latin idiom, Catholic means "one everywhere" or, as the more learned think, "obedience to all the Commandments of God."

St. Pacianus of Barcelona, Circa 360 A.D.

Christ instituted this new covenant, that is, the new testament in His blood, calling together a people from Jews and Gentiles, which would be. . .the new People of God.

Vatican II

According to the rabbis of the talmudic era, the creation of a human being is regarded as another creation of the world. A human being is conceived in the image of God and leads a beatific existence in the womb. During this period, the embryo learns the entire Torah from God. At the moment of birth, however, an angel arrives and strikes him on his mouth, and he forgets everything. Life after birth is a process of relearning, rather than learning, the entire Torah that the embryo once knew.

David S. Ariel

Choose life.

Moses

There is an absolute right of all innocent persons *not* to be killed.

Kevin T. McMahon

Beware of the naked man who offers you the shirt off his back.

Ralph McInerny

The world will not entertain you!

Evelyn Nigro

In every creature there is a spark of God.

Leos Janacek

No community whether family, village, or state is really strong if it will not carry its weak and even its very weakest members. They belong to it no less than the strong, and the quiet work of their maintenance and care, which might seem useless on a superficial view, is perhaps more effective than common labor, culture, or historical conflict in knitting it closely and securely together. On the other hand, a community which regards and treats its weak members as a hindrance, and even proceeds to their extermination, is on the verge of collapse.

Karl Barth

Woe betide any man who depends on the abstract humanity of another for his food and protection.

Michael Ignatieff

You can really do nothing about judges, lawyers, leaders, rulers, editors, entertainers, or theologians. In the long run, you can do nothing but *save yourself* while you try to help others.

Samuel A. Nigro-

Free choice does not extend to violating the necessary metaphysical principles of our very essence.

Peter Kreeft

Whatever — do not give them your children!

Name Lost

My God, make me see things as they really are.

St. Therese of Lisieu

The universe is not a democracy.

Peter Kreeft

A "uni-verse" is a unity-of-diversity.

Peter Kreeft

Everyone knows that Nature abhors a vacuum. Less recognized, nay even denied, is that Nature also abhors equality. Nature is a hierarchy wherein each being has its/his/her role to be transcendentally present. Period.

Samuel A. Nigro

Nature is a multiple of hierarchies. . .equality does not exist and cannot be completely forced in nature.

Samuel A. Nigro

Angelic minds have simple and blessed intelligence, not gathering their knowledge of Divine things from visible things as is the case with the human soul.

St. Thomas Aquinas

Human souls know by sensation and reasoning, while angels are purely intuitive; and human souls are essentially forms of bodies, and therefore incomplete without their bodies, while angels have no tendency to inform bodies.

Peter Kreeft

I pray to St. Anthony — of Padua — everyday — protect me, guide me, cure me, console me, aid me, assist me, help me, save me all the way through, right there and then, help me find the answer and control the solution, no time wasted if the pills are wasted. . .and he reminds me to take my pills too. . .and what to do. . .and I tell him, if you're tired of helping me just tell me. . .and I will try to get God for you. . .no time wasted.

Retarded and mentally ill adult patient
(Doing quite well, thank you!)

The laws of God are no more escapable in the longrun by any creature than the law of gravity is escapable by anybody.

Peter Kreeft

Natural things depend on the divine intellect as artificial things on the human.

St. Thomas Aquinas

Women aren't stupid; they have always known there was a life there. . .

Fay Wattleton, Director of Planned Parenthood on abortion

Dirty tricks are being played by anti-abortionists including prayer and fasting. . .

British abortionist and member of Parliament

You have a body. No question about that. But there are other parts of you which are just as important. You have an identity which ought to be considered as much as your body. You have truth which you must think of as much as your body. You have oneness, which you must think of as much as your body. You have goodness and beauty, each of which must be thought of as much as your body. Your body is one-sixth of your being. You should only be thinking of it one-sixth of the time.

Samuel A. Nigro

The invisible things of God are clearly seen being understood by the things that are made.

Romans 1:20

Life did not need you before. . .and it does not need you now. So don't get a big head.

Charles C. Nigro

The body is what we get to do with our soul in the temporal order.

Samuel A. Nigro

It's not a rock. It's not a Coke bottle. It is a human baby and it is standing on my bladder.

Mary Suma, pregnant Republican Convention delegate defending the Right-to Life plank in 1992

Asses would rather have refuse than gold.

Heracleitus

I have come to this pulpit in order to say clearly what I have to say to you. I am the voice of Christ crying in the desert (of this island). It is essential that you listen to it attentively: not just with any kind of attention, but with your entire heart and your entire being. It is the newest word ever addressed to you; the harshest, the hardest, the most surprising and awesome you would ever expect to hear.

The message of Christ, here it is: You are all in a state of mortal sin. You are living in mortal sin and will die in it, because of your cruelty and your tyrannical attitude towards innocent people. Tell me: By what right and in virtue of what justice do you keep the unborn (Indians) in such cruel and horrible treatment (servitude)? In the name of what authority have you waged your loathsome wars against the unborn (people) living in peace and tranquility, unborn (people) you have killed in infinite numbers, sowing unheard-of-death and terror? How could you — though your excessive demands — oppress them and wear them out to the point of exhaustion, not giving them food, not treating the illnesses they developed? They die of them — rather, you kill them — in order to procure your daily gold. Did you take care to ensure that the faith would be (was) preached to them so that they would know their God and Creator, would be baptized, hear Mass, observe Feast-Days and Sundays? Are they too not human beings? Are they not to be endowed with reason? Are you not obliged to love them as yourself? Do you not understand this? Do you not feel this? How can you remain asleep, buried in lethargic slumber?

Fray Antonio de Montesinos, Dominican priest on the Island of Hispaniola on the First Sunday of Advent 1511 preaching about the mistreatment of the Indians — which applies today concerning the unborn.

For he became man that we might become divine; he revealed himself through a body that we might receive an idea of the invisible Father.

St. Anthanasius

Thus man, so great and precious, fell from the value he had and fell into the mud of sin and clothed himself with clay and mortality. This is the image we counsel him to remove in the water of Christian life.

St. Gregory of Nyssa

The soul is the total transcendental actuality of a human being. Its *ens* (act of being) contains:

1. The *res* which is the corporal body, i.e. the most visible dimension for those in the material world. Naturally, Nature rules, neurochemistry and all, how the soul manifests in Nature.
2. The *aliquid* which is the identity or form of the being, i.e. for human beings, the achievement in fact of total humanity (not ethnicity, not color or anything else but *human beingness*).
3. The *verum* which is the truth of the being, i.e. the confluence of the human with reality (instead of with television, movies, magazines and newspapers).
4. The *unum* which is the oneness of the being, i.e. the conforming of the being with itself and all related to it.
5. The *bonum* which is the good of the being, i.e. the confluence of the being with Natural Law.
6. The *bella* which is the beauty of the being, i.e. its confluence with ascendancy or the "bringing out the best" of itself and of all around it.

The soul contains all these including (contrary to common misunderstanding) the body which is a mere one-sixth of it.

Samuel A. Nigro

She is full of grace, proclaimed to be entirely without sin. . . God's grace fills her with everything good and makes her devoid of all evil. . . God is with her, meaning that all she did or left undone is divine and the action of God in her and, moreover, God guarded and protected her from all that might be hurtful to her.

Martin Luther on Mary

Media appeal? Media appeal? To hell with media appeal! It has no staying power. . .

Anonymous

The Roman Catholic church is the mediator and cheerleader for the Transcendentals. She does this by its books (the Bible and libraries everywhere), by the Sacraments, and by a bewildering array of special people (Mary, the Apostles, the Popes, the Saints, and others) and their amazing to amusing stories. All activities of the Roman Catholic church promote, simplistically to profoundly, the dimensions of the soul.

Samuel A. Nigro

The best we can do is know, preserve, project and live out our Transcendentals, and without doing such, the soul cannot be saved (and that includes the body).

Samuel A. Nigro

The soul is the total personified custody for and living out of Transcendentals (and if you do not know your Transcendentals, you will not save your soul — which includes your body).

Samuel A. Nigro

Your soul is that part of the universe which is you, you jackass, and you had better do good by it!

Anna Marie Nigro to her mischievous grandson

. . .the good or evil of an action, as of other things, depends on its fullness of being or its lack of that fullness.

St. Thomas Aquinas

("Fullness of being" can only be the Transcendentals.)

The error is in always treating the soul as a product and never treating it as an origin.

G.K. Chesterton

We are in earnest — we will not equivocate — we will not excuse — we will not retreat one single inch — and we will be heard!

William Lloyd Garrison on the evil of his day (slavery)

. . .things that can be altered will be altered again.

G.K. Chesterton

Conversion is the whole process by which people constantly examine their own life, each measuring it against the values of the Gospel, and act accordingly. . . This is the *metanoia* to which we are called: that by changing for the better what is within my grasp, I can change the world!

James Potin

O you, who are beyond anything, are not these words all
 that can be sung about you?
What hymn could tell about you, what language? No word
 can express you.
What could our mind cling to? You are beyond any intelligence.
Only you are unutterable, for all that is uttered comes from you.
Only you are knowable, for all that is thought comes from you.
All beings, those who speak and those who are silent, proclaim you.
Universal desire, universal groaning calls you.
All that is prays to you, and to you any being who thinks
 in your universe, raises a silent hymn.
All that remains, remains through you; through you is sustained
 universal motion.
For all beings, you are the end; you are all beings and
 you are none of them.
You are not one sole being, you are not the totality of beings.
Yours are all the names, and how will I call you, you, the
only one who cannot be named?
What celestial spirit could penetrate the clouds covering
 the sky itself?
Have mercy, O you, who are beyond everything,
Isn't this all that can be sung about you?

St. Gregory Nazienzean (5th Century)

When, in Genesis, the serpent told Adam and Eve that they would be like God and that they would acquire the knowledge of good and evil, he told *two* lies. The first was that they would be like God — when they already were like God, having been made in the image of Him. But second, it was a lie that they would acquire the knowledge of good and evil because they already had it too. What happened when they ate the fruit was that the knowledge of good and evil became *unconscious*. It is this unconscious dimension of mankind's existence that is Original Sin. It is the unconsciousness of our knowledge of good and evil which is the cause of all our troubles.

Samuel A. Nigro

For the scientist who has lived by his faith in the power of reason, the story (the quest for origins) ends like a bad dream. He has scaled the mountains of ignorance; he is about to conquer the highest peak; as he pulls himself over the final rock, he is greeted by a band of theologians who have been sitting there for centuries.

Robert Jastrow

To a wise man, the whole earth is open, for the native land of the good soul is the whole earth.

Democritis

You cannot be fully human by being just yourself or just your own kind.

Name Lost

God is grasped only through Natural Law.

Samuel A. Nigro

We baptize our children because of a spiritual and moral imperative that arises from our faith in Christ, our obedience to His command, and our trust in His promises. Our profoundest desire as a community of faith and divine life is to share our most precious gift and values with the offspring God grants us. To do less is to betray our parental love.

John H. Miller, C.S.C.

Yahweh, what variety you have created, arranging everything so wisely!

Psalms 104:24

The soul is weighed down by the body. . .but lightened by the sacraments, virtue and the transcendentals.

Name Lost

You are your own best doctor. . .take care of yourself.

Charles C. Nigro

There is a point beyond which natural human feelings cannot be violated for the supposed good of the state and have any actual good for the state result.

Warren H. Carroll

It mus is!

Enthusiastic Believer

Then was fulfilled that which was spoken by Jeremiah the prophet, saying: A voice was heard in Rama; lamentation and great mourning: Rachel bewailing her children; and she would not be comforted, because they are not.

Matthew 2:17-18

Gird thyself with sackloth, O daughter of My people, and sprinkle thyself with ashes; make mourning as for an only son, a bitter lamentation, because the destroyer shall come suddenly upon us.

Jeremiah 6:26

Our task, if possible, is to understand nature objectively on the basis of logic and the experience of our senses.

Galileo

Dear Jesus, I am not sure of what to say. But I come to You in prayer for my friend. . . is hurting badly, Lord. Reach down and touch her/him. Let her/him know that You are the salvation. Let her/him not despair. She/He is my good friend, and I care about her/him so much. I know that You are the Almighty. You can do all things. And you can help him/her.

Jeanie's prayer for Susan made available for everyone

For some of us, there is not much left inside. Someone's got to start building us up again.

Aborted Woman

When you're out of synchrony with Natural Law, you are rejecting your Creator however you conceive creation.

Samuel A. Nigro

The Universe repeats itself, with the possible exception of history. . .which is the only science the conclusions of which are always wrong.

G.K. Chesterton

. . .nature. . .is inexorable and immutable. She never transgresses the laws imposed upon or cares about whether her abstruse reasons and efforts of operation are understandable to man.

Galileo

If we value the condor, we will value a condor not yet hatched, for we already know what it is.

James G. Hanink

Mary, console the children of the land sprinkled with blood and tears. . .

Our Lady of Siluva, 1608

What is cannot not be.

Parmenides

Not even an unborn baby.

Original sin is manifest by the fact that people end up believing the craziest things. Only by reason and the transcendentals can such be overcome.

Samuel A. Nigro

We can affirm without hesitation that science cannot affirm anything whatever about what animals were made *for*.

G.K. Chesterton

Even if I were a Eugenist, then I should not personally elect to waste my time locking up the feeble-minded. The people I should lock up would be the strong-minded.

G.K. Chesterton

Existence is the unity in which all essences are annealed in being.

Frederick D. Wilhelmsen

How is it that you, a Jew, have been baptized a Catholic? "Well, you know, there are just too many Jews for me among the Protestants."

Simplicissimus, 1898

The only way to proceed through a complex situation is to start with the right first principle.

G.K. Chesterton

If you wish to enter into life, keep the commandments.

Matthew 19:16-17

Surely I was sinful at birth, sinful from the time my mother conceived me.

Psalm 51:5

All attempts to apply the parallel of physical evolution to our ethical progress end on one of two things: They end in cutting ethics to fit evolution, which means immorality; or they end in cutting evolution to fit ethics, which means unscientific balderdash.

G.K. Chesterton

There can be no legitimate compromise which gives away what does not belong to any of the parties that compromise.

Damian Fedoryka

To God Alone Be the Glory.

J.S. Bach's inscription on all his compositions

What Is All This Race Stuff Anyway?

Those who talk about race generally do not know what race is. When people think they are talking about race, they usually are talking about color or slavery, which is to miss the forest for the trees and therefore get nowhere in understanding. A brief course on race follows:

The Nine Broadest Historical Geographic Races	*The Five Generic Races*	
American Indian }	Mongoloid	
Asiatic }		
Australian }	Australoid	
Melanesian }		
Micronesian }		
Polynesian }		
African }	{ Congoid }	Called "Negro" in 1555
	{ Capoid }	
Indian (South Asian) }	Caucasian	Label Originated c. 1800.
European }		

The above racial terms are valid and accurate for contemporary use. Interestingly enough, there is no color mentioned. And, simple enough, almost everyone can trace back to his geohistorical and generic racial origin. However, the significance of one's placement into any of these races is generally limited to a few genetically-inherited traits in teeth, blood, bone, hair and skin. But even those differences are not absolute and almost always overlap in one way or another.

However, as far as *living* goes, these hereditary linkages are secondary and subordinate to the family and society into which one has been born. That is, *how one lives* is more important than *hereditary composition* when studying the differences between the races. It is the "luck of birth" and/or family life into which one has been raised that determines almost everything rather than one's geohistorical or generic racial background.

Prior to 1500, people born into any of the before mentioned races found themselves fairly well separated and confined to their own racial group. This resulted in each race developing social, political and economic inbreeding to cope with their specific environment, the available resources, God, self and others. These social, psychological and cultural ways of relating provide the genuinely human component to each race, and the presence of this human component is what is important not only to humanity but to the ability to adapt to contacts with other races. Even though a case can be made that the ways of relating are merely matters of habit and reinforcement which, with exposure to others, can be changed, it is the way of relating which determines events. The cultural spheres dwarf the biological, even in race.

Geographically separated and culturally endogamous, the beneficial ways of relating for each listed race became relatively fixed and reflective of each race's successful adaptive thinking style. Furthermore, the peoples involved tended to ally politically into allegiences and relationships resulting in different types of governing methods varying from tribe to nation state peculiar to each setting. And because of geopgraphic separation, each race had little experience with others unlike themselves.

However, with Christopher Columbus and improved seafaring developed by Caucasians, increasing contact occurred between these geographically separated races. With this increased contact, confused efforts began as those races engaged and related for the first time in quantity in the years after Columbus proved one would not sail off the edge of the world. No longer afraid, Caucasians were going to sail everywhere and begin to break down geographic barriers between races. Cultural endogamy was going to end.

The word "Caucasian" was coined in the early 1800's by an anthropologist who erroneoualy claimed all "white" people derived from Caucasus Mountain area. He applied the term to a swath of peoples from Scandinavia across Europe through the Middle East and Northern Africa concluding with the Indian subcontinent. Thus "Indo-European" came to be "Caucasian."

At bottom, heady in their superiority of science and thinking levels because of the power of Western Civilization (self-reflection, linear rather than circular thinking, reasoned emotiveness, emphasis on virtue and low tolerance for its lack), Europeans were still confused about, and very impatient with, what they perceived to be inferior (lesser developed) races if only in so far as they could not sail as well. . . and who discovered whom? Basically, it was all too new. The confused and tense uncertainty we sometimes feel today in relating to people looking different is minuscule to what occurred in the sixteenth century, when different races first began to interact in large numbers. No one knew what "they" (the discovered or the discoverers) were.

Witness the first recorded use of the word "Negro" in 1555: "They are not accustomed to eate such meats as doo the Ethiopians or Negroes" (from Oxford Dictionary). The bewilderment of finding such different people did not stop the Europeans from trying in their ignorance to even "wash" the Negro (Oxford Dictionary) simplistically believing that they could be made more like Europeans. Failing that, the word "Negro" stuck and it was a good word because it identified those human beings having genetically-based thinker melanin layers with geographic roots to Africa. Over the centuries, the word maintained its own separateness and integrity, and generally everyone came to know the Negro was another human being. Overall, it is fair to say that these first experiences with Negroes facilitated a better understanding of common human beingness for other geographically separated races soon to be engaged in greater numbers also.

In a real sense, *today*, as is appropriate to the human species, race should devolve more to nationality (with or without hereditary commonness) than to actual biological genetic composition from one's generic or geohistorical race. Nationality with cultural development is a species-specific evolutionary quality peculiar to *homo sapiens*. It is how we have and are socially evolving. We should embrace it and understand it as our contemporary race.

With that background, the following are the four racial types relevant to all today. Each person can figure out his own race in a real way and draw his own conclusion as to what is important.

1. Primary Racial Type (current geographic origin) is the birth origin and citizenship of the person (ethnicity from *ethnos*, Greek meaning "nation"). Examples are Nigerian, American, Italian, Ethiopian, Egyptian, Japanese, et cetera. The national cultural spheres dwarf the biological. If a Negro-American returned to Africa and an Italian-American returned to Italy, both would be called "American" before anything else regardless of observable genetic traits.

2. Secondary Racial Type is the remote genetically-based national linkage which can be any of the primary nations. It is a single, double or multiple qualification of one's primary geographic origin. Examples are: Italian-American, American-Vietnamese, Nigerian-American, English-South African, et cetera.

3. Tertiary Racial Type is one's generic and/or geohistorical genetically-based origin which can be any of the five major generic or nine geohistorical races already mentioned. This has special significance if the primary or secondary national origins and roots are not known. Examples are European-American, Asian-American, Mongoloid-Amercian, Caucasian-American. Negro-

American is especially appropriate because Congoid and Capoid designations are now so blurred as to be obsolete.

4. Quaternary Racial Type is the biological hereditary description which is the use of biological characteristics for personal identification. Examples are blue eyed, black haired, brown skinned, et cetera. To use these terms in a broad way other than specific personal identification is actually to give them power which they do not deserve and is to achieve a racist type of designation, the primary examples of which are "black" and "white" as referring to groups. Biological descriptions are irrelevant except for personal description. Indeed, in all anthropology there is no rational use of any descriptive term in reference to race as a race itself. There is no "white"race. There is no "black" race. The use of color or other biological designation in substitution for race perpetuates unnatural and destructive distinctions possibly excluding one from being a part of his cultural race and country. And any society allowing such to occur will never provide the transcendental substance needed to sustain and advance.

What all this race stuff is about is essentially a matter of cultural understanding and recognition of the differences in mankind's past as part of variations within a *single* biological species. Therefore, biology is irrelevant even when present as far as human relationships go. A genuine understanding of race is to know man's unity and observed diversity — and this is cultural expectation of oneness rather than a biological commitment to division. The "inbreeding" is now global. There is *one* human family. There is one race. . . the human race.

Samuel A. Nigro

We're not animals.

Ray Nitschke, middle linebaker for the Vince Lombardi Green Bay Packers in an after-game interview

Dead children don't cause no problem.

Planned Parenthood social worker

Are there some rules? Yes: The transcendentals, virtues, and the Sacraments.

Samuel A. Nigro

Abortion is the denial of the Declaration of Independence.

Name Lost

The Catholic faith obliges us to hold that souls are immediately created by God.

Pope Pius XII

Religious freedom is not a pretext for moral anarchy.

John Courtney Murray

I call heaven and earth to record this day against you, that I have set before you life and death, blessing and cursing: therefore choose life, that both thou and thy seed may live.

Deuteronomy 30:19

Let not your rage or malice destroy a life, for, truly someone who does not esteem life does not deserve it.

Leonardo DeVinci

I ain't white. . .I'm Catholic!

Samuel A. Nigro

We love Man because Mankind consists of members of the animal kingdom and inhabitants of the planet who are thinking units of the universe. We cannot love Man when less.

Samuel A. Nigro

A healthy animality exists for humans in contrast to a grimy animality. Healthy animalness is in concert with nature consistent with the principle that morality cannot be separated from nature. Environmentalism gets it only partly right when it states we should respect the envelope of water, land, plants, and animals — it must also add human personal behavior consistent with nature.

Name Lost

All that exists, because it exists, is toward a knowing mind, even toward the finite human mind. This means: Not only is the eye sun-related, the sun as well is eye-related; all that has being is mind-related in its most intrinsic core. Mind and being are interconnected.

Josef Pieper

All things. . .linked are
That thou canst not stir a flower,
Without troubling of a star.

Francis Thompson

The work of St. Thomas Aquinas is deep and unique because it is an analysis of *Being*. Physics and metaphysics are combined gloriously. Natural law is defined from nature. St. Thomas grasps reality and focuses on the distinctions between beings and their most intrinsic *Beingness*. No one has ever, as St. Thomas, leaped mentally into the reality of the environment to define Natural Law which governs all we perceive through our senses as he did. St. Thomas is the ultimate analyzer and protector, the most magnanimous counter-culturalist, and the deepest-thinking environmental revolutionary of all time. Through St. Thomas' thought, natural liberty occurs rendering faith and reason to be consistent, compatible and not contradictory. His thoughts stand above any and all explanations or systems of world understanding and operation. People only pretend to know the universe unless they know something of the thought of St. Thomas Aquinas.

Samuel A. Nigro

Transcendental analysis is to ask six questions:
1. What is the material dimension (of matter) — the *res* of this?
2. What does this do to your identity (*aliquid*) as a complete human being (essence/form)?
3. What is the truth (*verum*) of this phenomenon as it relates to reality?

4. What is the oneness (*unum*) established for you by this with your family, your neighborhood, your community, the world?
5. What is the good (*bonum*) of this in concert with your personal evolution as well as that of the universe?
6. What is the beauty (*bella*) of this in terms of your personal ascension and uplifting those around you?

Samuel A. Nigro

Blessed is he who expecteth nothing, for he shall enjoy everything.

St. Francis of Assisi

Feminists reveal, *in vivo* so to speak, that cavemen were really kind folk in comparison to contemporary women who actually are more brutal than any archeologial evidence demonstrates about those scurrilously-slandered old guys who scratched pictures on the walls of caves.

Samuel A. Nigro

See G. Grisez's, J. Boyle's, J. Finnis' and W.E. May's article "Open to the New Life. . ." in *The Thomist* 52.3, July 1988, p. 370. The authors use the strong term of "pratical hatred" for describing the attitude toward the possible new human being coming to be, explaining that it is not necessarily emotional. While the word "hatred" can seem shocking to those spouses who believe in the goodness of contraception, because they had a chance to examine it deeply enough, nevertheless it truly describes the neglect of a possible new person at the moment of taking a pill or similar contraceptive.

Gintautas Vaitoska

Whence arrives the order and harmony of the world?

Isaac Newton about God

The essential is always invisible.

St. Exupery

Nothing really matters except a transcendental commitment which is Catholicism.

Samuel A. Nigro

The way things are is the only reliable basis for the way we should respond to them.

John Polkinghorne

Angels can fly because they can take themselves lightly.

G.K. Chesterton

God whispers to us in our pleasures, he speaks to us in our conscience, and he shouts to us in our pain.

C.S. Lewis

A liberal is a person with such grandiose ideation that he thinks he can solve everyone's problems himself even without considering nature.

Samuel A. Nigro

When mankind offends nature, all nature, including flora and fauna, screams. This is the case for the atmosphere, the air, the waters, the earth and soil, and plants and animals. They can be seen and heard in agony when mankind offends nature. But man is a part of nature too, and even man screams (usually belatedly) when nature including man is offended. This is nowhere more true than anent nature's marvelous procreative process. In all nature, sex is not recreation but is procreation, so when man deforms sex to recreation, all nature screams and suffers once again. In the final analysis, much of the negative happening to humans and the planet is a result of mankind's deformation of natural sexuality. Such is the proof of the wisdom of nature and of the folly of man.

Samuel A. Nigro

Divinity and infancy do definitely make a sort of epigram which a million repetitions cannot turn into a platitude. Bethlehem is emphatically a place where extremes meet. That tense sense of crisis which still tingles in the Christmas story and even in every Christmas celebration accentuates the idea of a search and discovery.

G.K. Chesterton

Nothing happens to anybody which he is not fitted by nature to bear.

Marcus Aurelius

So follow natural law.

The world is *charged* with the grandeur of God.

Gerard Manley Hopkins

To fish or cut bait. . .that is the question.

Paul Quinnett

It's nice to have a moral understanding that does not simply depend on the opinion of one's friends.

Hadley Arkes

Intellectual freedom cannot exist without complete objectivity.

Name Lost

No doctor, no parent, no court has any power to determine that the life of any child, however disabled the child will be, will be deliberately taken from it. I want this proposition clearly understood by all concerned.

Australian Supreme Court Justice Vincent

Inequality is present in the universe and handled in sub-human animals by the instincts. Humans handle their inequalities by virtues and the sacraments.

Samuel A. Nigro

No other story, no pagan legend or philosophic anecdote or historical event, does in fact affect any of us with that peculiar and even poignant impression produced on us by the word Bethlehem. No other birth of a god or childhood of sage seems to us to be Christmas or anything like Christmas.

G.K. Chesterton

The land is always stalking people.

Apache Elder

We recognize our mutual humanity in our differences, in our individuality, in our history, (and) in faithful discharge of our particular culture of obligations.

Michael Ignatieff

Man has no natural rights in opposition to his social duty.

Thomas Jefferson

Historically demonstrable, psychologically valid, and psychiatrically confirmed, are the irreplaceable benefits of an intact family unit with a pro-social value system. Indeed, the best deterrent to sleeping problems, the best deterrent to medical problems, the best deterrent to drug abuse, the best deterrent to heroin addiction, the best deterrent to inadequate school performance, the best deterrent to under-performance in work, the best deterrent to crime, the best deterrent to sexual perversion, the best deterrent to mental illness, and the best deterrent to human suffering, can all be summed up in two words: the family — specifically the family with a pro-social-moral value system which is lived by meaningful male/female relationships in which the children participate and wherein rights, duties, rules are openly discussed in mutual give-and-take with growth, respect, balance, gentleness, and self-sacrificing personal commitment. There is no equality. There has been no equality. There is only complementarity, and without complementarity, there is neither family nor society.

Every so often, apples are claimed to be oranges and men and women are claimed to be the same. In reference to human gender, unisexist pseudofeminist proclamations periodically occur demanding "person-entered language" among other things which generally prove to be private impositions masquerading as "equality" and "justice" (respectively, the latter two actually become "chivalry" and "role reversal" in practice).

The appeal of such unisexist ideas is intriguing and psychologically has much to do with the less energy and effort needed to float along pretending sameness rather than working to embrace one's natural role.

Often accompanying the unisexist demands is the theologically-correct perception that God is neither masculine nor feminine. However, Scripture and tradition emphasize the imagery given by God which clearly distinguishes male and female. Perhaps, just perhaps, the words and images Jesus gave with precision and passion contain more truths and greater capacity for love than some of the contemporary petty, inefficient and selfish proposals coming from unisexist people.

Indeed, the way social trends appear, Jesus might have known what He was saying and the images of "God the Father," etc. may have more bearing upon our lives according to natural law than we realize. When these images are removed, chaos becomes evident.

Samuel A. Nigro

Talking about relevant issues with deep transcendental understanding changes your chemistry. It is the soul impacting on the body.

Samuel A. Nigro

Show me a safe abortion and I will show you a safe electric chair.

George Rutler

The neurons must be stimulated. The neurons must be coded. The more the better. The brain's lexical axis must acquire the word of God and the words of prayers. Over and over! Prayers must be memorized. Early. It stimulates the neurons.

Samuel A. Nigro

It is better to find God by not finding Him than by finding not to find Him.

St. Augustine

It is clear that the influence of the Spirit is not confined to those levels of consciousness we take to be signs of maturity.

Colman E. O'Neil

The basic usefulness of faith lies precisely in the fact that a person believes and entrusts himself. . .Through faith, man achieves the good of his rational nature. . .Man must cooperate with God.

John Paul II

In every singular person, the humanity of all is present.

Peter J. Riga

And when ye shall come into the land and ye shall plant. . .

Leviticus 19,23

Nobody sings in an abortion clinic

Name Lost

In the depression things were so bad that I saw a rat sitting in the corner eating an onion crying like a newborn child.

Betty Howard

Brush your teeth twice a day and they will last one hundred years — and that is important when you're older so be sure and do it when you're younger.

Samuel A. Nigro

I hear but lack the faith and yet the sound calls me to life again. Earth's child I am again.

Faust

SONS OF GOD

"Blessed be the Peacemakers for they will be called sons of God."

Matthew 5:9

The phrase is "sons of God." This is obviously not a gender-specific use of the word "sons." In fact, other places in the Gospels reveal the use of a gender term in a non-gender way.

So what is the meaning of this? Are there any insights to be derived from deeper reflection on the use of such phrasing?

First of all, it seems obvious that being a "son of God" is not limited to males only. Indeed, in what used to be known as The Last Gospel, the phrase "son of God" obviously applies to all who profess belief in Jesus. But the gender word remains.

This brings up the second point: that Jesus is the Son of God. Obviously, we can become "sons of God" and participate in the mysteries of the universe as participating members in the Mystical Body of Christ. Somehow we become one with Him and participate in the divine process itself as part of Jesus' Son-ness by being a member of the Body of Christ. Our sex does not matter — we (male or female) become "sons of God."

The third point is to ask: "Why not `daughters of God'?" Is this sexism? Or is there a significance to "son" that is neither sexist nor negative but conveys a message and a mystery?

Well, a case can be made that it is clearly a message and mysterious only insofar as one must remember that male and female are different. The differences are apparent in creation — in all creation in terms of the transcendental distinctions between maleness and femaleness. That is, the masculine transcendentals are matter, truth, and goodness — they mean you will die in sacrifice. The feminine transcendentals are identity (form), oneness, and beauty — they mean you will give life.

While all created being has all of the transcendentals, the distinctions between male and female are real, complimentary, practical, and mysterious. It is totally unnatural to deny them.

So, in terms of the language with which humans must communicate, the concept of "son of God" conveys an existential grasp of good-promoting, truth-enhancing, and matter-organizing which are transcendentally operative in the existential sense rather than in a gender sense. Now this is how Nature is. And this is the phraseology that was *given to us*.

To interpret it negatively would seem to be an anomalous interpretation which conveys some sort of inferiority only if the transcendentals are incompletely applied. This is another way of saying that only those less embracing the transcendentals would be interpreting the gender components in a gender way and as an indication of inferiority. In other words, one is only "inferior" if one misses the whole point and begins to complain by saying "son" is gender and that it is a negative use rather than existential, explanatory, mysterious use of the word "son." It may be that we (male or female) all are "sons of God" because all must die in sacrifice as Jesus did to be a full member of the Body of Christ!

Thus, to be a "son of God" is gender irrelevant, but it is existential in the professed participation materially, truthfully, and with goodness in reated beingness sacrificing to death. this is not gender speific and it does not diminish but actually enhances the feminine transcendentals.

In fact, a case can be made that the feminine transcendentals of identity (form), oneness, and beauty complement a complete identification with Jesus as married to the church. That somehow the Mystical Body of Christ is a marriage with Christ as head and the church as Body with each "component" having its particular dimensions to be embraced fully consistent with different "members of the Body." The church is the Bride of Christ.

The church existentially conveys the feminine transcendentals: form (identity), oneness, and beauty.

A case can further be made that the Holy Spirit may convey the feminine (form/identity, oneness, beauty) transcendentals and male transcendentals (matter, truth, goodness) interrelating synthetically, although there is no reference in Scripture which would support such an interpretation even if it can be symbolically formulated.

But the embracing of humans as "sons of God" implies a more clear identity with Jesus as "Son of God" in a way that is not gender except insofar as the message conveys an identifiable Scriptural support for distinction of sexes which should never be denied.

Remember that God sent his Son to draw us into communion with Him. There is nothing gender about this except in the existential transcendental understanding of a specific embracing of good-promoting, truth-enhancing, and matter-organizing enabled by the belief in Jesus. And to be in the church, one embraces the feminine — forming, unifying and ascending. "For this is a great mystery, I mean in reference to Christ and the church. . ." (Ephesians 5:22-33) — Transcendentals, not gender. This is how to embrace Being — all of it!

Samuel A. Nigro

Angels are events more real than (or minimally at least as real as) any of the emotional, flashing, flickering light charlatans in television and movies. Angels are natural operations. If witnessing and transcendental confluence is desired, more faith can be placed in angels!

Samuel A. Nigro

The mind of man is divine, even in the unfathomable nature of its darkness. Men can think anything seriously, however absurd it is. Men can believe anything, even the truth.

G.K. Chesterton

A person is any created being actually or potentially capable of understanding and defending his own beginnings. In other words, if you will not defend your natural origins, you are not a person.

Samuel A. Nigro

Yesterday is the past, tomorrow is the future, but today is a gift — that's why they all it *the present*!

Richard Nero

To fear love is to fear life.

Italian proverb

We cannibals must help these Christians.

Queequeg

Conception

The pro-aborts have managed to change the meaning of the word "conception." Most of us were taught that it is equivalent to fertilization by union of sperm and egg. Recently, the pro-abortionists have made it equivalent to "implantation."

This verbicide of "conception" by the pro-aborts needs to be corrected. We must always state our meaning of "conception" to be the "traditional and accurate meaning of fertilization rather than implantation."

The reproductions below are from my *Dorlands Illustrated Medical Dictionary*, 23rd Edition, 1957. Later dictionaries may have been ruined by abortionists.

conception (kon-sep'shun) [L. *conceptio*]. 1. The fecundation of the ovum. 2. The image of a thing in the mind. **imperative conception**., a false idea which dominates a person"s actions.

fecundate (fe'kun-dat) [L. *fecundere* to make fruitfull]. To impregnate or fertilize.

fecundation (fe'kun-da'shun) [L. *fecundatio*]. Impregnation or fertilization. **artificial fertilization.**, artificial insemination.

fertilization (fer'ti-li-za-shun) The act of rendering fertile; fecundation. It consists of the fusion of a spermatozoon with an ovum, this being the natural stimulus which starts the development of the zygote thus formed. It results in inheritance, the determination of sex, and the initiation of cleavage. **cross fertilization**., the fertilization of one flower by the pollen of another.

Samuel A. Nigro, M.D.

Animals have no second thoughts. Man alone is able to see his own thoughts double.

G.K. Chesterton

It is called conscious-of-consciousness or C^2

The most important thing in life is to love life and to love life is to love God.

Pierre

For man and other rational creatures attain their end by knowing and loving God. Other creatures are not capable of this; they attain the ultimate end insofar as they participate in some likeness to God according to which they exist, or live, or even know.

St. Thomas

The greatest theoretic mistakes have arisen from the idea that the six days of creation are over.

G.K. Chesterton

For the object of the will, which is the human appetite, is universal good, just as the object of the intellect is universal truth. From this it is clear that nothing is able to satisfy the human will except universal good. But this is not found in anything created, but in God alone, because all creatures have a participated goodness.

St. Thomas

I can rejoice in my life because I did not swear false oaths, defended what was mine, did not pick quarrels, and can never be accused of the worst of all crimes: the murder of my own kin.

Beowulf

The religious hypothesis of the nature of the universe is actually much more rational, postulating a First Principle (God), the Source of energy which does not "run down," is not measurable, and is manifest to our rational faculties in both eternal and temporal aspects, by the measurable phenomena of inorganic matter, and through the rational faculty itself, which is of the non-measurable order, indicating a divine element in man, the immortal soul.

Isabel Paterson

We each began life as a single cell. 45 generations of doubling of number of cells by growth divisions were needed to reach the 30 trillion cells of an adult. Of these 45 generations of divisions, eight or nearly one-fifth have occurred by the time we were eight weeks old (in utero), 39 by 28 weeks' gestation, and 41 by the time we were born. The remaining tedious four occupy the whole of childhood and adolescence, and then there were no more.

Professor Sir Albert William Liley

In my boyhood it was common to say that many a man was a Great Might Have Been. To me it is a more solid and startling fact that any man in the street is a Great Might-Not Have Been.

G.K. Chesterton

And a lot of men are Have-Not-Been because of abortionists.

Those who oppose and resist nature are those who will lose.

Thomas Hardy

Gentlemen, in applied mathematics, you must describe your unit.

Sir Isaac Newton

No group is as intelligent as an individual. No group, as a group, has any intelligence; all intelligence is an individual's.

Isabel Paterson

No race nor creed can love exclude
If honored be God's name;
Our family embraces all
Whose Father is the same.

Ubi Caritas 6th verse

Behold the virgin shall conceive and bear a Son, in His name and shall call his name Emmanuel.

Isaiah 7:14

For a child is born to us, a son is given to us, and the government shall be on his shoulder, and they will call his name wonderful counselor, mighty God, everlasting Father, Prince of Peace.

Isaiah 9:5-6

Behold the days are coming, says the Lord, and I will make a new covenant with the house of Israel and the house of Juda. Not like the covenant I made with their fathers, on the day I took them by the hand to bring them out of the land of Egypt. My covenant they broke, and I was a master over them, says the Lord. But this is the covenant. . . I will place my law within them and write it upon their hearts. And I will be their God and they shall be my people.

Jeremiah 31:31-33

When God crowns your merits, He crowns nothing other than His own gifts.

St. Augustine

The cosmos is exceedingly specific and therefore has to be contingent on a choice among a great number of possibilities.

Paul Haffner

I implore you, my child, observe heaven and earth, and consider all that is in them, and acknowledge that God made them out of what did not exist.

2 Maccabees 7:28

Through the grandeur and the beauty of the creatures we may by analogy contemplate their Author.

Wisdom 13:1-5

All religion is in two categories: In one there is the Judeo-Christian religion with its belief in a linear cosmic story running from in the beginning to a new heaven and earth. In the other are all the pagan religions, primitive and sophisticated, old and modern, which invariably posit the cyclic and eternal recurrence of all, or rather the confining of all into an eternal treadmill, the most effective generator of the feeling of unhappiness and haplessness.

S.L. Jaki

Neither the eternity, nor the temporality of the universe can be demonstrated on the basis of reason alone.

St. Thomas

If the universe is not necessary, that is not necessarily what it is, then it is contingent. If, however, it is contingent, its actual shape and its very existence are dependent on a choice which transcends the entire universe. Such a choice or power can only be the creative omnipotence of God.

S.L. Jaki

If existence is defined in any way except by the transcendentals we are in trouble.

Samuel A. Nigro

We are born between feces and urine.

St. Augustine

While the leopard, the great whale, and the forests are to be protected by restraining mankind to a proper sense of things, man as a natural being is to be given no protection? There are aspects of the cheetah's existence which ought not to be violated, but none of man's? Other animals are to be protected in their natural habitats and in their natural function, but man is not. . .?

Paul Ramsey

Abortion is the rape of the womb.

Debra Evans

If this is not in your doctor's office, LEAVE!

A.D. 1995 Restatement of the Oath of Hippocrates (Circa 400 B.C.)

I SWEAR in the presence of the Almighty and before my family, my teachers and my peers that according to my ability and judgment I will keep this Oath and Stipulation:

TO RECKON all who have taught me this art equally dear to me as my parents and in the same spirit and dedication to impart a knowledge of the art of medicine to others. I will continue with diligence to keep abreast of advances in medicine. I will treat without exception all who seek my ministrations, so long as the treatment of others is not compromised thereby, and I will seek the counsel of particularly skilled physicians where indicated for the benefit of my patient.

I WILL FOLLOW that method of treatment which according to my ability and judgment, I consider for the benefit of my patient and abstain from whatever is harmful or mischievous. I will neither prescribe nor administer a lethal dose of medicine to any patient even if asked nor counsel any such thing nor perform act or omission with direct intent deliberately to end a human life. I will maintain the utmost respect for every human life from fertilization to natural death and reject abortion that deliberately takes a unique human life.

WITH PURITY, HOLINESS AND BENEFICENCE I will pass my life and practice my art. Except for the prudent correction of an imminent danger, I will neither treat any patient nor carry out any research on any human being without the valid informed consent of the subject or the appropriate legal protector thereof, understanding that research must have as its purpose the furtherance of the health of that individual. Into whatever patient setting I enter, I will go for the benefit of the sick and will asbstain from every voluntary act of mischief or corruption and further from the seduction of any patient.

WHATEVER IN CONNECTION with my professional practice or not in connection with it I may see or hear in the lives of my patients which ought not be spoken abroad I will not divulge, reckoning that all such should be kept secret.

WHILE I CONTINUE to keep this Oath unviolated may it be granted to me to enjoy life and the practice of the art and science of medicine with the blessing of the Almighty and respected by my peers and society, but should I trespass and violate this Oath, may the reverse be my lot.

It takes an incredible act of faith to believe in science — because science has no staying power.

Name Lost

I will ask the Father and he will send you another Advocate to be with you always, the Spirit of truth which the world cannot accept, because it neither sees nor knows it. But you know it, because it remains with you, and will be in you. I will not leave you orphans.

John 14:6-18

AH, THE NOBLE SAVAGE

They live. . . in a "chronic state of warfare." Wife-beating, chest-pounding matches and club-fighting duels were common. Abduction of women in murderous intervillage raids were a fact of life. . . Even among members of the same band, arguments and fights — usually over women — were frequent and often resulted in the village "fissioning" that characterized Yanomama settlement patterns and kept the groups from expanding to more than 100 or 150 individuals. . . . What made the piture that much more disturbing was that the Yanomama were probably the most pristine society in the world.

Brandeis Review, Winter 1991

Everything short of thee, oh Lord, is changeable, but Thou endurest. . . The creature changes, the Creator never. Then only the creature stops changing, when it rests on Thee.

Cardinal Newman

We are Christians only insofar as we believe in Jesus and keep His word.

Father Solanus Casey

The metamorphosis of animals is incredibly unbelievable for the creatures themselves and actually impossible for us humans to have preconceived without observing, say, the five metamorphoses of shrimp to adulthood. For humans, this amazing phenomenon in Nature is known as Christianity, and each sacrament is a metamorphosis.

Samuel A. Nigro

The sole test to apply to an evolutionist is to ask: What will be the last product of human evolution?

Anonymous

Reality and individuality are only known by the transcendentals.

Samuel A. Nigro

Catholicity recognizes in Nature something sacred and inviolable, which even the church must respect. . .

Eric Voegelan

A man knows himself only insofar as he knows the world.

Goethe

If I do not believe in God, I should still want my doctor, my lawyer, and my baker to do so.

G.K. Chesterton

Hell's work is purely spiritual, you know; hell cannot produce a single atom of that blessed creation of God, matter.

Peter Kreeft

I was not born to be free. I was born to adore and to obey.

C.S. Lewis

Happiness can come only from being, not having.

Peter Kreeft

All being is either the supremely good Creator or else His creation, which He himself solemnly pronounced "very good" after creating it.

Peter Kreeft

There are three kinds of people in the world: those who have sought God and have found him and now serve Him, those who are seeking Him but have not yet found him, and those who neither seek Him nor find Him. The first are reasonable and happy, the second reasonable and unhappy, the third unreasonable and unhappy.

Paschal

The principal mark of genius is not perfection but originality, the opening of new frontiers.

Arthur Koestler

Call me anything but late for dinner.

Sylvian Smith

Cross an oyster with an owl, and you'd get pearls of wisdom.

Milton Segal

Cross a camel with a cow, and you'd get a dromedary.

Ellis Steward

Cross a mosquito with a rabbit, and you'd get a bug's bunny.

Pam, Lois & Allison Roberts

Cross a giraffe with an ostrich, and you'd really be sticking your neck out.

Jim Goodwin

Spring is God's way of saying, "One more time!"

Robert Orben

To prevent birth is anticipated murder. . . The one who will be a man is already one.

Tertullian

The ordinary modern progressive position is that this is a bad universe, but will certainly get better. I say it is certainly a good universe even if it gets worse.

G.K. Chesterton

Right is right, even if nobody does it. Wrong is wrong, even if everybody is wrong about it.

G.K. Chesterton

If a thing is worth doing, it is worth doing badly.

G.K. Chesterton

Except a man be born again, he cannot see the Kingdom of God.

John 3:3

She was baptized, with all her household.

Acts 16:15

Yes, and I did baptize the household of Stephanas.

I Corinthians 1:16

The chief message I handed onto you, as it was handed onto me, was that Christ, as the Scriptures foretold, died for our sins. . . That is our preaching, mine or theirs as you will; that is the faith that has come to you.

1 Corinthians 15:3-11

Rise up, and receive baptism, washing away your sins at the invocation of his name.

Acts 22:16

When one party is removed to a great distance, as God is, the possibility of friendship ceases.

Aristotle

But Aristotle did not know Christ.

Samuel A. Nigro

We have found the one of whom Moses wrote in the Book of the Law and of whom the prophets also wrote. He is Jesus, the Son of Joseph, from Nazareth.

John 1:45

Beauty is as beauty does.

old proverb

And whoever welcomes in my name one such child as this, welcomes me.

Matthew 18:5

Watch out for false prophets; they come to you looking like sheep on the outside but they are really like wild wolves on the inside. You will know them by the way they act.

Matthew 7:15-16

But I belong to that race of people who, born to Catholicism, realize in earliest manhood that they will be within it forever and ever. They are inundated with light; they know that it is true.

Francois Mauriac

PLEASE, TELL ME ABOUT OUR CHILD
Please tell me about our child.
Don't tell me you haven't thought about it.
I know it's been on your mind a lot.
So tell me.
Please.
I need to know.

Was our baby a little boy or a little girl?
What would he have looked like?
Would she have smiled when you held her to your breast?
Would she have reached out with tiny hands with that warmth in her eyes that comes from knowing that she was safe and loved?
How much did she weigh?
Was carrying her all that hard as you both grew larger and larger?
Did you feel full again and alive, like a woman?
What color was her hair, her eyes?
Did she kick inside you?
don't tell me you haven't thought about it.
I know you have.
I know it's probably been on your mind a lot since then.
So please tell me.
I need to know.
I need to know because I am a man and I have thought about it a lot.
Every day.
Since before you left me.
And I know that if our baby's going away has torn out of me as much as it has, it tore out of you, too, only more.
She was inside of you.
And she was torn out.
I know that what I say is true.
So please don't deny that.
I need to know.
And so do you.

This poem was written by a young single man whosegirlfriend decided to have an abortion without consulting him

Now a child is the very sign and sacrament of personal freedom. He is a fresh will to the wills of the world; he is something that his parents have freely chosen to produce and which they freely agree to protect.

G.K. Chesterton

If you are pro-choice, why are you not pro-abortion?

Samuel A. Nigro

You tear off the mask of nature and you find God.

G.K. Chesterton

Humans are the only creature in the animal kingdom which wastes energy having sexual intercourse when fertility is not possible.

Name Lost

Matter repels man and matter rejects man, especially when man abuses it. In a way, matter is foreign to man except that small part of matter called the body which is included in the soul. So, no wonder we have such a hard time. The soul is eternal and matter is bitter about it. . .unless baptized and kept holy by the sacraments.

Samuel A. Nigro

The soul soaks the body.

G.K. Chesterton

Get a new soul.

G.K. Chesterton

Aren't you glad you're a people?

Kristin Nigro Kranz -4 years old looking at a large eel in the Cleveland Aquarium

Abortion is the symbol, the supreme act and ultimate achievement of a modern, sophisticated tyranny. It is a moral bomb exploding one's own skull as sure as it destroys the future of the universe, intolerantly crushes the brains of a human adversary and expands the beastly ability of mankind to new immanity.

Samuel A. Nigro

If "choice" is more important than life, then anything goes if you choose it.

Name Lost

It is more dignified to act through an intermediary than to act directly. Sharing in causality gives a being the dignity of a cause.

Leon J. Podles

The supreme adventure is being born. There we do walk suddenly into a splendid and startling trap. There we do see something of which we have not dreamed before. Our father and mother do lie in wait for us, and leap out at us, like brigands from a bush. Our uncle is a surprise. Our aunt is, in the beautiful common expression, a bolt from the blue.

G.K. Chesterton

A baby is God's opinion that the world should go on.

Carl Sandburg

The underlying force that creates and unites humanity is the love that moves the sun and the other stars.

Dante leaving Heaven

Abortion is essentially *unnatural selection* diametrically opposed to the evolutionary theory.

Name Lost

Having spent half a lifetime working at the forefront of fundamental physics, I have found the use of words like "design," "meaning," and "purpose" irresistible. How can one accept a scheme of things so cleverly arranged, so subtle and felicitous, simply as a brute fact, as a package of properties that just happens to be? Of course, science cannot prove the existence of a design, or a designer, but it an reveal the sheer depth of ingenuity that goes to make up this marvelous universe, our home.

Paul Davies

Your eyes beheld my unformed substance.

Psalm 139:16

Abortion is killing like throwing a pebble in a pond. There is an immediate and obvious splash: the death of an unborn child — relief for the mother. But there are ripples that go out in all directions. Try as you may, morality can never be privatized: our choices inevitably affect others.

Anthony Fisher

Much of the essence of psychotherapy and analysis is what a patient told me: "I tell them all about me and they repeat it with a few words I don't understand." This is not enough.

Joseph Mauceri

People who support environmental security and natural processes but deny the same for behavior, are fooling themselves. Animals are not "free" to violate behavioral norms in nature — and just as with the environment, neither should humans choose to be contrary to natural behavior.

Name Lost

Abortion is legal amnesty for murder.

Samuel A. Nigro

It is exactly when we regard man as an animal that we know he is not an animal.

G.K. Chesterton

Every human has his right to possess himself, his life, and that which contributes to it.

John Paul II

Believe in it? *Madam, I've seen it done.*

William James to a woman who asked
him if he believed in Baptism

Where there is nothing, there is Satan.

G.K. Chesterton

The acts and conduct as substantially charged in the indictment (enouraging and compelling abortions) constitute crimes against humanity. . .and. . .war crimes.

Nurenberg Military Tribunal

The river of human nonsense flows on forever.

G.K. Chesterton

All reality is magic! All life is a miracle! Each individual came from nothing! And everything can be sacramental and therefore everything can save. Jesus touches all lives through the Incarnation.

Samuel A. Nigro

Life is a mystery to be lived, not a problem to be solved.

Adrian Van Kaam

Clothes are natural to man because man is not merely natural.

G.K. Chesterton

I will give them a new heart and put a new spirit within them; I will remove the stony heart from their bodies, and replace it with a natural heart, so that they will live according to my statutes, and observe and carry out my ordinances.

Ezekiel 11-19-20

Abortion kills the Golden Rule.

— Samuel A. Nigro

Violent energy is always needed to sustain that which is not real.

— Samuel A. Nigro

But gramercy, what of those Godpossibled souls that we nightly impossibilize, which is a sin against the Holy Ghost, Very God, Lord and Giver of Life. In her lay a Godframed Godgiven preformed possibility which thou hast fructified with thy modicum of man's work. Cleave to her! Serve! And let all Malthusiasts go hang Herod's slaughter of the innocents were the truer name.

— Stephen Dedealus

If the laws of the planet, the environment and nature have created us, then we MUST always be trying to know, love and serve natural law principles. To do otherwise is to repudiate our being which is crazy. To do otherwise is to violate the environment itself, to soil the planet and betray nature, and at the same time, we are obviously are, if God is, rejecting God!

— Samuel A. Nigro

Abortion seems harmless enough and helpful enough but it is killing innocent human individuals at a stage all human beings went through once and only once.

— Samuel A. Nigro

If a man does not talk to himself it is because he is worth talking to.

— G.K. Chesterton

Without me, there could be no everybody.

— Ashleigh Brilliant

Why am I me?

— burning question since 4 years old

God made man in his own image and man returned the compliment.

— Blaise Pascal

You came from nothing. What more is there in this astonishing, awesome amazement? And what greater love is there than in Heaven!

— Name lost

I never believed in miracles, until I was born.

— Ashleigh Brilliant

Nature wins every battle in the end, so, whenever there's a choice, I side with nature.

— Ashleigh Brilliant

It is absurd for the evolutionists to complain that it is unthinkable for an admittedly unthinkable God to make everything out of nothing, and then pretend that it is more thinkable that nothing should turn itself into everything.

— G.K. Chesterton

A person is any unique, individual, rational creature with the potential and willingness to define, protect, and promote the origin and beingness of itself and its species as found in nature. (Obviously, this definition of "person" excludes those who would do or be for abortion.)

— Samuel A. Nigro

If your hearts were pure every creature would be to you a mirror of God and a book of holy teaching.

— Thomas à Kempis

Nature's tears are reason's never not.

— from Romeo & Juliet

. . .more than kin. . .less than kind. . .

— Hamlet

The unborn have as little or as much right to be enrolled in life as you and I. Those unborn babies deserve their chance to see if they can make it. Letting them live is the *sine qua non* for anyone who believes in "equality."

— Samuel A. Nigro

As Jesus gave us The Our Father, it goes without saying that somehow He would also give us The Hail Mary. . . if He believed in the Fourth Commandment.

— Samuel A. Nigro

The key to living well is human nature adequately understood.

— Raphael Waters

The Good News is that Original Sin is over, and we can live just as in the Garden of Eden but it requires us to choose the transcendentals.

— Samuel A. Nigro

There are no ordinary people. You have never talked to a mere mortal.

C.S. Lewis

The Jews gave us God. . .one God but in more ways than one. Jews are to be thanked, honored and prayed with.

Samuel A. Nigro

Babies are the voice of God.

Name Lost

Do not let anyone ruin your gene pool contribution. Protect the gene pool and let life happen.

Samuel A. Nigro

Neither love nor friendship will save us. I once thought they would, but now I realize that it is the other way around. Love and friendship are the results of salvation, not the cause.

James Schall

In the temporal order, an *event* is a point in space-time of something that happens at a certain place and a certain time. So is Baptism. This means you.

CHAPTER 4:

PENANCE

In the physical order, a *spectrum* is the splitting of energy into position-time relationships. Your human beingness is a spectrum.

In the spiritual order, *Penance* is a *spectrum* of *unity* (re-unity, really) wherein negative occurrences are "selectively ignored" and split to insignificance. Resulting is *hope* with trust in an ultimate positivity and capacity for ascending.

"Father, forgive them, for they know not what they do."

Penance makes you a spectrum — a splitting off of what disunites you so that one is unity and hope selectively ignoring entropy.

Live Penance — a reconciliation from willful disunion to restored oneness.

**Suffering converts entropy to synthesis.
To Ascend and to participate in the Incarnation.**

In physics, a *spectrum* is the splitting of energy into position-time relationships. So is Penance.

Penance is a Sacrament in which the sins committed after Baptism are forgiven. Penance is a *spectrum.*

Penance is wherein negative occurrences are to be "selectively ignored" and split to insignificance. This coincides in the physical-temporal world with *spectrum* wherein energies are split. For the human, the principle of *unity* is forthcoming, accompanied by *hope* in that the negativity will be selectively ignored and positivity will create ascension.

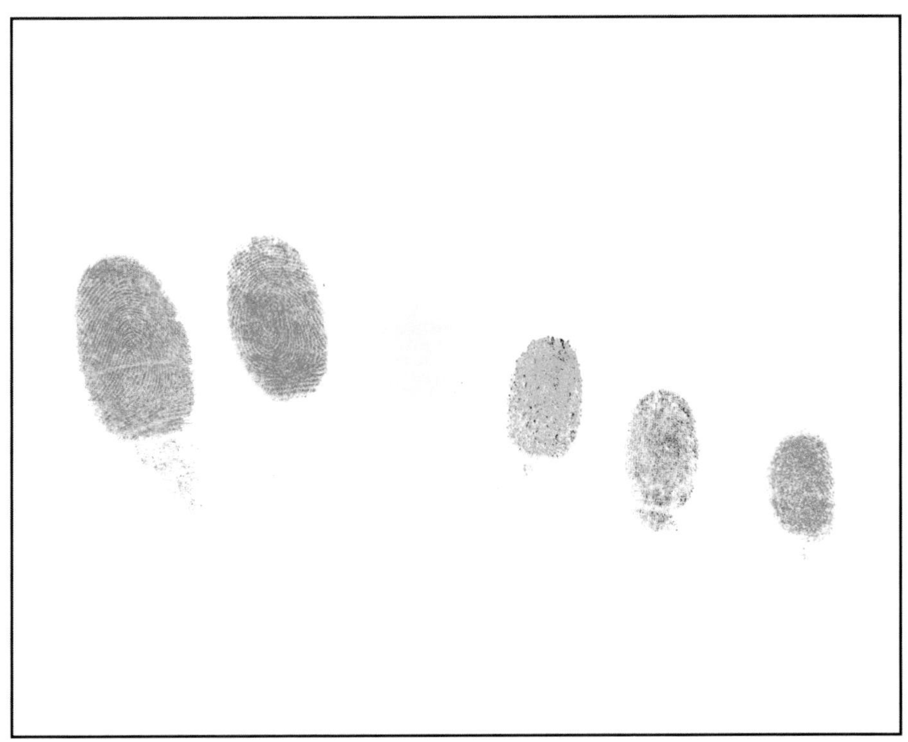

Selective Ignoring. . .

. . . One way to be a human being. Animals seldom ignore and often are indiscriminate. But a human being consciously selects those things to be overlooked in the interest of mutual respect. Ignoring those things removes antipathy which wastes human energy. Selectively ignore . . . so that nothing ruins relationship. Thus hate will be thwarted, and love will personalize whatever confronts you.

SELECTIVE IGNORING

There are times it's best to look the other way. This does not mean that one does not identify or take note of what has been said or done, but it is appropriate, for the time being, to ignore such. This may be coupled with: "I really don't want to see that — so let's try it again and do it right."

* * * * *

Tears are at the heart of things.

Virgil

Make lemonade out of it. . . .

Anna Marie O'Hare (after listening too long to someone's troubles)

Sin is willful entropy — the increasing of disorder by conscious decision.

Samuel A. Nigro

If it weren't for the rocks in its bed, the stream would have no song.

Carl Perkins

I was what people called a "troublesome boy."

Sir Winston Churchill

Happy the man who has a good wife; he lives twice as long.

J.W. Goethe

She dies so young?

No life is so hard that you can't make it easier by the way you take it.

Ellen Glasgow

Everyone goes through the I-have-the-answer stage which is a manifestation of Original Sin when not transcendentally sound. Only by transcendental analysis can we recognize the know-nothings from those who really have something to offer.

Samuel A. Nigro

Good works are always accompanied by entropy which we know as suffering, and suffering as "offered-up" entropy can *de novo* create good works.

Samuel A. Nigro

Your liberty to swing your arm ends where my nose begins.

Stuart Chase

The mind is its own place, and in itself can make a heaven of hell, a hell of heaven.

John Milton

Pain nourishes courage. You can't be brave if you've only had wonderful things happen to you.

Mary Tyler Moore

Democracy may not prove in the long run to be as efficient as other forms of government, but it has one saving grace: It allows us to know and say that it isn't.

Bill Moyers

For evil to exist, it must have something "good" to parasitize — evil depends on us.

Samuel A. Nigro

The reason most people are unhappy is that they focus on what they do not have rather than what they do have.

Anthony de Mello

"Family" is learning to fight fair.

Samuel A. Nigro

. . .The odious unctuous vituperative rabble-cooking villainous hate-mongering sanctimonious pseudo-sophistical satanic bellowing barbarous pandering lizard-eyed. . . .

NH Representative Gregg

(This beats swearing!)

Refusing to have an opinion is a way of having one, isn't it?

Luigi Pirandello

A fanatic is someone who can't change his mind and won't change the subject.

Sir Winston Churchill

There's no dealing with a cat who knows you're awake.

Brad Solomon

Most of what we all disagreement is merely confusion.

John Courtney Murray

Too much caution is bad for you. By avoiding things you fear, you may let yourself in for unhappy consequences. It is usually wiser to stand up to a scary-seeming experience and walk right into it, risking the bruises or hard knocks. You are likely to find it is not as tough as you had thought. Or you may find it plenty tough, but also discover you have what it takes to handle it.

Norman Vincent Peale

Don't lend people money. It gives them amnesia.

Robert Barrett

Greed has the insidious feature of not knowing how much is enough.

Donald DeMarco

It is the toy box, all these people and things we play with, which keeps us from Christ.

St. Augustine

The most grievous and detrimental sin is from pride wherein we need to proclaim something is "right" *because* we are doing it.

Samuel A. Nigro

People *must* proclaim what they do is right — regardless of what they do.

Samuel A. Nigro

We must accept finite disappointment, but we must never lose infinite hope.

Martin Luther King, Jr.

You can't be afraid of stepping on toes if you want to go dancing.

Lewis Freedman

The test of courage comes when we are in the minority. The test of tolerance comes when we are in the majority.

Ralph W. Sockman

Premarital sex is nothing but trouble.

Samuel A. Nigro

When someone says "I love you," do they mean: "I love me and take off your clothes?"

Reverend Paul Marx

"Well-adjusted" means you can make the same mistakes over and over again, and keep smiling.

George Bergman

We love those who know the worst of us and don't turn their faces away.

Walker Percy

It is not the man who has too little who is poor, but the one who craves more.

Seneca

The Bible tells us to love our neighbors and also to love our enemies; probably because generally they are the same people.

G.K. Chesterton

A CHURCH FOR SINNERS EXISTS

The church tells what we *need* to know rather than what we want to hear. We need a church that refuses to allow us to feel good while we are doing bad. We need a church that helps us to do good and avoid evil. We need a church that leads instead of follows. That challenges rather than complies — no "democracy of sin" here. A church of hard sacrifice before easy answers. A church for sinners rather than the righteous who never do anything wrong! A church that stands for something. A church that has been through the centuries as a bulwark of sanity. A church able to shunt off the crazy schemes of each given era. A church that knows and promotes Truth and Love and keeps us from being engulfed in the latest madness which leads, regardless of the era, to a grimy animality. Yes, we need a church that offers confession or an efficient method of forgiveness for our sins.

Given that such a church exists, the reasonable conclusion is that its members ought to use the gift of the sacrament of confession.

The reason is clear: To participate in a church which stands for something means that we must undergo a grace-obtaining self-examination in order to have everlasting life because none of us is perfect.

Confession requires a serious self-reflection which is indeed a cleansing of the mind. It helps set one's priorities in order. It can re-establish self-integrity. It places one in touch with the realities of the world rather than the fantasies. It is a formalized grappling with real truth, with naked truth, and with the personal truth about ourselves. Confession helps inform the conscience — a great necessity because a conscience is not truly functional if it is mere impulse uninformed about Truth and Love.

Confession is the time to look at oneself closely and take ownership for all that has gone wrong without blaming others.

A thoughtful examination of behavior and conscience together with confession itself is the least expensive and most promising positive mental health promoting process every devised or more accurately given by God.

But be not confused. Confession is not mental health counseling. It is not psychotherapy. It is not a mental health promoting process in the primary sense — but only as a secondary spinoff. It is not a replacement for psychotherapy or counseling. Nevertheless, to the average person, it is more helpful than psychological and psychotherapeutic approaches.

The open face-to-face style never stays the dispensation of grace, but it does seem to imitate or simulate mental health counseling. Though the result may be therapeutic, confession is not therapy. At present, most priests are not sufficiently trained for the counseling which purportedly goes on. Choice of style may still be up to the penitent — however, the church is not *per se* in the therapy business.

In addition, confidentiality is not as simple for the penitent in face-to-face confessions. In the psychological sense, anonymity helps confirm confidentiality. Granted that the confidentiality of the confession is absolute and protected by law, but anonymity makes it easier for most.

Furthermore, people who go to confession are not necessarily seeking mental health, but rather are searching for forgiveness and new grace.

People attending confession are desiring to look truth in the eye and not some man who will be recognized at the next church event — and who may recognize you.

Face-to-face confession creates some discomfort when the confessor and the penitent meet by chance at a later time. The problem is that you know that he knows — or at least you believe such, even though you are not immediately identified among the hundreds of confessions the priest has heard. You "know that he knows" — and should he at some level recognize you, there occurs a distance and awkwardness that was not ever a problem when confessions had the one-way anonymity and the absolute confidentiality which goes with anonymity.

On the other hand, in the darkened confessional, the very impersonality of secret anonymity personalizes as no other way can. When personal confidences are revealed, positive mental health results which is intrinsic to the *anonymity* of confession and essential for the good mental feeling which accompanied actual reconciliation by grace. Confidential and anonymous confession puts us in touch with God and not with another man.

In the darkness of the closed confessional, in an atmosphere of profound absolute secrecy, in an *unique interational relationship never duplicated anywhere else ever in the annals of human history*, comes the willingness to reveal one's self to Jesus' successor in the person of the priest. One senses the presence of the Divinity under those circumstanes rather than a mere human interaction with a person who looks not much different from you or me — but who looks through the blurring screen of the dark confessional as someone superhuman rather than merely "like me." Indeed, the priest is God's Divine representative empowered by the Holy Spirit.

The Roman Catholic Church is for us sinners. We must get back to using the Sacrament of confession in order to "get right with God."

Confession, in the Roman Catholic tradition, is a singularly unique process which allows in an anonymous setting an intense personal introspection and a salubrious renewal to do what is right. The tendency today of interpreting it as a psychological process has made it into a mundane interaction, gutting it of its uniqueness and meaning. The power of the priesthood is enhanced by a return to the truth-confronting, grace-seeking, personal contact with God as mediated through the priest who is not just "another human being." Restoring this power might even attract vocations whereas being an inadequate counselor will not.

Name Lost

Dr. Nigro, you need a phrenologist.

angry patient

The difference between a pessimist and an optimist is that the pessimist has more experience.

Clare Boothe Luce

No good deed goes unpunished.

Clare Boothe Luce

Sex is the *ersatz*, or substitute, religion of the 20th century.

Malcolm Muggeridge

When are you going to stop making yourself miserable and blaming it on everyone else?

Samuel A. Nigro

The capacity to inflict pain.

Harvard University President's answer when asked to name the fundamental quality of leadership.

False pride is pride in anything other than what you are doing right now.

Samuel A. Nigro

We make our friends; we make our enemies; but God makes our next door neighbor.

G.K. Chesterton

If there were no God, there would be no atheists.

G.K. Chesterton

There are only three things in the world that women do not understand; and they are liberty, equality, and fraternity.

G.K. Chesterton

I believe in preaching to the converted; for I have generally found that the converted do not understand their own religion.

G.K. Chesterton

It is a holy and wholesome thought to pray for the dead that they may be loosed from their sins.

2 Maccabees 12:46

So much has been written down that you may learn to believe Jesus is the Christ, the son of God, and so believing find life through his name.

John 20:31

Everything in scripture has been divinely inspired, and it has its uses; to instruct us, to expose our errors, to correct our faults, to educate in holy living.

2 Tim 3:17

Receive the Holy Spirit; when you forgive men's sins, they are forgiven; when you hold them bound, they are held bound.

John 20:22-23

I tell you, you will not get out till you have paid the very last penny.

Luke 12:59

Do you know that the unjust will not inherit the Kingdom of God? Do not be deceived; neither fornicators nor idolaters, not adulterers nor boy prostitutes nor praticing homosexuals. . .will inherit the Kingdom of God.

1 Corinthians 6:9-10

No studies are needed any longer to determine if masturbation makes one stupid. The evidence is in: just observe a gay and lesbian parade.

Name Lost

Men die only once, and after that comes judgment.

Hebrews 9:27

There is no forgiveness either in this world or in the world to come.

Matthew 12:32

He will be the loser, and yet he himself will be saved, though only as men are saved by passing through fire.

1 Corinthians 3:15

Repent, Peter said to them, and be baptized, every one of you, in the name of Jesus Christ, to have your sins forgiven: then you will receive the gift of the Holy Spirit. This promise is for you and your children, and for all those, however far away, whom the Lord our God calls to himself.

Acts 2:38-39

Now the works of the flesh are manifest, which are immorality, uncleanness, licentiousness, idolatry, witchcraft, enmities, contentions, jealousies, anger, quarrels, factions, parties, envies, murderers, drunkness, carousings, and such like. . . I have warned you that they who do such things will not attain the kingdom of God.

Galatians 5:19-20

He breathed on them, and said to them, receive the Holy Spirit; when you forgive men's sins, they are forgiven, when you hold them bound, they are held bound.

John 20:22-23

Be it known therefore to you, brethren, that through Him (Christ) forgiveness of sins is proclaimed to you, and in Him everyone who believes is acquitted of all the things of which you could not be acquitted by the Law of Moses.

Acts 13:38-39

This, as always, is God's doing; it is He who, through Christ, has reconciled us to himself, and allowed us to minister this reconciliation of his to others.

2 Corinthians 5:18

If we go on sinning willfully, when one the full knowledge of truth has been granted to us, we have no further sacrifice for sin to look forward to; nothing but a terrible expectation of judgment, of fire that will eagerly consume the rebellious.

Hebrews 10:26

Not all sin is deadly.

1 John 5:17

Jesus exercised the power to forgive sins as *man*, "to convince you that the Son of Man has authority to forgive sins while he is on earth."

Mark 3:10

Only, brethren, I entreat you by our Lord Jesus Christ, and by the love of the Holy Spirit, to give me the help of your prayers to God on my behalf.

Romans 15:30

Not everyone who says to me, "Lord, Lord" shall enter the Kingdom of Heaven.

Matthew 7:21

These things I have written to you who believe in the name of the Son of God, that you may know that you have eternal life, and that you may continue to believe in the name of the Son of God.

1 John 5:13

I buffet my own body, and make it my slave; or I, who have preached to others, may myself be rejected as worthless.

1 Corinthians 9:27

Do you only take a bath once a year too?

Reverend Paul Marx

Beloved, you have always shown yourselves obedience; and now that I am at a distance, not less but much more than when I am present, you must work to earn your salvation, in anxious fear.

Philippians 2:12

All of us have a scrutiny to undergo before Christ's judgment seat, for each to reap what his mortal life has earned, good or ill, according to his deeds.

2 Corinthians 5:10

An indulgence is the remission in whole or in part of the temporal punishment due to sin. The word "indulgence" means a favor or concession, and it obtains by a very slight penance the remission of penalties that would otherwise be severe.

The Baltimore Catechism

Yelling: "I have been saved!" is not a real indulgence even though it goes far beyond any indulgence ever offered in history.

Samuel A. Nigro

God will award to every man what his acts have deserved.

Romans 2:6

There is graciousness, then, in God, and there is also severity. His severity is for those who have fallen away, his graciousness is for thee, only so long as thou doest continue in his grace; if not, thou too shalt be pruned away.

Romans 11:22

They shall confess their sin which they have done.

Numbers 5:7

Thou shalt call his name Jesus for He shall save his people from their sins.

Matthew 1:21

Thy sins are forgiven thee. . . Go in peace.

Luke 7:48-50

If your sins be as scarlet, they should be made as white as snow. And if they be as red as crimson, they shall be white as wool.

Isaiah 1:18

They that are in health need not a physician, but they that are ill. Go then and learn what this meaneth, I will have mercy and not sacrifice. For I am not come to call the just, but sinners.

Matthew 9:11-13

I say to you, that even so there shall be joy in heaven upon one sinner that doth penance, more than upon ninety-nine just who need not penance.

Luke 15:7

As the Father hath sent me, I also send you. When he had said this, he breathed on them; and he said to them: Receive ye the Holy Spirit. Whose sins you shall retain, they are retained.

John 20:21-23

Many of them who believed came confessing and declaring their deeds (to the Apostles).

Acts 19:18

The foolish things of the world hath God chosen that He might confound the wise; and the weak things of the world hath God chosen that He might confound the strong. And the base things of the world, and the things that are contemptible, hath God chosen, and the things that are not, that He might bring to nought things that are. That no flesh should glory in His site.

1 Corinthians 1:27-29

Nothing unclean shall enter Heaven.

Revelations 21:27

Who made you without you, will not justify you without you.

St. Augustine

Sin is the punishment of sin.

St. Augustine

If you squander your existence, there literally will be hell to pay.

Samuel A. Nigro

Love your enemies, bless them that curse you, do good to them that hate you, and pray for them which despitefully use you, and persecute you.

Matthew 5:44

Forgive us our debts, as we forgive our debtors.

Matthew 6:12

If ye forgive not men their trespasses, neither will your Father forgive your trespasses.

Matthew 6:15

Father, forgive them; for they know not what they do.

Luke 23:34

Be ye kind one to another, tenderhearted, forgiving one another, even as God for Christ's sake hath forgiven you.

Ephesians 4:32

If we confess our sins, he is faithful and just to forgive us our sins, and to cleanse us from all unrighteousness.

1 John 1:9

Then he began to upbraid the cities wherein most of his mighty works were done, because they repented not.

Matthew 11:20

Woe unto you also, ye lawyers! for ye lade men with burdens grievous to be borne, and ye yourselves touch not the burdens with one of your fingers.

Luke 11:46

. . .out of the heart proceed evil thoughts, murders, adulteries, fornications, thefts, false witnesses, blasphemies: These are the things which defile a man.

Matthew 15:18

So shall it be at the end of the world: the angels shall come forth, and sever the wicked from among the just, and shall cast them into the furnace of fire: there shall be wailing and gnashing of teeth.

Matthew 13:43-50

And whosoever shall offend one of these little ones that believe in me, it is better for him that a millstone were hanged about his neck and he were cast into the sea.

Mark 9:42

He who is not with me is against me, and he who does not gather with me scatters.

Matthew 12:30

Be not overcome by evil, but overcome evil with good.

Romans 12:21

Lord, do not hold this sin against them.

Saint Stephen at his Martyrdom

I will never say I do not know you even if I have to die with you!

Mark 14:31

Let the punishment for his death fall on us and on our children.

Matthew 27:25

The modern world shows its cynicism when it prefers to present its young with images of brokenness rather than images of beauty.

Donald DeMarco

Good advice usually works best when preceded by a bad scare.

Al Batt

Then Jesus said to him, "Listen! Don't tell anyone but go straight to the priest and let him examine you; then offer the sacrifice that Moses ordered, to prove to everyone that you are now clean."

Matthew 8:4

I tell you this: On the Judgment Day everyone will have to give account of every useless word he has spoken. For your words will be used to judge you, either to declare you innocent or to declare you guilty.

Matthew 12:36-37

As words are inflated along the superhighway of high-tech wordprocessing, they are correspondingly deflated in the moral universe that binds a person to what he says. . . . Words are now so disconnected from their human authorship that they offer little solace for those who feel the alienating chill of a heartless bureaucracy.

Donald DeMarco

Unless you make them angels.

I think I'll quit putting on my glasses, because everybody looks so beautiful the other way.

Jimmy Durante

The function of guilt is civilization. Guilt can be too much. . . rarely. Usually it merely means one has a conscience. . . which is good for the person and the world. Where there is no guilt, there is no civilization.

Samuel A. Nigro

History is important to study, but even more important is not believing it.

Samuel A. Nigro

He who is not willing to suffer with and for Christ will also not share in His Resurrection.

Franz Jagerstatter

If you do not protest evil, evil will engulf you.

Samuel A. Nigro

Tragedies such as untimely deaths, earthquakes, floods, and such, cannot be explained except as vivid demonstrations that evil is the absence of good.

Samuel A. Nigro

Every actual state is corrupt. Good men must not obey the laws too well.

Ralph Waldo Emerson

Faith in the heart leads to justification, confession on the lips to salvation.

Romans 10:10

If something is worth doing, it is worth doing well.

Homer Hill

We are never justified in being "bitter" toward anyone except ourselves.

Father Solanus Casey

Mr. Rikenbaker advises us that me meant exactly the reverse of what he wrote.

William F. Buckley, Jr.

Then Peter opened his mouth and said, "Of a truth I perceive that God is no respecter of persons. But in every nation he that fears him and worketh righteousness, is accepted by him."

Acts 10:34

Any press called "free" *belongs to the people* and it should be "free" for all except editors and journalists, whose job is not freedom but *truth* in all its dimensions. And the proven, willful disregard of truth should be the only crime for which capital punishment is exacted.

Samuel A. Nigro

Jesus Christ, Son of God, have mery on me, a sinner.

Meditation Prayer of Russian Monastery
(Prayer of Jesus)

Having seen the legal defense of "insanity" at work, it should be obvious that at least one-half of our lawyers, three-fourths of our politicians, and almost all the judges are not responsible for their behavior.

Anonymous

Original Sin is manifest by that which distinguishes humans from the rest of the animal kingdom: the mind. Thus, Original Sin is in the mind and it is actually *the unconscious* — the mental component of human life which out of self-love objects that we are not *all* that there is. How the unconscious presents and copes with our differences and limitations is the unconscious source of all mankind's troubles. It is the mark of Original Sin.

Samuel A. Nigro

Remember, no one wishing to follow our Lord can escape sorrows and persecutions.

Father Theodore Ushakoff

You can never tell one lie — there is always another.

Arthur Ashe

And whispering, "I will ne'er consent" — consented.

Lord Byron

Orthodoxy can only be secured by a cooperation of which free controversy is an essential part.

W.H. Auden

. . .if it (an unjust law) is of such a nature that it requires you to be the agent of injustice to another, then I say, break the law.

Henry Thoreau

Cults engage in deception to pursue their ends.

Steven Hassan

Most of life's evils arise from man's being unable to sit still in a room.

Paschal

We cannot grasp nature's bare blade without shedding our own blood.

Camille Paglia

A 13-year study of television demonstrates that viewers become more drowsy, sad, bored, lonely, and hostile the longer they watch.

Name Lost

Sports participation by activity or as spectator is an opportunity to improve oneself and others. If it does not do both, then to hell with it.

Samuel A. Nigro

Every kid should have an opportunity to play every position in every type of sport possible for no other reason than it is an opportunity to participate and be able to say that one did "try."

Name Lost

One more such victory and I am undone.

Pyrrhus

I have loved justice and hated inequity; therefore I die in exile.

Pope Gregory VII

Justice? There isn't enough to go round.

Arthur Balfour

It is charateristic of human nature to hate the one whom you have offended.

Tacitus

The witching spell of things that are little, makes it hard to see the good things.

Wisdom 4:12

This body of ours has one fault: The more you indulge it, the more ailments and needs it discovers.

St. Theresa of Avila

Satan transformed himself into an angel of light.

2 Corinthians 11:14

Beware of flickering lights. . .like television and movies.

They (evil-doers) do not know the penalty of wrongdoing. . . It is not stripes in death. . .evil-doers often escape these, but a penalty that cannot be escaped. . .that they lead a life like the pattern into which they are growing.

Socrates

. . .if the souls of tyrants could be laid bare, one could see wounds and mutilations — swellings left on the spirit like lashmarks on a body, by cruelty, lust, and ill-will.

Tacitus

Every sin brings with it a disturbance of the universal order, which God arranged in His inexpressible wisdom and infinite love. . . So it is necessary for the full remission and reparation of sins. . . .

Pope Paul VI

Expiate your sins by acts of mercy, and your inequity by benefience to the poor.

Daniel 4:24

Alms giving delivers from death, and does not let one go into darkness.

Tobit 4:10

If you can't accept "no" pleasantly, you should never hear "yes."

Mom

Anytime you have to explain a victory, you have lost.

William McGurn

An error committed at the beginning of a process only becomes intensified and compounded as the process goes on.

St. Thomas Aquinas

When women do not say "no," the world becomes no good — that is the story of Adam and Eve.

Samuel A. Nigro

Nothing great is ever done without much enduring.

Catherine of Sienna

He that covereth his sins shall not prosper; but whoso confesseth and forsaketh them shall have mercy.

Proverbs 28:13

A friendship without disruption of one's daily life is unthinkable.

Franz Kafka

I have a little yard where there grows a fig tree on which many citizens have hanged themselves. And, because I mean to make some building on the place, I thought it good to let you all understand that, before the tree be cut down, if any of you be desperate, you may there go hang yourself.

Timon as quoted by Plutarch

Uncivilized people cannot mind their own business.

Name Lost

Our mistake is in supposing men better than they are. They are bad, and will act their character out.

Fisher Ames

The people! The people, sir, are a great beast!

Alexander Hamilton

What other form of civil rules so irresistibly tends to free vice from restraint and to subject virtue to persecution?

Fisher Ames on democracy

I have rarely opened a door by mistake without discovering a spectacle which made me look upon humanity with pity, disgust, or horror.

Anatole France

To be a Gringo in Mexico — ah, that is euthanasia!

Ambrose Bierce

The saddest thing about oppression is that it makes its victims unfit for anything but to be oppressed. . . In the end they turn out to be fairly energetic oppressors themselves.

Ambrose Bierce

The connection between vice and vicious act does not occur to us. We would be shocked at ourselves if we ever realized that crime is nothing more than the dividend that vice has always promised.

Donald DeMarco

Sweet are the uses of adversity.

Shakespeare

If you are disabled physically, you cannot afford to be disabled psychologically.

Stephen Hawking

Hedge in thy ears with thorns, hear not a wicked tongue, and place doors and bars on thy mouth.

Sirach 28:24-25

Heal, oh Lord, my soul, for I have sinned against thee.

Psalm 41:4

What can be made clean by the unclean? And what truth can come from that which is false?

Sirach 34:4

There are five paths of repentance: condemnation of our own sins, forgiveness of our neighbor's sins against us, prayer, alms-giving and humility.

St. John Chrysostom, 407 A.D.

Only those will be offended who deserve to be.

Walker Percy

Guilty, but not so dern awful guilty.

Old frontier verdict

Judges and legislators are to our generation as standing armies were to the generation of 1776.

Patrick Riley

I have never helped you, so why do you hate me?

Name Lost

Many owe their renown to the lying reports spread among the people.

Boethius

Evil is relative to good but good is not relative to evil.

Peter Kreeft

Evil is like a parasite which destroys its good host. If it could totally destroy its host, it would also destroy itself. So, evil is inherently self-destructive.

Peter Kreeft

The sinner who dies unrepentant for the abuse of his freedom is stuck with it. . .is stuck with the self he has made, and that is the hell of it.

Ralph McInerny

Men love truth when it enlightens, they hate it when it reproves.

St. Augustine

The *more* someone tells the truth, the more enemies, and the more passionate enemies, he will make.

Peter Kreeft

In a very real sense, the degree to which any group calls attention to itself or needs special help, the group is, in a sense, inferior.

Name Lost

An effect cannot possibly escape the order of the universal cause.

St. Thomas Aquinas

Sin is an escape from the universal truth of conforming to the creative plan.

Peter Kreeft

God neither wills evil to be done, nor wills it not to be done, but wills to permit evil to be done; and this is a good.

St. Thomas Aquinas

Sin is privation of right order to divine good.

St. Thomas Aquinas

The greatest evil is not done in those sordid dens of crime that Dickens loved to paint. . .it is conceived and moved, seconded, carried, and minuted in clean, carpeted, warmed, and well-lighted offices by quiet men with white collars and cut fingernails and smooth-shaven cheeks who do not need to raise their voices.

C.S. Lewis

The *one thing necessary* is seen in the light of eternity to be our love of God. . .which means that we do not offend Him by sin and that we direct toward Him all the other manifestations of our love.

Dietrich von Hildebrand

The concept of guilt and sin does not in the deepest sense emerge in paganism.

Soren Kierkegaard

Confessing to injustices we have not committed can only deaden us to those we have. Surely there is enough genuine wickedness of which we are guilty, and which deserves to be remedied, without feigning remorse for sins we can't see, even after reflection. . . If I can only appease my accuser by an act of dishonesty or a soothing falsehood, I have failed. . . .

Paul Mankowski

God does not need my lie.

St. Augustine

What is worthwhile is never easy.

Plato

Work out your salvation with fear and trembling.

Philippians 2:12

Even the demons believe — and tremble.

James 2:19

I am not aware of anything against myself, but I am not thereby acquitted. It is the Lord who judges me. Therefore do not pronounce judgment before the time, before the Lord comes.

1 Corinthians 4:4-5

I do not run aimlessly, I do not box as one meeting the air; but I chastise my body and bring it under subjection, lest after preaching to others I myself should be disqualified.

1 Corinthians 9:27

For if a man believe rightly in the Father and in the Son and in the Holy Spirit but does not live rightly, his faith will avail him nothing towards salvation.

St. John Chrysostom, 391 A.D.

"My soul is sorrowful even unto death" (Matthew 26:38). Therefore, sorrow is compatible with virtue.

St. Thomas Aquinas

He who made you without your consent does not justify you without your consent. He made you without your knowledge, but does not justify you without your willing it.

St. Augustine, 400 A.D.

Whoever dies in his sins. . .even if he professed to believe in Christ, does not truly believe in Him; and even if that which exists without works be called Faith, such Faith is dead in itself. . . .

Origen, 230 A.D.

Wounds tend to heal better without scarring if you stop picking at them. This is as true psychologically as it is physically.

Samuel A. Nigro

. . .everything guards its unity as it guards its being.

St. Thomas Aquinas

Never tell the truth to a pollster. . .it is none of his business.

Samuel A. Nigro

Woe to those who live a lie — and more to those who let them!

Name Lost

Their end will correspond to their deeds.

2 Corinthians 11:15

Then another scroll was opened, the book of life. The dead were judged according to their deeds, by what was written in the scrolls. The sea gave up its dead; then Death and Hades gave up their dead. All the dead were judged according to their deeds.

Revelations 20:12-13

To be wise is to suffer.

Teiresias in *Oedipus Rex*

The pessimist is half-licked before he starts. . . .

Thomas A. Buckner

When I see somebody helpless just being picked on, I feel sick to my stomach. If I had just stood there, I would have puked.

Ed Stivender, 5th grader

We never lose, but some days we run out of time.

Green Bay Packers

Oh, my God, I am sorry for all my sins because you are so good.

The Perfect Act of Contrition

Oh, God, be merciful to me, a sinner.

Desperation Prayer

When you impose your suffering onto others it becomes a violence to them. Kept to yourself, it is a penance.

Anonymous

Just as in the body the stronger the movement against the order of Nature, the greater the weakness, so likewise, the stronger the movement of passion against the order of reason, the greater the weakness of the soul.

St. Thomas Aquinas

> The soul is weak when reason focuses on the body more than on identity, truth, goodness, oneness, and beauty.

. . .self-love is the cause of every sin. . .inordinate love of self is the cause of every sin.

St. Thomas Aquinas

I'm not giving up a lifetime habit for your personal convenience.

Evelyn Waugh after a reprimand by his commanding officer upset that Waugh, tipsy, had spilled his drink onto the commanding officer's lap.

Never trust a politician or a celebrity when you do not know him personally. If you know him personally, you already do not trust him.

Samuel A. Nigro

When it comes to politicians, celebrities, entertainers, journalists, and teachers, if you cannot say anything bad, then say nothing at all.

Samuel A. Nigro

Police methods would only be perfect if men were perfect. And if men were perfect, there would be no police methods at all.

G.K. Chesterton

I didn't know I was so poor until I read your book.

Dr. Martin Luther King, Jr. to Michael Harrington about the latter's book, *The Other America*, which converted victimhood into a vocation

. . .freedom of conscience is never freedom "from" the truth but always and only freedom "in" truth. . . .

John Paul II

I do not know you.

Matthew 25:12

Do not stifle the spirit. Do not despair peoples. Test everything; retain what is good. Avoid any semblance of evil.

1 Thessalonians 5:17-19

If we boast of our best, we must repent of our worst.

G.K. Chesterton

All men are capable of all crimes.

G.K. Chesterton

The finest type of learning is from *other's* mistakes!

Samuel A. Nigro

[A]nd you will be hated by all for my name's sake. But he who endures to the end will be saved.

Matthew 10:22

For whoever would save his life will lose it; and whoever loses his life for my sake and the gospel's will save it.

Mark 8:3-5

Besides this you know what hour it is, how it is full time now for you to wake from sleep. For salvation is nearer to us now than when we first believed.

Romans 13:11

If any man's work is burned up, he will suffer loss, though he himself will be saved, but only as through fire.

1 Corinthians 3:15

Memory is a form of revenge.

Martin Bergman

A ghetto. . .a ghetto is as much a state of mind as a place.

Louis Wirth

Don't look at the ground when you say, "I'm sorry." Hold your head up and look the person in the eye, so he'll know you mean it.

Susan Jacoby

There are no accidents.

Joseph Meissner

If this is how you treat your friends, God, it's no wonder you have so few of them.

St. Theresa of Avila when her carriage got stuck in the mud

Once one begins to understand, one begins to forgive, and once one begins to forgive, there is no end, one rewrites the story. . . .

Barbara Grizzuti Harrison

What is wrong with the world is the devil.

G.K. Chesterton

Beware of thyself, old man.

Starbuck to Captain Ahab

Sammy, I think you've peaked already — so don't even bother calling if this happens again.

A father to his 16-year-old son after picking him up from the police station for the third time in nine days.

Take what you want, says God, but pay for it.

Greek proverb

The most difficult part of retirement is the haunting realization that for the first forty-five years of my practice, I was doing it all wrong.

85-year-old Freudian-trained psychiatrist

To render the highest justice to corruption, you must retain your innocence. You have to be conscious all the time within yourself of treachery to something valuable.

Graham Greene

You go brute me, you go scorn me
You go scandalize my name.
Since my soul got a seat up in the Kingdom,
That's all right.

Guy and Candie Carawan

The question is not, "Can they reason? Nor can they talk? But, can they suffer?"

Jeremy Bentham

Not everyone who says to me "Lord, Lord," shall enter the kingdom of heaven; but he who does the will of my Father in heaven shall enter the kingdom of heaven. Many will say to me on that day, "Lord, Lord, did we not prophesy in Thy name and cast out devils in Thy name and work many miracles in Thy name?" And then I will declare to them, "I never knew you. Depart from me, you workers of inequity!"

Matthew 7:21-23

One thing alone I call my own — the obligation to distribute to my brethren the possessions with which God has entrusted me.

St. Thomas of Villanova

If any man would come after me, let him deny himself and take up his Cross and follow me.

Matthew 16:34

For the measure you give will be the measure you get back.

Luke 6:38

If I have told you earthly things and you do not believe, how can you believe if I tell you heavenly things? No one ascended into heaven but he who descended from heaven, the Son of Man.

John 3:12-13

You, therefore, must be perfect, as your heavenly Father is perfect.

Matthew 5:48

. . .whoever does the will of my Father in heaven is my brother and sister, and my mother.

Matthew 12:48

. . .many that are first will be last, and the last first.

Matthew 19:30

And do not fear those who kill the body but cannot kill the soul; rather fear him who can destroy both soul and body. . . .

Matthew 10:27-28

God is at work in you, both to will and to work, for his good pleasure.

Philippians 2:13

For we have not a high priest who is unable to sympathize with our weaknesses, but one who in every respect has been tempted as we are, yet without sinning.

Hebrews 4:15

Friend, how did you get in here without a wedding garment?

Matthew 22:12

Lo, when the wall is fallen, shall it not be said unto you, where is the mortar wherewith ye should have daubed it?

Ezekiel 13:9-12

How free are you? Are you free enough to forgive?

Samuel A. Nigro

He who abides in me, and I in him, he it is that bears much fruit, for apart from me you can do nothing.

John 15:5

Or what shall a man give in return for his life?

Matthew 16:25

If you do not take pride in what you do for all Mankind, then you take false pride in what you do for your selfish self.

Name Lost

Afterward the other maidens came along also, saying, "Lord, Lord, open to us." But he replied, "Truly, I say to you, I do not know you." Watch therefore, for you know neither the day nor the hour.

Matthew 25:11-13

The Apostle likewise bears witness and says: . . .Whoever eats the bread or drinks the cup of the Lord unworthily will be guilty of the body and blood of the Lord. But [the impenitent] spurn and despise all these warnings; before their sins are expiated, before they have made a confession of their crime, before their conscience has been purged in the ceremony and at the hand of the priest. . .they do violence to his body and blood, and with their hands and mouth they sin against the Lord more than when they denied him.

Cyprian, A.D. 251

Not all moral virtues are about delight and sorrow, as their proper matter, but. . .every virtuous person delights in the act of virtue and is saddened by an act contrary to virtue.

St. Thomas Aquinas

God has created you without your cooperation, but he won't save you without your cooperation.

St. Augustine

If you don't forgive, you cannot forget.

Anna Marie Nigro

Lawyers are people who feed off other people who do something meaningful.

Anonymous

God forgives always; man forgives sometimes; nature forgives never.

Name Lost

The Fall is a view of life. It is not only enlightening, but the only encouraging view of life.

G.K. Chesterton

One of you will be crying in a minute. . .and then I will make you both cry.

Evelyn Nigro

Luxury is the great enemy of liberty.

Stephen J. Tonsor

If we must suffer, let us suffer nobly.

Victor Hugo

Suffering makes you choose between right and wrong — but only when you choose right, are you free.

Name Lost

Have you seen the fool that corrupted his own live body? Or the fool that corrupted her own live body? For they do not conceal themselves, and cannot conceal themselves.

Walt Whitman

To be capable of living well and free from social restraint (rules, rules and rules), one must have formed a Nature-and-Humanity-valuing conscience.

Name Lost

To hate or be bitter because of the past is to continue the past into the present. Sometimes remembering the past is not to prevent it from recurring but is to actually bring its reoccurence about.

Anonymous

Every problem that occurs in childhood between the parent and child is an opportunity for intellectual growth by learning something or is an opportunity for conscience-formation (moments to strengthen the will). The latter is the more important of the two. The two most common names for this are "consequences" and "punishment." If too weak, they unleash massive selfishness and inability to care for others. If too strong, they crush the child's sense of self-worth, turning him into a broken, withdrawn, or retaliating violent person.

Samuel A. Nigro

The wages of sin is death, but the gift of God is eternal life through Jesus Christ our Lord.

Romans 3:22

The most important step in trying to solve problems is to look for the lie.

Name Lost

Untruths always create problems, and to solve any problems, one must look for and correct the untruths causing them.

Samuel A. Nigro

Confess your sins in church, and do not go up to your prayer with an evil conscience. This is the way of life.

Didache, 1st century

On the Lord's Day gather together, break bread, and give thanks, after confessing your transgressions so that you may be pure.

Didache, 1st century

Put to death therefore what is earthly in you: fornication, impurity, passion, evil desire, and covetousness, which is idolatry. On account of these, the wrath of God is coming. In these you once walked, while you lived in them. But now put them all away: anger, wrath, malice, slander, and foul talk from your mouth. Do not lie to one another, seeing that you have put off the old nature with its practices and have put on the new nature, which is being renewed in knowledge after the image of its Creator.

Colossians 3:5-10

It is all the work of His hands. Me? I always needed everybody's help!

St. John Bosco

Don't feel bad. Think of Our Lord's hands.

Father Solanus Casey

We all have strength enough to endure the misfortunes of others. . . .

La Rochefoucauld

He that is without sin among you, let him cast a first stone.

John 8:7

We are guilt-laden; we have been faithless; we have robbed, and we have spoken basely; we have committed iniquity, and caused unrighteousness; we have been presumptuous, done violence, framed falsehoods; we have counselled evil, we have failed in promises, we have scoffed, revolted and blasphemed. We have done wickedly, we have corrupted ourselves and omitted abominations; we have gone astray, and we have led others astray.

Orthodox Jewish prayer recited repeatedly on Yom Kippur

. . .what good is it to profess faith without practicing it? Such faith has no power to save one, has it?

James 2:14-16

Sin when it is full grown brings forth death.

James 1:15

The press and media make their living by creating tension.

Anonymous

Don't worry about the press and media — they are simply mercenaries for homosexuals.

Name Lost

If my fellow citizens want to go to hell, I will help them. It's my job.

Oliver Wendell Holmes

Never allow yourself to be a glazed, blurry-eyed, zombied man debrained by the diarrhea of insignificant morphemes and desenitizing photons from television, movies or newspapers, all of which are most accurately called *psychochezia* (mind defecation.) That IS our press and media today. Almost anything suggested by the press and media should be rejected. *Suggestibility* is a disease! Do not be suggestible about buying things, judging people and especially sex!

Samuel A. Nigro

. . .if we walk in the light, as He is in the light, we have fellowship with one another, and the blood of Jesus, his Son, cleanses us from all sin. If we say we have no sins, we deceive ourselves, and the truth is not in us. If we confess our sins, He is faithful and just, and will forgive our sins and cleanse us from all unrighteousness.

1 John 1:7-10

Corrupters of families will not inherit the Kingdom of God. And if they who do these things according to the flesh suffer death, how much more if a man corrupt by evil teaching the faith of God, for the sake of which Jesus was crucified? A man become so foul will depart into unquenchable fire; and so will anyone who listens to him.

St. Ignatius of Antioch, 110 A.D.

If we do the will of Christ, we shall obtain rest; but if not, if we neglect his Commandments, nothing will rescue us from eternal punishment.

Clement of Rome, 150 A.D.

Give studious attention to the prophetic writings (the Bible) and they will lead you on a clear path to escape the eternal punishments and to obtain the eternal good things of God. . . God will examine everything and will judge justly, granting recompense to each according to merit. To those who seek immortality by the patient exercise of good works, he will give everlasting life, joy, peace, rest and all good things. . . For the unbelievers and for the contemptuous and for those who do not submit to the truth but assent to inequity, when they have been involved in adulteries, and fornications, and homosexualities, and avarice, and in lawless idolatries, there will be wrath and indignation, tribulation, and anguish; and in the end, such men as these will be detained in everlasting fire.

Theophilus of Antioch, 181 A.D.

Beware of allowing a tactless word, a rebuttal, a rejection to obliterate the whole sky.

Anais Nin

Do not be in a hurry to tie what you cannot untie.

English Proverb

Do not measure another's coat on your own body.

Malay Proverb

The best way to knock the chip off your neighbor's shoulder is to pat him on the back.

Anonymous

Never do anything against conscience even if the state demands it.

Albert Einstein

An informed conscience, that is.

One cannot weep for the entire world. It is beyond human strength. One must choose.

Jean Anouilh

Money is human happiness in the abstract; he who can no longer enjoy happiness in the concrete devotes himself entirely to money.

Shopenhauer

A harmful truth is better than a useful lie.

Arthur Koestler

He who is unaware of his ignorance, will only be misled by his knowledge.

Richard Wately

Man can overlook anything provided it is big enough.

G.K. Chesterton

They are so crooked, you're going to have to screw them in the ground when they die.

Louisiana barber on U.S. Congressmen

Never criticize a man until you've walked a mile in his moccasins.

American Indian Proverb

Let the truth and right by which you are apparently the loser be preferable to you to the falsehood and wrong by which you are apparently the gainer.

Moses Maimonides

Let not your tongue say what your head may pay for.

Italian Proverb

Make peace with man and war with your sins.

Russian Proverb

Wash your soiled linen in private.

Napoleon I

What you dislike in another take care to correct in yourself.

Thomas Sprat

So live as if you were living already for the second time and as if you had acted the first time as wrongly as you are about to act now!

Victor E. Frankl

Sin has a big "I" in the middle of it.

Steve Wood

Our pilgrimage on earth cannot be exempt from trial. We progress by means of trial. No one knows himself except through trial, or receives a crown except after victory, or strives except against an enemy or temptations.

St. Augustine

If a person is tempted by such trials, he must not say, "This temptation comes from God." For God cannot be tempted by evil, and He himself tempts no one.

James 1:13

When one sups with the devil, one must use a long spoon.

C.S. Lewis

Be compassionate as your Father is compassionate. Do not judge, and you will not be judged yourselves; do not condemn, and you will not be condemned yourselves.

Luke 6:36-37

When you are behaving as if you loved someone, you will presently come to love him. If you injure someone you dislike, you will find yourself disliking him more. If you do him a good turn, you will find yourself disliking him less.

C.S. Lewis

Readiness is all.

Hamlet

Keep clear of psychiatrists unless you know that they are also Christians. Otherwise they start with the assumption that your religion is an illusion and try to "cure" it: and this assumption they make not as professional psychologists but as immature philosophers.

C.S. Lewis

Search others for their virtues, thyself for the vices.

English Proverb

For children are innocent and love justice; while most of us are wicked and naturally prefer mercy.

G.K. Chesterton

Perfect love, we know, casteth out fear. But so do several other things — ignorance, alcohol, passion, presumption, and stupidity.

C.S. Lewis

Do not look where you fell, but where you slipped.

African Proverb

Remember, even monkeys fall out of trees.

Korean Proverb

No matter how far you have gone on a wrong road, turn back.

Turkish Proverb

When evil men plot, good men must plan. When evil men shout ugly words of hatred, good men commit themselves to the glories of love.

Martin Luther King, Jr.

He who is devoid of power to forgive is devoid of the power to love.

Martin Luther King, Jr.

When you fall, pick something up.

Oswald Avery

Break the legs of an evil custom.

Italian Proverb

Hanging is too good for a man who makes puns; he should be drawn and quoted.

Fred Allen

Accept things as they are, not as you wish them to be.

Napoleon I

Thou hypocrite, first cast out the beam out of thine own eyes; and then shalt thou see clearly to cast out the mote out of thy brother's eye.

Luke 6:42

Always put off until tomorrow what you shouldn't do at all.

Author Unknown

A Man consumes the Time you make him Wait thinking of your Faults — so don't be late.

Arthur Guiterman

Distrust all men in whom the impulse to punish is powerful.

Friedrich Nietzsche

Monkey see, monkey do.

Aunt Rose

One door closes and another door opens.

Evelyn Nigro

Never look back; something might be gaining on you.

Satchel Paige

Man cannot live without joy; therefore when he is deprived of true spiritual joys it is necessary that he become addicted to carnal pleasures.

St. Thomas Aquinas

Reeling and writhing of course, to begin with, and then the different branches of arithmetic — ambition, detraction, uglification, and derision.

Education according to the Mock Turtle

There are only two kinds of people: Fools, who think they are wise, and the wise, who know they are fools.

Peter Kreeft

Every sin says to God, "*My* will be done."

Peter Kreeft

In order to overcome their pride, God punishes certain men by allowing them to fall into sins of the flesh, which though they be less grievous are more evidently shameful. . . From this indeed the gravity of pride is made manifest.

St. Thomas Aquinas

Pride has ingrown eyeballs.

Peter Kreeft

We're taught to climb to the top of the heap. What we're not taught is that the heap is a garbage heap.

Peter Kreeft

How blessed is poverty, suffering, and anything that destroys the most deadly thing in the world, the quiet drift to hell! Dissatisfaction is the second best thing there is, because it dissolves the glue that entraps us to false satisfactions, and drives us to God, the only true satisfaction. The road home is the next best thing to home. God is home and dissatisfaction is the road, hunger and thirst for God is the road. Blessed are those who hunger and thirst for God's righteousness, for they shall be filled.

Peter Kreeft

Long ago, Aristotle taught that there are three reasons for seeking knowledge. The most important one is truth, the next is moral action, and the last and least important is power, or ability to make things: Technique, technology, know-how. Bacon and modernity have turned Aristotle upside down.

Peter Kreeft

St. Thomas defines "sloth" as "sorrow about spiritual good," or joylessness when faced with God as the supreme joy. . . sloth refuses to work at our *heavenly* task. . .it denies meaning to our lives. . .as St. Thomas further describes it as "an oppressive sorrow which so weighs upon a man's mind that he wants to do nothing.

Peter Kreeft

The times are never so bad but that a good man can live in.

St. Thomas More

Insofar as he is of science, he will doubtless be exact, impartial, and veracious. Insofar as he is a *man* of science he will be loose, partial, and a liar.

G.K. Chesterton

. . .if such men are not held answerable for doing such things, such men will do them again; and myriads of such men will do myriads of such things, again and again until the rack of doom.

G.K. Chesterton on tyrants

. . .weariness. . .is the enemy of all noble things.

G.K. Chesterton

Evil is a privation of the Transcendentals. Evil is manifest by *pain* when we are withdrawn from immanentals (form, oneness and beauty). Evil is manifest by *sin* when we withdraw from our transcendentals (matter, truth and good). Sin is the greater evil.

Samuel A. Nigro

The most important characteristic for a sane person will be an immunity to lies.

Samuel A. Nigro

Children must learn firsthand the reasoned pain of appropriate punishment when they are young, because it is too late when they are older.

Name Lost

The scientific conclusions are in: Free will does not exist. Spinoza started this idea mindlessly supported by scientists ever since. Free will does not exist, so it is impossible for the lucid person to have it. So what does it mean that I chose *not* to believe in the scientific blather that free will does not exist? In fact, the following is undeniable: "I choose, therefore I have free will."

Name Lost

That people should not be forced to do or not do anything and be able to follow their own conscience without demands from others who believe otherwise, is a self-contradictory statement of the first magnitude — because it actually prohibits those who feel there are moral absolutes from following their consciences. "Live and let live," may approximate a mean for some behavior, but as a moral principle, it is good for nothing because it fails logic and abuses reason.

Samuel A. Nigro

. . .printing exists to conceal the truth.

G.K. Chesterton

Don't be such a sourpuss, you jackass!

Charles C. Nigro to his moping son

Only those who hold something as true are in a position to be tolerant. Skeptics cannot be tolerant, only permissive.

G.K. Chesterton

Conflicts within oneself, family, society, and the church remind of the need for forgiveness and forgiveness of sins. Logic demands the Good News have a method to undo that which we do wrong.

If you attend a church which tells you what you want to hear, you will not be in conflict or have much to worry about nor will you ever have need for confession or Reconciliation or Penance.

Some churches seem to be meant for the "perfect," wherein members proclaim salvation loudly with little attention to good works or misdeeds. "Perfection" is pretended. For them, neither confession nor even a church is needed except perhaps for socializing and song-fests.

If some are always healthy (the bored, unhappy Struldbrugs of *Gulliver's Travels*), what need have they for a hospital or, in the moral sphere, a healer? On the other hand, if you are a sinner or belong to a church which tells you right from wrong, then confession becomes a necessity.

That God reached out to humanity and created a church for sinners seems to have been forgotten. Before the church of Jesus, no efficient salvation was possible. Since Original Sin, therefore, confession was needed for eons more than the past 2000 years. Thankfully, we live now. We have a special channel to Salvation. We came from God. With confession, we will return to God.

By Original Sin, humanity acquired the "capacity to choose wrongly." And "choosing wrong" seems to be rampant nowadays, resulting in an ocean of chaos, wrong-doing and conflict. So there must be something for sinners!

Samuel A. Nigro

Of two bad things, it is better to be the barbarian who destroys something for some reason he dislikes or does not understand rather than to be the vulgarian who erects something exactly expressive of what he likes. . . .

G.K. Chesterton

Guilt is an objective state of a broken relationship with God. . .it is not a mere subjective feeling but the mental awareness of the rejection of mere being.

Name Lost

Vengeance is mine sayeth the Lord.

Jeremiah

He thinks too much: such men are dangerous.

Julius Caesar

When rational engagement is not used, there will have to be violence.

Samuel A. Nigro

Woe to you that call evil good, and good evil; that put darkness *for* light and light *for* darkness; that put bitter for sweet and sweet for bitter. Woe to you that are wise in your own eyes, and prudent in your own conceits. Woe to you that are might to drink wine, and stout men at drunkenness. That justify the wicked for gifts, and take away the justice of the just from him.

Isaiah 5:20-23

God, the Father of mercies,
through the death and resurrection of His Son,
has reconciled the world to himself
and sent the Holy Spirit among us for
the forgiveness of sins:
through the ministry of the church
may God give you pardon and peace,

and I absolve you from your sins
in the name of the Father, and of the Son,
and of the Holy Spirit.

Absolution Formula

I almost had an idea but it got away.

Virgil Romager

If you always do what you always did, you'll always get what you always got.

Name Lost

The business of every God-fearing man is to disassociate himself from evil.

Ghandi

All human history is a mere tissue of the partialities, pious frauds, government persecutions and hack butcheries of the hired judge on the bench.

G.K. Chesterton

The strongest man is weak to his own conscience.

G.K. Chesterton

It is not always wrong to go to the brink of the lowest promontory and look down on hell. It is when you look up at hell that a serious miscalculation has probably been made.

G.K. Chesterton

Sin is the failure to grow.

St. Gregory of Nyassa

If a man settles in a certain place and does not bring forth the fruit of that place, the place itself casts him out.

Saying of the desert Monks

The charities of the modern rich man are not meant to atone for his sins; they are meant to deny them. In old times a bequest was taken as proving a sinner to be penitent; in our time it is taken as proving a sinner to be sinless.

G.K. Chesterton

Vanity is active. It desires the applause of infinite multitudes; pride is passive, desiring only the applause of one person.

G.K. Chesterton

Sin is the primary manifestation of the acquired transcendental deficiency syndrome.

Samuel A. Nigro

The cat in a hurry may give birth to blind kittens.

Italian Proverb

The men who really believe in themselves are in lunatic asylums.

G.K. Chesterton

Philanthropy is the recognizable mark of a wicked man.

G.K. Chesterton

Eye for eye, tooth for tooth, hand for hand, foot for foot, burning for burning, wound for wound, stripe for stripe. . . .

Exodus 21:24-25

It is as hard to tell the truth as to hide it.

Baltasar Graian

Sin maketh nations miserable.

Proverbs 14:34

We instruct you, brothers, in the name of (our) Lord Jesus Christ who shuns any brother who conducts himself in a disorderly way and not according to the tradition they received from us. . . .

2 Thessalonians 3:6

Anyone who supports contraception and abortion should be forced to limit themselves to both. Euthanasia too.

Samuel A. Nigro

Only inferior people believe they can be decreed equal.

Samuel A. Nigro

"Self esteem" is actually an oxymoron for most of us.

Samuel A. Nigro

Fanatics are always the unconscious caricatures of their cause.

G.K. Chesterton

So have a good cause!

I *had* learned a lot: You couldn't trust anybody.

T.O. Madden, Jr.

How hollow and full of trash is the heart of man.

Paschal

I keep asking myself: If that's what they say about me, how can I believe what they're saying about others?. . . As a child I enjoyed going to amusement parks where I could see myself deformed by strangely-shaped mirrors. Now with the amount of press coverage I receive, I get the same funny results for free.

Cardinal Giacomo Biffi on trustability in the media

Resentment for being a mere creature *is* a rejection of the need for Penance.

Name Lost

In the darkness of the closed confessional, in an atmosphere of profound, absolute secrecy, in an *unique interactional relationship never duplicated anywhere else ever in the annals of human history*, comes the willingness to reveal one's self to Jesus' successor in the person of the priest. One senses the presence of the Divinity under these circumstances rather than a mere human interaction with a person who looks not much different from you or me — but looks through the blurring screen of the dark confessional as someone superhuman rather than merely "like me." Indeed, the priest is God's Divine representative empowered by the Holy Spirit. This is the way to understand oneself — to have genuine humility instead of the fraudulent "self-esteem" which most often is if not undeserved then exaggerated. This is the way to "get right with God."

Samuel A. Nigro

A community is infinitely more brutalized by the habitual employment of punishment than by the occasional appearance of crime.

Oscar Wilde

Perhaps so if it is only an "occasional" appearance of crime. . . .

Guilt is the awareness of transcendental rejection. Lack of guilt therefore is a major deficiency of being rather than a type of freedom.

Samuel A. Nigro

I chose to become a bowler rather than a golfer because you seldom lose a bowling ball.

Don Carter

In a 1912 boxing match, Joe Rivers and Ed Wolgast KO'd each other simultaneously. Wolgast was delared the winner because he fell on top of Rivers.

Name Lost

A good Catholic is always apologetic.

Name Lost

What happens when there is no Penance? Well, what happens is the same as when traditional, conservative, strict consequences for wrongdoing are mocked and prevented: The atmosphere first becomes one of liberal tolerance which *seems* okay; then occurs more and more openness to more and more daring and flaunting under the aegis of fraudulent freedom; followed quickly by the taunting lack of inhibitions about everything; which turns, in no time at all, to a lack of responsibility about anything because explanations become excuses at which time "anything goes" and almost everything goes unpunished. Such are the chaotic and violent consequences, obvious today, of the absence of traditional, conservative strictness. Without Penance, there is no guilt about anything; no one is responsible for anything; and there are excuses for everything.

Samuel A. Nigro

Oh, I can't do that. That's my bad side.

Yogi Berra to a photographer who asked
Yogi to look straight at the camera

The usual pretext of those who make others miserable is that they want to do them good.

Vauvenargue

Everything has an end, only the sausage has two.

Viennese Coffeehouse Philosopher

De-constructionists and re-constructionists have nothing new to add or say — they really give nothing new — and are so sterile and impotent that, pathetically, they can only attack and attempt to rewrite what was done by those before.

Name Lost

I want you to know that I love you very much. We are family. I want you to know that I am sorry for anything and everything I ever did to hurt you. And if I ever hurt you in the future, I hope it's not much and I apologize for it already. I'll try not to let anything wrong happen.

universal phone call to all family members
after Easter Penance

There is no pluralism as far as crime is concerned. If society cannot decide what is good, then there is no society left.

Jerome Lejeune

Flawed principles will inevitably lead to flawed programs, even with the best intentions.

John Miller, C.S.C.

When you know a real specialist, he knows quite everything about nothing.

Jerome LeJeune

A conscience does not decide what is right or wrong. A conscience discovers what is right or wrong.

Janice Smith

The man who claims "I know him," without keeping his Commandments, is a liar. . . .

1 John 2:4

Modern broad-mindedness benefits the rich; and benefits nobody else.

G.K. Chesterton

An optimist is a happy imbecile, while a pessimist is an unhappy imbecile.

Jerome LeJeune

Guilt is a puzzling phenomenon, but let no one make you believe that it is always nonfunctional or counterproductive. In fact, the only type of guilt which is wrong and truly negative is guilt *about* guilt.

Samuel A. Nigro

A transcendental God would condemn what? Anti-transcendental acts, of course. We sin when we act against matter, form, good, one, truth, and beauty. The transcendentals are how we live with nature and within our own nature. Violation of the transcendentals offends God.

Samuel A. Nigro

Of what must we be afraid. . .? . . .Of one thing only: Our own conscience..

Nico Rost — Atheist Concentration Camp Survivor

(Our times have) ended by placing the impulse of the will at the heart of reason, and reason has therefore become murderous.

Camus

Salvation: You can't earn it but you can blow it.

William Most

. . .the wickedness of human beings is insatiable.

Aristotle

When I get my doorstep perfectly clean, I'll worry about someone else's.

Florence Hill

. . .a little error in the beginning will lead to a large error in the end. . . .

Aristotle

Evil is a matter of active choice whereas disease is not.

G.K. Chesterton

You can say that again and again and again!

The people sit next to the devil and don't even know it.

Faust

It is common knowledge to every schoolboy and even
every bachelor of Arts,
That all sin is divided into two parts.
One kind of sin is called a sin of commission, and that
is very important,
And it is what you are doing when you are doing
something you ortant.
And the other kind of sin is just the opposite and is
called a sin of omission and that is equally bad
in the eyes of all right-thinking people, from
Billy Sunday to Buddha,
And it consists of not having done something you
shuddha.

Ogden Nash

I'll moider de bum.

Two Ton Tony Galento before his title fight with
Joe Lewis in 1939. Lewis ended the fight in the fourth
round to keep Galento from committing any crimes.

If you run when light is turned on, you are probably a cockroach.

Name Lost.

It's a great life if you don't weaken.

Aunt Justina

After the dead are buried, and the maimed have left the hospitals and started their new lives, after the physical pain of grief has become, with time, a permanent wound in the soul, a sorrow that will last as long as the body does, after the horrors become nightmares and sudden daylight memories, then comes the transcendent and common bond of human suffering, and with that comes forgiveness, and with forgiveness comes love.

Andre Dubus

And why not say, as some slanderously claim that we *do say*, "Let's do evil that good may come of it!" Those who say such things are justly condemned!

Romans 3:8

. . . conscience is an instrument for *detecting* moral truth. Conscience interprets a norm, but *it does not create it.*

John Henry Newman

The love of money is the root of all evil.

2 Timothy 6:10

All evil comes from enjoying what we ought to use and using what we ought to enjoy.

G.K. Chesterton

The specialist learns more and more about less and less until, finally, he knows everything about nothing; whereas, the generalist learns less and less about more and more until, finally, he knows nothing about everything.

Donsen's Law

A mediator stands in the middle, separated from either extreme, uniting them by carrying things across from one to the other. Christ as man, set apart from God in nature and from the rest of men by the eminence of His grace and glory, communicates the commandments and gifts of God to men and makes amends and intercedes for men to God. So in the truest sense of the word He is, as man, a mediator. The personal power to take away sin belongs to Christ as God, but making amends for mankind's sin belongs to Him as a man; and it is in this respect that He is called the Mediator between God and man.

St. Thomas Aquinas

While there are many ways to put a clock back together, only one way works.

Rabbi Lapin

I have been vilified, I have been crucified — I have even been c*riticized.*

Chicago Mayor Richard Daley

"Pardon my sin for admiring my beauty every morning in the mirror. . ." That is no sin, my dear. It is just an error of judgment.

Name Lost

An eye for an eye makes the whole world blind.

Gandhi

The church won't let you do wrong without feeling bad and that is good.

Samuel A. Nigro

A joke is not a joke unless the person on whom it is played laughs first.

Name Lost

Oh God, give me not poverty lest I steal. . . .

Moll Flanders Prayer

One of the first unpleasant learning experiences which prove dramatically to you that you cannot have your own way is when you realize that you *have* to go to the bathroom like everyone else. And the next thing you learn is that you need close to eight hours of sleep every night. In neither instance can one fool oneself for very long.

Name Lost

At last we emerged again to see the stars.

Dante leaving hell

"Your defect is a propensity to hate everybody."

Said Elizabeth

". . . And yours is willfully to misunderstand them."

Said Darcy from *Pride and Prejudice*

That is a failing indeed. . . Implacable resentment is a shade in a character but you have chosen your fault well. I really cannot laugh at it. You are safe from me.

Elizabeth in *Pride and Prejudice*

The lamp dies down, a vapor grows, red quivering dart 'round my head.

Faust

Angels are split energy forms intellectually required by and for the unity of the universe. If all relate through a spectrum of unrecognizable interrelating, more hope can be placed in angels!

Samuel A. Nigro

AN OPEN LETTER

"You cannot call every bastard, a bastard. Some bastards cannot take it."

James Schall, S.J.

"For good priests and religious, we will never do better than 11 out of 12."

A hurting pilgrim

"Unless you forgive, you cannot forget."

A healed pilgrim

This letter is written to apologize for the deficiencies of our Church and to ask your forgiveness for the pain we of the Church have caused you. We just are not as good as we should be.

While the specifics are not certain to us, we are sure that you have experienced something from the Church that falls into the following categories:

— erratically obnoxious, insensitive priests and religious;
— dogmatism without reason;
— noncontemporary dogma;
— failure to keep allegiance to Jesus and the Apostles;
— too much or too little of just about everything.

Part of living the Sacrament of Penance is by selective ignoring, which must be done every day to maintain unity and oneness and to prevent fragmentation. The splitting of our energies occurs often to the detriment of many, and when we have to *selectively ignore* anything, sorrow and contrition automatically accompany it, whether we know it or not. This is how the Sacrament of Penance occurs within us in our daily lives.

This letter is an effort to confess the recognition of your injury even though the specifics are not known. In what we have done and in what we have failed to do, forgiveness is needed. . .probably both ways, to and from the Church.

We hope you will live the sacraments and rejoin the Church. We take sustenance from your presence and prayers in the church community. Please let no one drive you away from the ancient secrets of the Church and salvation. Please do not bring your checkbook back to Church. Just bring yourself. Please rejoin. Promises cannot be made that things will be very different, but after Penance comes Holy Eucharist and the other Sacraments — and the pleasure of living all the Sacraments provides a positive engagement with all on earth. Please rejoin us.

Name Lost

We're fighting friends but remember this: No matter how bitter things get, they're still our own friends and this is still our home.

Atticus Finch

Nonsense happens.

James Schall

. . .the best man can be as bad as he chooses.

G.K. Chesterton

Little white lies to help one's beliefs along when people with power do not understand, rigorously increase the risk of inappropriate condemnation and anti-transcendental adjuration.

Samuel A. Nigro

Existence is itself a contradiction in terms.

G.K. Chesterton

Detestation of the high is the involuntary homage of the low.

Marquis de Evremonde

It is extraordinary to me that you people cannot take care of yourselves and your children. One or the other of you is forever in the way. How do I know what injury you have done to my horses.

Marquis de Evremonde after his carriage
ran over and killed a child

Why can't I learn to keep quiet!

Jo of *Little Women*

Lies are not the ways to get out of being common.

Joe in *Great Expectations*

People of New England, ye that have loved me, ye that have deemed me holy behold me here the one center of the world. At last, at last I stand upon the spot where seven years hence I should have stood here with this woman whose arm sustains me at this dreadful moment from groveling down upon my face. Lo, the scarlet letter which Hester wears. Ye have all shuddered at it, but there stood one in the midst you at whose brand of sin and infamy you have not shuddered. Now, at the death hour, he stands up before you. He bids you look again at Hester's scarlet letter. He tells you that with all its mysterious horror it is but the shadow of what he bears on his own breast and that even this, his own red stigma, is no more than the type of what has feared his innermost heart.

Dimmsdale in *Scarlet Letter*

The scars don't bother me because you were always ugly anyway.

Jane Eyre

. . .their image problem is that they're a bunch of communists who have a bunch of Cubans there.

Admiral Daniel Murphy as a public relations representative for Angola's military government

Gentlemen don't read other people's mail.

Henry Stimson, F.D.R.'s Secretary of War, when he closed down a secret intelligence service before World War II

If you think X belongs here, why did you leave X? If you left X, why are you trying to bring X with you? If you want to dress like you are in X, why do you not go back to X? If you act as if you are in X, why did you leave X? If you can only think about X, is that the reason you are unable to get along with Y? Is it caused by you? If you are for diversity, how come you only think of your own kind, X? If your identity prevents your getting along with Y, are you not obligated to avoid Y and not complain when Y throws his hands up at the impasse you have created? If you want someone not to care about your X, why and how can you only care about your X? If you want to care only about your X, how can you be that diverse? Truly, if X is so great, why don't you go back.

Samuel A. Nigro on immigration

You cannot be for diversity if all you care about is your own kind.

Samuel A. Nigro

I have lost the path that does not stray. . . .

Dante

Unless a man is doomed beforehand, fate is likely to be favorable to the courageous.

Beowulf

. . . there was no way for him to behave well. He had only a choice of behaving badly in different ways.

Isabel Paterson

Well, what's today's gravamen?

Franz Josef

He makes his sun rise on the evil and the good and sends his rain on the just and the unjust.

Matthew 5:45

Why does the sun shine on the just and the unjust alike?

Tess of the D'Urbervilles

Cry about one thing in life; cry about all; one thread runs through the whole piece.

Mrs. Yeobright

The first duty in life is to be as artificial as possible; what the second duty is, no one has yet discovered.

Oscar Wilde

Most of the harm in the world is done by good people, and not by accident, lapse, or omission. It is the result of their deliberate actions, long persevered in, which they hold to be motivated by high ideals towards virtuous ends.

Isabel Paterson

And the answer is in the transcendentals.

ADULT CONFESSION

Childhoods are outgrown. What is good and positive as children will often be insufficient for us as adults. This applies to entertainment, games, and to general activities and interests in all other areas including religion. Cap pistols and jacks are replaced by bicycles, then cards and jobs, just as nursery rhymes are replaced by opera.

In the same manner, the formula used for confession as a child must change to be of significance for mature adults.

The absence of guidelines to clarify this leads many adults to avoid going to confession, because the only pattern known is what was learned in the first and second grades. This being so for many, it is small wonder that going to confession holds little interest and makes adults feel uncomfortable because it seems "childish."

A suggested adult formula is the following:

Bless me, Father, for I have sinned. It has been *(duration)* since my last confession.

Now, the penitent would not list one's offenses in categories as children and youths do but would focus on the theological and cardinal virtues as well as the capital sources of sin. The confessor could define and help with introspective analysis of adult sin (turning away from God) and clarifying, thereby reinforcing, the positive intellectual and moral virtues needed to counteract negative impulses and feelings.

THEOLOGICAL & CARDINAL VIRTUES	CAPITAL SINS
Faith	Pride
Hope	Covetousness
Charity	Lust
Prudence	Anger
Justice	Gluttony
Fortitude	Envy
Temperance	Sloth

For these and all my sins, I am heartedly sorry. (Act of Contrition)

The shift from the childhood listing of wrongdoings is to a reflective renewal of what constitutes virtue as it applies to one's personal life. Considering the current culture, this may be the only opportunity for an individual to hear about virtues, because they are almost totally ignored in today's culture except by sensational descriptions of actions violating these virtues. Yet, these very virtues remain the underlying structure upon which all societies depend.

By focusing on the virtues and the traditional sources of sin, a more adult mode of confession is provided.

A final thought. Church bulletins should advertise what confession is all about: "In conflict? You want to feel good? Make a good confession! Be a better person. Get right with God. Search your soul. Anonymous — confidential — the way to salvation."

Thus, conflict can be resolved, and man can be forgiven to live on earth in joy. The Good News really is good news — because it is Loving Truth. There can be a happy ending.

Samuel A. Nigro

COMMUNAL PENANCE

When is the last time you took a bath? The church says we ought to bathe at least one a year. . .or was that confession at least one a year? No doubt we ought to bathe our souls more frequently.

When is the last time you went to confession old style? Whatever, you ought to try the new communal penance liturgy. It is sacramental. It is good chemistry for the body. It is introspective for truth in the mind. It secures humility for self-awareness and one's identity. It reinforces oneness with each other and the universe. It shouts goodness for activities. It uplifts to be beautiful in the eyes of God again. In summary, it is redemptive for the soul.

When asked why he became a Catholic, G.K. Chesterton said: "To get my sins forgiven!" Indeed!

If you have not participated in communal penance liturgy, you do not know what you are missing. It just may be salvation.

Samuel A. Nigro

Scandal is gossip made tedious by morality.

Ocsar Wilde

Teachers must have sufficient authority for any necessary discipline.

Isabel Paterson

We are being rebarbarized.

Herbert Spencer

The popular idea of revolution being made by "masses" ground down for a long period into abject penury is fallacious. Slavery has never been abolished by a slave insurrection, but only by the exertions of free men.

Isabel Paterson

Don't expect anything original from an echo.

Anonymous

Truly great men and women are never terrifying. Their humility puts you at ease. If a very important person frightens you, he is not great; he only thinks he is.

Elizabeth Goudge

Nothing worse could happen to one than to be completely understood.

Carl Jung

Every closed eye is not sleeping, and every open eye is not seeing.

Bill Cosby

A half-truth, like a half-brick, an be thrown twice as far.

William Smith

Much of good manners is about knowing when to pretend what's happening isn't happening.

Mrs. Falk Feeley

We protest against unjust criticism, but we accept unearned applause.

Jose Narosky

A trip to nostalgia now and then is good for the spirit, as long as you don't set up housekeeping.

Dan Bartolovic

Man has become as intelligent as he is because he did not go where he wished. If he had been allowed to follow his innate emotions or to do what he likes he would certainly not have achieved the powers which his intellect now confers on him.

Friedrich Hayek

Don't burn all your bridges — unless you have a boat.

Bill Cosby

The power to do wrong does not give me the power to do wrong.

Rupert J. Ederer

A harmful truth is better than a useful lie.

Thomas Mann

Penance is a Sacrament in which the sins committed after Baptism are forgiven.

Baltimore Catechism

Know thyself.

Socrates

To participate in a church which stands for something means that we must undergo a grace-obtaining, self-examination in order to have everlasting life because none of us is perfect. Penance requires a serious self-reflection which is indeed a cleansing of the mind. It gets one's priorities in order. It reestablishes self-integrity. It places one in touch with the realities of the world rather than the fantasies. It is a formalized grappling with real truths, with naked truths, and with the personal truth about ourselves. Penance helps inform the conscience — a great necessity because a conscience is not truly functional if it is mere impulse uninformed by Truth and Love.

Samuel A. Nigro

That each human needs someone to hate is the clearest evidence of Original Sin.

Samuel A. Nigro

Without entertaining, this Church welcomes sinners and eats with them.

A hungry sinner

Pretending to be good is good, because at some point you will no longer be pretending.

Samuel A. Nigro

Do penance (repent) because the kingdom of heaven is at hand.

Matthew 3:2

It is the lesson of our daily experience that when a man seriously resolves to amend his life, he begins at once to be more fiercely assaulted by the concupisence of the flesh; he is, as it were, like the Israelites of old, more cruelly oppressed in works of brick and clay for attempting to flee out of Egypt and from the power of King Pharo.

St. Bernard

As wax melteth before the fire, so should the wicked perish before the face of God.

Psalm 68:2

Unless one gets to confession. . . .

There is no sin committed by any man which another would not also commit unless restrained by the grace of God.

St. Augustine

Confession is the broom, so to speak, by means of which the prisonhouse puts off its forbidding aspect and reassumes its former home-like appearance, being first "swept and garnished" (Matthew 12:44) afterwards with the beautiful green rushes of regular observances.

St. Bernard

The greatest treason: to do the right deed for the wrong reason.

T.S. Eliot

A furious and fighting penal code is perfectly natural when the robbers are as strong as the police.

G.K. Chesterton

When I am in really great trouble, as anyone who knows me intimately will tell you, I refuse everything except food and drink.

Algernon

Be a good boy. We don't want any bad boys around here.

Dad

Let he who is without sin cast the first stone?? No, let *she*. . .the feminists need this more than anyone.

Samuel A. Nigro

Victimhood (playing the poor me role) excuses people from having to think and allows them to escape responsibility for some of their actions.

Samuel A. Nigro

An error is more menacing than a crime, for an error begets crime.

G.K. Chesterton

As on an autumn day when Zeus sends down the most violent waters in deep rage against mortals after they stir him to anger because in violent assembly, men pass decrees that are crooked and drive righteousness from among them and care nothing for what the gods think. . . .

Homer on the just indignation of Zeus

Haughtiness and a high hand of disdain tempts and outrages God's holy law, and any mortal who dares hold no immortal power in awe, will be caught up in a net of pain.

Chorus from *Oedipus Rex*

Academic freedom like all so-called unlimited "genuine" freedom is internally contradictory and therefore a fiction. That is, academic freedom cannot embrace without violating itself those academics who teach that there IS a limit on freedom. Those who preach unlimited freedom of any kind are unaware at least and grossly scheming at worst.

Samuel A. Nigro

Dialogue is not possible without living Penance. In order to have a oneness with the other person, the acceptance of criticism is an absolute requirement. All dialogue depends on the acceptance of criticism with intention of exchanging ideas until there is either a mutual agreement or a mutual understanding that one's continued disagreement has no bearing upon the personhood of either party. It is the mistaking of criticism for depersonalization which breaks off communication and togetherness. The inability to accept criticism, therefore, even if harsh, brutal and wrong, prevents one from being able to relate further. All people must learn to accept criticism *as if* it were intended to reestablish oneness (even if it was not) because only by such penitential attitude can oneness be maintained in the face of disagreement.

Samuel A. Nigro

The most prejudiced people in the world are people who are always looking for prejudice.

Samuel A. Nigro

Make yourself useful to your oppressors, until you're strong enough to overthrow them.

Ashleigh Brilliant

I should have gone to Wittenberg. . .

Hamlet's afterthought

The plays the thing wherein I'll catch the conscience of the king.

Hamlet

My thoughts be bloody or nothing works.

Hamlet

Comfort is relative to what you are comparing yourself to. . .

Name Lost

Morality is what we *ought* to do. We seek the ought so we won't be naughty.

Raphael Waters

This is, I suppose, the whole subtlety of the sin of pride; all other sins attack men when they are weak and weary; but this attacks when men are happy and valuable and nearer to all the virtues.

G.K. Chesterton

Those who think they have no sin are always throwing stones.

Name Lost

Save yourselves from this corrupt generation.

Acts 2:40

It's strange, but wherever I take my eyes, they always see things from my point of view.

Ashleigh Brilliant

Whatever betrayals, sellouts, schemes, cynicisms, falsehoods and unprincipled show business comes from politicians, all of it pales to that of the press, because the press is not a mere user of show biz but IS all of the above without anything "once-removed". . .and one cannot get any more fake and unreal that the press in such regards.

Name Lost

It has taken me thirty years to understand that the admission and forgiveness of sin is the essence of the New Testament.

Sebastian Moore

The greatest sin is to lose the sense of sin.

Paul Claudel

Give me strength to face my weaknesses.

Ashleigh Brilliant

How high you are depends entirely upon what you consider to be the bottom.

Ashleigh Brilliant

When seen from the distance, your problems are somehow much smaller than mine.

Ashleigh Brilliant

Where are people who seek the highest compliment to pay themselves?

Samuel A. Nigro

Unless you were a slave yourself, you have no right to claim special victimhood status or special consideration for yourself because of those who were.

Name Lost

The power of Jesus Christ, the power of healing forgiveness simply means, "I will not succumb to the hatred and the bitterness, but move on with life."

Helen Prejean

Gene mapping efforts will, by focusing on journalists, discover the gene for lying, and by focusing on politicians will discover the gene for dishonesty.

Samuel A. Nigro

I am guilt-laden; I have been faithless; I have robbed, and I have spoken basely; I have committed iniquity, and caused unrighteousness; I have been presumptuous, done violence, framed falsehoods; I have counselled evil, I have failed in promises, I have scoffed, revolted and blasphemed. I have done wickedly, I have corrupted myself and committed abomination; I have gone astray, and I have led others astray. I have sinned by pride, covetousness, lust, anger, gluttony, envy and sloth.

what to say at confession when you do not know what to confess. . .the Yom Kippur Prayer and the seven capital sins — also what to recite repeatedly on Good Friday

Violence is always needed to maintain that which is not true nor good nor one nor beautiful. Without the transcendentals, violence is almost automatic.

Samuel A. Nigro

Ninety-nine percent of people on movie and television screens are fakes.

Name Lost

Will power is not a problem if you have a lot of good things to do. Keeping busy doing the good takes care of will power.

Name Lost

Halitosis is better than no breath at all!

Red Skelton

I will only evil but I do only good.

The devil in Faust complaining about how things turn out with God

Forgive and forget other people's foolishness. That way it does not bother you anymore.

Name Lost

People attack and lie about the Roman Catholic church to keep themselves from converting.

Samuel A. Nigro

You will never go wrong doing right.

Joseph Mauceri

Repentance is. . .a clearing of the ground, the establishment of a clean basis in preparation for further moral actions — what in the life of the individual is called "reform." And if in private life what has been done must be put right by deeds, not words, this is all the more true in the life of a nation.

Alexander Solzhenitsyn

I do not believe in a parsimonious world. There are friends and relatives whose depth and beauty and intelligence and generosity are so overwhelming that we can only react with a kind of awe. If we react with envy, it is because we only want our own world.

James Schall

Where evil abounds, grace abounds more fully. This is the only sense in which we are created equal.

James Schall

In the temporal order, a *spectrum* is the splitting of energy into position-time relationships. So is Penance. Reconcile yourself to a place in the Universe.

CHAPTER 5:

HOLY EUCHARIST

In the physical order, a *field* is a matrix existing throughout space and time. Your human beingness is a field.

In the spiritual order, *Holy Eucharist* is *field* of *integrity* of "subdued spontaneity and non-self excluded" (genuineness). Resulting is *charity* with conscious commitment to perfection of all beings.

"Father, into thy hands I commend my spirit."

Holy Eucharist makes you a field — an integrated sacrificing suffering charity intersticing with all the universe.

Live Holy Eucharist — a resignation about suffering to salvation without ever giving up.

To be in the Body of Christ.
To enter the Statimuum and
to participate in the
Incarnation.

In physics, a *field* is a matrix existing throughout space and time. So is Holy Eucharist.

Holy Eucharist is the Sacrament which contains the body and blood, soul and divinity of our Lord Jesus Christ under the appearances of bread and wine. Holy Eucharist is a *field.*

Holy Eucharist is a pattern of "spontaneity and genuineness" which coincides in the physical world with *field*, i.e. a matrix of space and time. The resulting human principle is that of *integrity* wherein *charity* results by the conscious suffering commitment to personal perfection, spontaneously and genuinely pervading the universe.

Subdued Spontaneity. . .

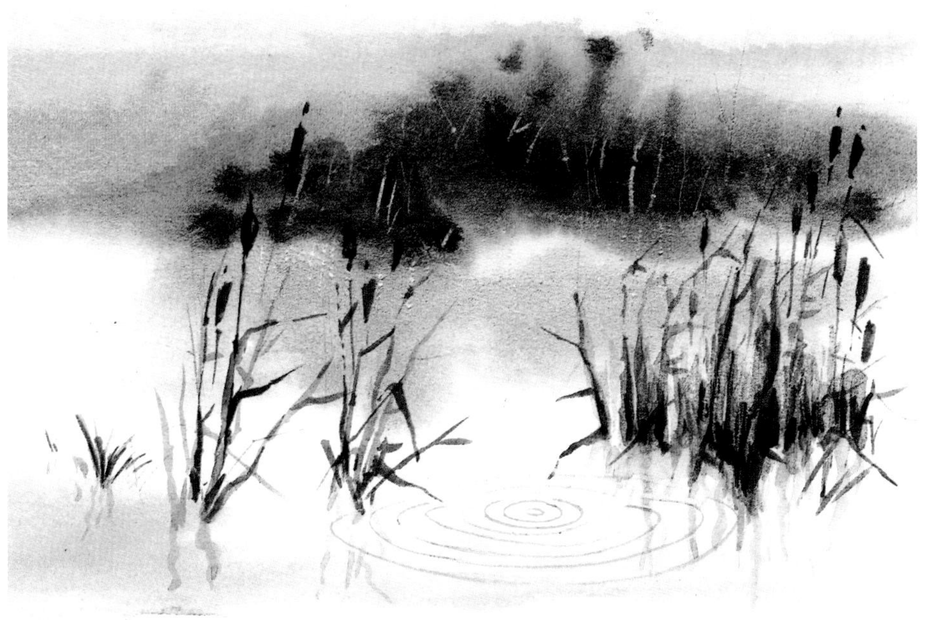

. . . One way to be a human being. Spontaneity is to be genuinely responsive (it is a kind of freedom!). However, subduedness is necessary to avoid raucous overbearingness. And deleting "nonself" is to be without affectation and, as well, is to play not a fraudulent role. In sum, a human being avoids artificial pretending, is free and open, but. . . is subdued so as not to offend others. Be yourself therefore, but keep it calm. . . and thereby dignity, truth, and respect-for others become a personalizing and pleasant way of life.

SUBDUED SPONTANEITY, NON-SELF EXCLUDED

Spontaneity is extremely important. One must be one's self when relating to others. But it must be done in a subdued, low-key way. Talk slowly. Create a relaxed interaction.

On the other hand, it is important to see humor in some of the situations into which we get. Add a humorous dimension with occasional low-key laughing. Enjoy the interchanges. Lighten up. And be yourself (gently).

* * * * *

The Body of Christ in the Eucharist has no need of garments but of a pure soul. The Body of Christ outside needs much care.

St. John Chrysostom in 400 A.D.

This is the biggest fool thing we have ever done. The bomb will never go off, and I speak as an expert in explosives.

Adm. Bill Leahy to President Truman in 1945
about the Manhattan Project

Space travel is utter bilge.

Astronomer Royal of Britain two years before Sputnik

They couldn't hit an elephant at this dis. . .

The last words of General Sedgewick during the Civil War

The passion of Christ is the radical liberation from evil, sin, and ultimately death in order to live a new life in genuine freedom and charity.

Pier Franco Beatrice

There is no psychiatrist in the world like a puppy licking your face.

Bern Williams

When you're hungry, sing; when you're hurt, laugh.

King David

Life begets life. Energy creates energy. It is by spending oneself that one becomes rich.

Sarah Bernhardt

The fragrance always stays in the hand that gives the rose.

Hada Bejar

"Celebrate" means "performed with due rite" and "solemnly held."
"Liturgy" means "public worship."

Oxford English Dictionary

The real secret of patience is to find something else to do in the meantime.

Dell Pencil Puzzles and Word Games

As soon as it's light, I start to eat.

Art Donovan, a 310-lb. former Colt defensive
lineman describing himself as a "light eater"

Christ took upon himself this human form of ours. . .so that men should be like him. And in the Incarnation, the whole human race recovers the dignity of the image of God. Henceforth, any attack even on the least of men is an attack on Christ. . . . Through fellowship and communion with the incarnate Lord. . .we are delivered from that individualism which is the consequence of sin, and retrieve our solidarity with the whole human race.

Dietrich Bonhoeffer

He's so tight, he don't even breath all the air he needs.

Anonymous

A few drinks of that and you're nine feet tall and bulletproof.

Anonymous

He's so ugly, he'd make a freight train take a dirt road.

Anonymous

It ain't that he's mean, but the mean ones don't mess with him.

Anonymous

Long as I got a biscuit, you got half.

Anonymous

Even Norman Vincent Peal has his low moments. After he wrote THE POWER OF POSITIVE THINKING, some pastors gave him a rough time, and he thought about quitting. So he went to see his father, a retired Methodist minister and by then an old man. His father said, "Norman, I've followed you all your life. You've always preached the Gospel and always remained true to Jesus Christ. You're sound. There's only one thing left to do." "What's that?" "Tell those people to go to hell."

Buddy Martin

When there's a lot of it around, you never want it very much.

Peg Bracken

What great thing would you attempt if you knew you could not fail?

Robert H. Schuller

Eventually it comes to you: The thing that makes you exceptional, if you are at all, is inevitably that which must also make you lonely.

Lorraine Hansberry

I never lose sight of the fact that just *being* is fun.

Katherine Hepburn

To learn how to be good to oneself is often more difficult than to learn how to be good to others.

Joshua Loth Liebran

If I knew what I know now, I wouldn't be thinking "If I knew then what I know now."

Harry Wayne Addison

We need a Son tan, not a sun tan.

Thomas Droleskey

Life is like bein' on a mule train. Unless you're the lead mule, all the scenery looks about the same.

Kathryn Jenson

There is no distance on this earth as far away as yesterday.

Robert Nathan

Incarnational intensity without eschatological finality is not salvific.

George A. Aschenbrenner

People often say that this or that person has not yet found himself. But the self is not something that one finds. It is something one creates.

Thomas Szasz

The man who insists upon seeing with perfect clearness before he decides, never decides.

Henri Frederic Amiel

Holy Eucharist is the Sacrament which contains the body and blood, soul and divinity of our Lord Jesus Christ under the appearances of bread and wine.

Baltimore Catechism

If you don't make waves, you're not under way.

Leonard Gollobin

To wait and do nothing is to be nothing.

Ed Marinak

Like watching television or movies.

Make your whole year's plans in the spring, and your day's plans early in the morning.

Chinese proverb

When you look at your life, the greatest happinesses are family happinesses.

Joyce Brothers

In most modern people there is a battle between the new opinions, which they do not follow out to their end, and the old traditions, which they do not trace back to their beginning. If they followed the new notions forward, it would lead them to Bedlam. If they followed the better instincts backward, it would lead them to Rome.

G.K. Chesterton

I myself am the bread that has come down from heaven. If anyone eats of this bread, he shall live forever. And now, what is this bread that I am to give? It is my flesh, given for the life of the world.

John 6:51-52

You can have no life in yourselves, unless you eat the flesh of the Son of Man and drink his blood. The man who eats my flesh and drinks my blood enjoys eternal life, and I will raise him up on the last day. My flesh is real food, my blood is real drink. He who eats my flesh, and drinks my blood, lives continually in me, and I in him.

John 6:54-57

Only the spirit gives life; the flesh is of no avail; and the words I have been speaking to you are spirit and life.

John 6:64

If you hate well, then you love; whereas if you love badly, you hate.

St. Augustine

. . .the easiest and the noblest way (to live) is not to be rushing others, but to be improving yourselves.

Socrates

Active participation in the Mass is to be in the Statimuum for a brief moment.

Samuel A. Nigro

So it is the Lord's death that you are heralding, whenever you eat this bread and drink this cup, until he comes. And therefore, if anyone eats this bread or drinks this cup of the Lord unworthily, he will be held to account for the Lord's body and blood. A man must examine himself first, and then eat of that bread and drink of that cup; he is eating and drinking damnation to himself if he eats and drinks unworthily, not recognizing the Lord's body for what it is.

1 Corinthians 11:26-30

Then he took bread, and blessed and broke it, and gave it to them, saying, This is my body, given for you; do this for commemoration of me.

Luke 22:19

We are confident in the hope of attaining glory as the sons of God.

Roman 5:2

Nothing unclean shall enter Heaven.

Revelations 21:27

You are no longer exiles, then, or aliens; the saints are your fellow citizens, you belong to God's household.

Ephesians 2:19

Stand firm, then, brethren, and hold by the traditions you have learned, in word or in writing, from us.

2 Thessalonians 2:14

I must praise you for your constant memory of me, for upholding your traditions just as I handed them onto you.

1 Corinthians 11:2

Christ was offered one for all, to drain the cup of the world's sin.

Hebrews 9:28

This cup is the New Covenant in my blood.

Luke 22:20

This is the New Covenant in my blood. . .for as oft as you eat this bread, and drink this cup, ye proclaim the Lord's death until he come.

1 Corinthians 11:25-26

I shall not drink from henceforth of the fruit of the vine until the Kingdom of God shall come.

Luke 22:18

From the rising of the sun even to the going down, my name is great among the Gentiles; and in every place there is a sacrifice and there is offered to my name a clean oblation.

Malachi 1:10-11

The blood of Jesus his son cleanses us from all sin.

1 John 1:7

So it is the Lord's death ye are heralding, whenever you eat this bread and drink this cup, until he comes.

1 Corinthians 11:26

Have you never read in the book of Moses how God spoke to him at the burning bush, and said, "I am the God of Abraham, and the God of Isaac, and the God of Jacob?" Yet it is of living men, not dead men, that he is the God.

Mark 12:26-27

Each of us has one body, with many different parts, and not all these parts have the same function; just so we, many in number, form one body in Christ, and each acts as the counterpart of another.

Romans 12:4-5

But Jesus told them, It is I who am the bread of life.

John 6:34-35

Amen, Amen, I say unto you: Except you eat the flesh of the Son of Man, and drink His blood, you shall not have life in you.

John 6:54

Custom is our nature.

Paschal

How is it that you don't understand that I was not telling you about bread?

Matthew 16:11

And while they were at supper, Jesus took bread and blessed and broke and gave to His disciples and said: Take ye and eat. This is my body. And taking the chalice, He gave thanks and gave to them, saying: Drink ye all of this; for this is my blood of the New Testament, which shall be shed for many unto remission of sins.

Matthew 26:26-29

But now I tell you: Love your enemies, and pray for those who persecute you, so that you will become the Sons of your Father in heaven.

Matthew 5:44-45

You must love the Lord your God with all your heart, with all your soul, and with all your mind. . . .You must love your fellow man as yourself.

Matthew 22:37-40

. . .Suddenly the Lord himself stood among them and said to them "Peace be with you."

Luke 24:36

Suffering is seasoning.

Anthony de Mello

Roman Catholic *Orthodoxy* is environmentalism for the mind, soul, family and society.

Samuel A. Nigro

Go save the world, and have a good time. But keep both feet firmly planted in mid air. . .

Anonymous

Agonies are one of my changes of garments,
I do not ask the wounded person how he feels,
I myself become a wounded person,
My hurts turn livid upon me as I lean on a cane and observe.

Walt Whitman

God does not intervene to stop suffering. To do so would remove freedom from mankind. Suffering is the result of the absence of the immanentals (identity, oneness and beauty) causing pain, or the absence of the transcendentals (matter, truth and good) causing sin. When the full community (humanity as a whole) does not fill the world with immanentals and transcendentals, innocents will suffer. God will not intervene. We must do it ourselves, in all things, at all times, forever. When all and all the world loves, all suffering will cease. Come on, Church!

Samuel A. Nigro

If you're not having fun, it's your own damn fault.

Anonymous

Freedom and joy are really synonyms insofar as you can only have both when you are projecting your transcendentals. This means that you get up early and leap into the day doing good.

Anonymous

So we, though many, are one body in Christ, and individually members one of another. . . .

Romans 12:5

The hours have wings and fly up to the Author of Time with reports of how we have used them.

John Milton

God's Commandments are not burdensome to someone who loves, but they are burdensome to someone who does not love.

St. Augustine

Human life is connected. No single virtue, or even a cluster of virtues can survive in isolation from others required for human existence.

Romanus Cessario

What matters is faith that expresses itself in love.

Galatians 5:6

Unless you turn and become children, you will never enter the Kingdom of Heaven.

Matthew 18:3

Did you not know that I must be in my Father's house?

Luke 2:49

. . .the kingdom of God is in the midst of you.

Luke 17:21

How do you know me?

John 1:48

Do you not know that your body is a temple of the Holy Spirit within you, which you have from God? You are not your own; you were bought with a price. So glorify God in your body.

1 Corinthians 6:19-20

One optimist says that is the best of all possible worlds. The other says that it is certainly not the best of all possible worlds, but it is the best of all possible things that a world should be possible.

G.K. Chesterton

A Christian should be an alleluia from head to foot.

Sister Dorothy Kazel

Some people have such open minds that their brains fall out.

Flannery O'Connor

Easier said than done, but never done unless said.

Samuel A. Nigro

I'm not going to diddle around with those jerks.

John Knowles

Jesus is a moral beacon in the twilight of the gods.

George W. Rutler

Dependence becomes pleasure in the presence of unspoilt love.

G.K. Chesterton

Hatred of truth is misanthropy to the full extent because it denotes a hatred of the human spirit at its most noble.

Florence King

Cannot you be more than just simply your stupid non-self?

Sister Mary Francetta

Honesty is the crucible. Justice cannot be served by injustice.

Betty Steele

Science is a mere trifling; nothing is real but love.

Pierre Simon

Nowhere does God, in His grace, reveal Himself to me more clearly than in some human form, which I love solely because it is a mirrored image of Himself.

Michelangelo

If I don't go to Mass, who will miss me?

Teenager

When it comes to "something to be excited about," nothing, once you know what it is, can beat the Holy Sacrifice of the Mass.

Samuel A. Nigro

Therefore I tell you, do not be anxious about your life, what you shall eat or what you shall drink, nor about your body, what you shall put on. Is not life more than food, the body more than clothing? Look at the birds of the air: they neither sow nor reap nor gather into barns, and yet your heavenly Father feeds them. Are you not of more value than they? And which of you by being anxious can add one cubit to his span of life?

Matthew 6:25-27

See the face of Christ revealed in
every person standing by your side,
Gift to one another, and temples of your love.

Marty Haugen

The Incarnation is an utterly supreme and fantastic idea which, if you think deeply about it, makes absolute sense and can never be decided as unreasonable.

Anonymous

If you want the Good Life, then follow virtues and project your transcendentals. If you are having the Good Life, then this is what you are doing whether you know it or not.

Anonymous

Faith is required by thee, and a sincere life, not loftiness and intellect, nor deepness in the Mysteries of God.

Thomas a Kempis

Love everybody, but trust no one.

Anonymous

Never deal with any group promoting something that the group itself does not exemplify.

Anonymous

Be not conformed to this world, but be transformed in the newness of your mind.

Romans 12:2

If you wish peace, defend life.

Pope Paul VI

For all that has been — Thanks!
To all that shall be — YES!

Dag Hammarskjold

What is good has been explained to you, man; this is what the Lord asks of you: only this, to act justly, to love tenderly and to walk humbly with your God.

Micah 6:8

Nature, which is the time-vesture of God and reveals Him to the wise, hides Him from the foolish.

Thomas Carlyle

God gave me this voice and He deserves to hear it. I am going to sing at church.

Father Wally Hyclak

The ultimate question for any undertaking: Is it consistent with human-animal nature at a rational level?

Anonymous

My son, mark all your actions with the sign of the life-giving Cross. Do not neglect that sign whether in eating or drinking or going to sleep or in the home or going on a journey. There is no habit to be compared with it. Let it be a protecting wall round all your conduct and teach it to your children that they may earnestly learn the custom.

Ephraim

In all travels, in our coming in and going out, in putting on our clothes and our shoes, at table, in going to rest, whatever employment occupies us, we mark our forehead with the sign of the Cross.

Tertullian

Amen, amen, I say to you, unless you eat the flesh of the Son of Man, and drink his blood, you shall not have life in you. He who eats my flesh and drinks my blood has life everlasting and I will raise you up on the last day. For my flesh is food indeed, and my blood is drink indeed. He who eats my flesh, and drinks my blood, abides in me and I in him. As the living Father has sent me, and as I live because of the Father, so he who eats me, he shall also live because of me. This is the Bread that has come down from heaven; not as your fathers ate manna, and died. He who eats this Bread shall live for ever.

John 6:54-60

For if the blood of goats and bulls and the sprinkled ashes of a heifer sanctify the unclean unto the cleansing of the flesh, how much more will the blood of Christ, who through the Holy Spirit offered himself unblemished unto God, cleanse your conscience from the dead, work to serve the living God?

Hebrews 9:13-14

Not only are we fools for the Lord but warriors for Loving Truth.

Anonymous

On that luminous night. . .Jesus, the gentle, little child of only one hour changed the night of my soul into rays of light. On that night when He made Himself subject to weakness, and suffering for love of me, He made me strong and courageous, arming me with His weapons. Since that night, I have never been defeated in any combat, but rather walked from victory to victory.

St. Therese of Lisieux

The art of conversation is to be prompt without being stubborn, to refute without argument, and to clothe grave matters in a motley garb.

Benjamin Disraeli

Take a deep breath of life and consider how it should be lived.
Call nothing thine, except thy soul.
Love not what thou art, only what thou may become.
Do not pursue pleasure; for thou might have the misfortune of overtaking it.

Don Quixote's Creed

The Incarnation happened, and everything else in God's creation takes on meaning and significance in the light of this singular event in which Eternity took unto itself time. Therefore, the Roman Catholic church will not bend.

Frederick D. Wilhelmsen

We do not great things — only small things with great love.

Mother Teresa of Calcutta

I don't know, I don't care, and it doesn't matter.

Jack Kerouac

We must know, we shall know!

David Hilbert

God knows; He cares; and it does matter.

Anonymous

It helps us to understand the term "first-born" and "only-begotten" when the Evangelist tells us that Mary remained a virgin "until she brought forth her first-born son" (Matthew 1:25); for neither did Mary, who is to be honored and praised above all others, marry anyone else, nor did she ever become the Mother of anyone else, but even after child birth she remained always and forever an immaculate virgin.

Dedimus the Blind, 390 A.D.

A Virgin conceiving, a Virgin bearing, a Virgin pregnant, a Virgin bringing forth, a Virgin perpetual. Why do you wonder at this, oh man?

St. Augustine

Live for another if you wish to live for yourself.

Seneca

Never talk for more than half a minute without pausing and giving others an opportunity to strike in.

Sidney Smith

Don't look over other people's shoulders. Look in their eyes. Don't talk at your children. Take their faces in your hands and talk to them. Don't make love to a body, make love to a person.

Leo Buscagllia

The probability of evolution as set by science is 1 x 10 to the power 4000. It is easier to believe in God.

British Scientist (name lost)

Keep company with those who may make you better.

English saying

Don't hurry, don't worry. You're only here for a short visit. So be sure to stop and smell the flowers.

Walter Hagen

SUFFERING: The bearing of a burden which contradicts our spontaneous will, inhibiting and redirecting the natural course of thought and action. The burden of sickness in ourselves or a loved one; the burden of putting aside our plans for the needs of another; the burden of imposed restrictions upon our liberty from whatever source and for whatever purpose.

John F. Downs

The habit of asking why has ruined the world.

Padre Pio

All who want to live godly lives in Christ will suffer persecution.

St. Raymond of Penyafort

Oh Lord, our hearts are restless and they shall never rest until they rest in Thee, because thou hast made them for Thyself and Thyself and Thee.

St. Augustine

Suffering is not useless! If it is united to that of Christ, human suffering acquires something of the redeeming value of the Passion itself of the Son of God.

Pope Paul VI

Love is a gift of one's self to another for the other's greater good.

John F. Downs

You shall love the Lord your God with your whole heart, your whole soul, and with all your mind. . . . You shall love your neighbor as yourself. On these two Commandments, the whole law is based. . . .

Matthew 22:37-40

There is no greater love than this: that one lay down his life for his friends.

John 15:12-13

If anyone will come after Me, let him deny himself, take up his Cross and follow Me.

Matthew 15:24-25

The rational creature is confirmed in righteousness through beatitudes given by the clear vision of God.

St. Thomas Aquinas

The only authentic option for the poor is one that fosters their own self-reliance.

Daniel Gordon

It is I who am the Bread of Life.

John 6:34-35

I myself am the Bread that has come down from heaven. If anyone eats of the Bread, he shall live for ever. And now what is this Bread that I am to give? It is my flesh given for the life of the world.

John 6:51-52

You can trust God not to let you be tried beyond your strength, and with any trial He will give you a way out of it and the strength to bear it.

1 Corinthians 10:13

Beauty always "ascends" — it means "helping people up." Beauty brings out the best.

Samuel A. Nigro

There is a season for everything, a time for every occupation under heaven:
A time for giving birth,
a time for dying;
a time for planting,
a time for uprooting what has been planted. . .
A time for healing;
a time for knocking down,
a time for building.
A time for tears,
a time for laughter;
a time for mourning,
a time for dancing. . .
A time for loving,
a time for hating;
a time for war,
a time for peace.

Ecclesiastes 3:1-8

Suffering is the only time when we have to choose how to live.

Anonymous

Love one another as I have loved you.

John 15:12

He died for us and that is some love.

Anonymous

My Lord Jesus Christ, I put all my affairs in your hands, and from You alone I ask protection and help.

Isabel Queen of Spain: The Catholic Queen,
The Greatest Woman Ruler in History

To grow, a lobster must shed its old shell numerous times. Each shedding renders the creature totally defensiveless until the new shell forms. When risk becomes frightening, think of the lobster: Vulnerability is often the price of growth.

Name Lost

Be fearless, be confident, for go where you will, the Lord your God is with you.

Joshua 1:9

I must often be glad that certain prayers of my own were not granted.

C.S. Lewis

Charity means love. It is called agape in the New Testament to distinguish it from eros (sexual love), storge (family affection), and philia (friendship). So there are four kinds of love, all good in their proper place, but Agape is the best because it is the kind of love God has for us and is good in all circumstances.

C.S. Lewis

Love, in the Christian sense, does not mean an emotion. It is a state not of the feelings but of the will; that state of the will which we have naturally about ourselves, and must learn to have about other people.

C.S. Lewis

Life is not easy for any of us. But what of that? We must have perseverance and above all confidence in ourselves. We must believe that we are gifted for something, and that this thing, at whatever cost, must be attained.

Marie Curie

Love all, trust a few. Do wrong to no one.

Shakespeare

Frame your mind to mirth and merriment,
Which bars a thousand harms and lengthens life.

Shakespeare

True love comes quietly, without banners or flashing lights. If you hear bells, get your ears checked.

Erich Segal

Evil is never the road to good. The cruel logic of violence leads nowhere. No good is obtained by contributing to its growth. Seek the roads of dialogue and not those of violence. Don't let your potential for generosity and altruism be exploited. Violence is not a medium of construction. It offends God, those who suffer and those who practice it.

Pope John Paul II

Beware that you do not lose substance by grasping at the shadow.

Aesop

He only earns his freedom and existence who daily conquers them anew.

Goethe

The Christian development does not appear something analogous to the regular evolution of a living germ which grows, expands, and dies — the Christian development presents an original and unique physiognomy. It is not subject to laws — nor is it left to chance. One cannot classify it either as arbitrary or necessary. It appears as something conditioned by an *infinity* of facts which, in last analysis, derive from man's free will and from the free grace of God.

Albert Dufourcq

God loved the world so much, he gave his only Son, that all who believe in him might not perish, but might have eternal life.

John 3:16

As food for the body, words do good things for the mind.

Name Lost

When one's expectations are reduced to zero, one really does appreciate everything that one does have.

Stephen Hawking

All will be well, and all will be well, and all manner of things will be well.

Julian of Norwich

The learned Buddhist said: Know the sufferings although there is nothing to know; relinquish the causes of misery although there is nothing to relinquish; be earnest in cessation although there is nothing to cease; practice the meanings of cessation although there is nothing to practice. In other words, pray the Rosary.

Ann, an elderly blind nun

Don't worry. Easter is coming.

Anonymous

The heart has its reasons of which reason knows nothing.

Paschal

We are like dwarfs seated on the shoulders of giants. We see more things than the Ancients and things more distant, but it is due neither to the sharpness of our sight nor the greatness of our stature. It is simply because they have lent us their own.

Bernard of Chartres

Whatever else may be taken away from us by rational criticism, Christ is still left, a unique figure, not more like all his precursors and all his followers.

John Stuart Mill

Human character, perfected through suffering and through resisting temptations, not through escaping it by mental apathy or moral numbness, that is the ideal of Christ, the cornerstone of Christian doctrine.

John L. Stoddard

What an abyss between my profound misery and the eternal reign of Christ, which is proclaimed, loved and adored, and is extending over all the earth!

Napoleon

Prayer is the Christian's vital breath.

John L. Stoddard

The Cross will still remain the Cross; and earth has not, and never will be, heaven.

John L. Stoddard

I hate and despise the animal called Mankind but I like the occasional Tom, Dick and Harry.

Jonathan Swift

And on the Lord's Day, after you have come together, break bread and offer the Eucharist, having first confessed your sins, so that your sacrifice may be pure.

The Didache

We hold our common assembly on Sunday because it is the first day of the week, because on that day our savior, Jesus Christ, rose from the dead.

St. Justine Martyr, 150 A.D.

If one cannot have too much of a good thing, one cannot have too little.

G.K. Chesterton

Whenever you eat this bread and drink this cup, you announce the death of the Lord until He comes.

1 Corinthians 11:26

The sky is the daily bread of the eyes.

Ralph Waldo Emerson

God may be subtle but he isn't mean.

Albert Einstein

The only way to look outward while you are looking inward is by focusing on your transcendentals and projecting them.

Name Lost

Pain and suffering are inevitable: misery is optional.

Lou Gehrig's disease patient
on respirator for 16 years

This is the Gospel I preach; in preaching it I suffer as a criminal. . . .

2 Timothy 2:8-9

You gotta wanna be on that tree!

Name Lost

. . .the mysterious and transforming power of suffering that is accepted and worked through. . . .

John E. Bamberger

(Suffering has value!)

Life is traditional.

Evelyn Nigro

The Holy Eucharist as a Sacrament is like a magnetic field or a coat of paint, only it is composed of genuine love connecting creatures created in God's image.

Samuel A. Nigro

If you would make a man happy, study not to augment his goods; but to diminish his wants. One of the greatest services Christianity has rendered to the world has been its consecration of poverty, and its elevation of labor to the dignity of a moral duty.

Orestes Brownson

Because there is one bread, we though many, are one body, all of us who partake of the one bread and in the one cup.

1 Corinthians 10:17

The man who has not suffered — what can he know, anyway?

Rabbi Abraham Heschel

If your heart is as mine is, give me your hand.

John Wesley

I consider that the sufferings of this present time are not worthy to be compared with the glory which shall be revealed in us.

Romans 8:18

If there is harmony in the heart, there will be harmony in the family. If there is harmony in the family, there will be harmony in the nation. If there is harmony in the nation, there will be harmony in the world.

Confucius

Because I *am* one of his fingers.

Corrie Ten Boom answering the question, "How can you be sure your Jesus won't let you slip through his fingers?"

The soul receives exactly what it expects of God.

St. Therese of Lisieux

Love is repaid by love alone.

St. John of Cross

Oh Jesus, ineffable sweetness, change all the consolations of this earth into bitterness for me.

Thomas a Kempis

Why?. . .to diminish the *res* and increase the other Transcendentals!

Christ is my love. He is my whole life.

St. Therese of Lisieux

"This is my body which will be given up for you" has implications for Transcendental (Sacramental) living. Indeed, we must give up our body (or *res*) as we embrace the remaining Transcendentals of identity, truth, oneness, goodness and beauty to establish our full act of being (*ens*). Truly, we must follow Jesus and "give up our body."

Samuel A. Nigro

All I can claim to have learned is that the only happiness is love, which is attained by giving, not receiving.

Malolm Muggeridge

To see the wounds of another person is a call to love him more.

Julie

Saintliness is more effective than eloquence.

Alice von Hildebrand

It has been granted to us that for the sake of Christ, we should not only believe in him, but also suffer for his sake.

Philippians 1:29

Suffering is the only thing that ever taught me anything. No catastrophe occurs that is not also an illumination. And we never would have heard of Christ if it had not been for the Cross.

Malcolm Muggeridge

The sacrifice of an offering unjustly acquired is a mockery; the gifts of impious men are unacceptable.

Ecclesiastes 34:18

. . .anyone who would not work should not eat.

2 Thessalonians 3:10

Do whatever He tells you.

Mary

Eternity is the simultaneously whole and perfect possession of interminable life.

St. Thomas Aquinas

I am God's wheat to be ground up by the teeth of wild beasts to become pure bread for Christ.

St. Ignatius of Antioch

I have not taste for corruptible food nor for the pleasure of this life. I desire the Bread of God which is the flesh of Jesus Christ, and for drink I desire his Blood which is love incorruptible. There is a living water within which speaks and says, "come to the father."

St. Ignatius of Antioch

The flesh is washed so that the soul may be made clean. The flesh is anointed so that the soul may be dedicated to holiness. . . . The flesh feeds on the Body and Blood of Christ so that the soul, too, may fatten on God. They cannot be separated in their reward when they are united in work.

Tertullian

. . .everyone must choose between God and self as the first object of love.

Peter Kreeft

What shall prevent me from putting forth my whole strength to defend whatever makes life worth living?

G.K. Chesterton's question to pacifists

All men are always being influenced, as every incident is an influence, the question is, which incident we allow to be most influential.

G.K. Chesterton

The whole of mankind is wonderfully helped by what you are doing in ways you do not understand.

Medieval mystical text on prayer

It's dangerous to wave raw meat around tigers.

Wallace Stegner

Mount calvary with your savior.

Name Lost

Even though Jewish authorities and those who followed their lead pressed for the death of Christ (cf. John 19:6), neither all Jews indiscriminately at that time, nor Jews today, can be charged with the crimes committed during his passion. . .as if they followed from Holy Scripture.

Vatican II

It is finished. . . Father, into thy hands I command my spirit (John 19:30 and Luke 23:43). The ground shivered. Across the valley and beyond the wall from Golgotha, the lintel of the great double-winged entrance to the sanctuary or "Holy Place" of the Temple, where stood the altar for incense, the table for the Shewbread, and the seven-branched gold candelabrum (the menorah) facing the Holy of Holies, cracked down the middle. The huge ornate curtain hanging from it — a Babylonian carpet in white, purple, blue, and red 82 feet by 24 — tore in two. A brass gate of the inner Temple building that normally required twenty men to move it, swung open by itself. The central light of the great candelabrum went out. Much of this information comes to us from Jewish, not Christian sources (Josephus and the Talmud), substantially and very significantly supplementing the brief reference to the rending of the Temple curtain in the gospels. The Talmud even dates the strange opening of the brass gate specifically to the year 30 A.D.

Warren H. Carroll

The new social order as it could be and would be if all men loved God and loved their brothers because they are all sons of God! A land of peace and tranquility and joy in work and activity. It is heaven indeed that we are contemplating. Do you expect that we are going to be able to accomplish it here? We can accomplish much, of that I am certain. We can do much to change the face of the earth, in that I have hope and faith. But these pains and sufferings are the price we have to pay. Can we change men in a night or a day? Can we give them as much as three months or even a year? A child is forming in the mother's womb for nine long months, and it seems so long. But to make a man in the time of our present disorder with all the world convulsed with hatred and strife and selfishness, that is a lifetime's work and then too it is not accomplished. We are never going to be finished!

Dorothy Day

To our bitterest opponents we say: We shall match your capacity to inflict suffering by our capacity to enduring suffering. We shall meet your physical force with soul force. Do to us what you will, we shall continue to love you. We cannot in all good conscience obey your unjust laws, because noncooperation with evil is as much a moral obligation as is cooperation with good. Throw us in jail, we shall still love you. Send your hooded perpetrators of violence into our communities at the midnight hour and beat us and leave us half dead, and we shall still love you. But be assured that we will wear you down by our capacity to suffer. One day we shall win freedom, but not only for ourselves. We shall so appeal to your heart and conscience that we shall win you in the process and our victory will be a double victory.

Martin Luther King, Jr.

To be fed by God! To feed on God! By instituting the Eucharist Jesus not only fulfilled the sacrificial types of old; He transcended them by far. Leaving behind animals formerly used in sacrificial meals, even cereals and breads and wines. He transubstantiates the latter two into His own body and blood, and by feeding us with Himself He floods our being with His own divine life. "He who eats my flesh and drinks my blood has life eternal" (John 6:54).

John H. Miller, C.S.C.

Martyrdom is not gallantly standing before a firing squad. Usually it is the losing of a job because of not taking a loyalty oath, or buying a war bond, or paying a tax. Martyrdom is small, hidden, misunderstood. Or if it is a bloody martyrdom, it is the cry in the dark, the terror, the shame, the loneliness, nobody to hear, nobody to suffer with, let alone to save. Oh, the loneliness of all of us in these days, in all the great moments of our lives, this dying which we do, by little and by little, over a short space of time or over the years. One day is as a thousand in these crises. A week in jail is as a year.

Dorothy Day

Compassion — it is a word meaning to suffer with. If we all carry a little burden, it will be lightened. If we share in the suffering of the world, then some will not have to endure so heavy an affliction. It evens out. What you do here in New York, in Harrisburg, helps those in China, India, South Africa, Europe, Russia, as well as in the oasis where you are. You may think you are alone. But we are members one of another. We are children of God together.

Dorothy Day

And the high priest said to him, "I adjure you by the living God, tell us if you are the Christ, the Son of God." Jesus said to him, "You have said so. But I tell you, hereafter you will see the Son of Man seated at the right hand of Power, and coming on the clouds of heaven." Then the high priest tore his robes, and said, "He has uttered blasphemy. Why do we still need witness? You have now heard this blasphemy. What is your judgment?" They answered, "He deserves death."

Matthew 26:63-66

Again the high priest asked him, "Are you the Christ, the Son of the Blessed?" And Jesus said, "I am; and you will see the Son of Man sitting at the right hand of Power, and coming with the clouds of heaven." And the high priest tore his mantle, and said, "Why do we still need witnesses? You have heard his blasphemy. What is your decision?" And they all condemned him as deserving death.

Mark 14:61-64

When the day came, the assembly of the elders of the people gathered together, both chief priest and scribes; and they led him away to their council, and they said, "If you are the Christ, tell us." But he said to them, "If I tell you, you will not believe; and if I ask you, you will not answer. But from now on the Son of Man shall be seated at the right hand of the power of God." And they all said, "Are you the Son of God, then?" And he said to them, "You say that I am." And they said, "What further testimony do we need? We have heard it ourselves from his own lips."

The whole company of them arose, and brought him before Pilate. And they began to accuse him.

Luke 22:66-23:2

So Jesus came out, wearing the crown of thorns and the purple robe. Pilate said to them, "Here is the man!" When the chief priests and the officers saw him, they cried out, "Crucify him, Crucify him!" Pilate said to them, "Take him yourself and crucify him, for I find no crime in him." The Jews answered him, "We have a law, and by that law he ought to die, because he has made himself the Son of God."

John 19:5-7

One would suffer a great deal to be happy.

Mary Wortly Montague

There is no way of telling people that they are all walking about shining like the sun.

Thomas Burton

The Mass is a beaming-up to God via Calvary.

Samuel A. Nigro

God put his kid (his Son, and in a mysterious way Himself) through a horrible death on the Cross. The most obvious message therefrom is that death under the most vile conditions is really not a problem, especially if one has committed oneself to the transcendental life. Such is the meaning of the Mass and such is the significance of participating in the Eucharist.

Samuel A. Nigro

If something is bound to be, we do not choose it, and if we do not choose it, it is not really ours.

James Schall

Persuasion is an act that begins in charity, not in righteousness.

Reid Buckley

To ecstasy, I prefer the monotony of sacrifice.

St. Therese of Lisieux

Suffering is the pain of *choosing how to behave* when that choice of how to behave is the only choice left except to accept the alternative when the alternative is wrong or bad. Suffering, therefore, is the awareness of freedom at its most elementary. Suffering and freedom are tautologies. That is, only when dealing with those pains which accompany difficult choices, are we really free in making the choices. If it is easy, then there is no choice really. Suffering is staring the most basic freedom eye-to-eye and the fundamental choice of deciding how you are going to behave over that which you have no control. Suffering is the mental awareness of genuine freedom. Suffering is the essence of freedom when we choose to be good, when we choose to ascend, and when we make the proper choices. Genuine freedom and suffering are hand and glove.

Samuel A. Nigro

Look, going to mass and confession and church is not fun. It is too serious to be fun. You get your fun later. Yes, it is not new — it is old — it is ancient secrets, hundreds of them, and those secrets will give you mastery of the universe. Going to church is also not entertainment. It is history in the making, and it will give you your past and your future. So go to mass, communion, confession once in a while, and pray.

a father to his children

Paradise has nothing to do with Heaven!

Erik von Kuehnelt-Leddihn

You are not exercising your freedom unless you are choosing the good against odds that make you suffer. Anything less is to be following some kind of a reflex or conditioned stimulus which can never be called freedom.

Samuel A. Nigro

I am willing to receive what you send, to lack what you withhold, to relinquish what you take, to suffer what you inflict, to do what you command, to be what you require.

Name Lost - about accepting God's will

What good does it do to give offense?

John Miller

For us, there is only the trying period. The rest is not our business.

T.S. Eliot

I only stood at the gate and looked upon the dark stage. . . . But the spokes of the terrible wheel had begun to turn already, and blood and horror drift out of its shining circle.

Ernst Wiechert about his experience in the
Buchenwald Concentration Camp in 1939

Oh Lord, remember not only the men and women of good will but also those of ill-will. But do not remember all the sorrow and suffering they inflicted on us. Remember the fruits we have bought thanks to that suffering: Our comradeship, our loyalty, our humility, our courage, our generosity, the greatness of heart that has grown out of all this. And when they come to judgment, let all the fruits that we have borne be their forgiveness.

note left by a woman killed at Ravenbrook Camp in World War II

The let us love one another and laugh. Time passes, and we shall soon laugh no longer — and meanwhile common living is a burden, and earnest men are at siege upon us all around. Let us suffer absurdities, for that is only to suffer one another.

Hilaire Belloc

. . .Power is made perfect in weakness.

2 Corinthians 12:9

So the grape is crushed underfoot and becomes wine, so the olive is pressed and. . .leaving behind its dregs, becomes rich oil. . . . The more the fire of tribulation rids us of our rust, the cleaner will we be when we come before Christ.

St. Gregory

How else but through a broken heart can the good Lord enter in?

Oscar Wilde

The distance from our pain is our distance from God.
All suffering prepares the soul for vision.

Martin Buber

You can only find peace out of pain by walking into your grief and accepting the Mystery, knowing that He is with you.

Ram Dass

There's nothing wrong with pain except that it hurts.

Name Lost

I believe in justice
And in playin' it clean
And in treatin' my neighbor
Like a human bein'.
But if for people like me
This world don't care
I wash my hands
Of the whole affair.
(couldn't do it.
couldn't do it.
couldn't do it
If I tried 'til I died.)
Used to be a dreamer
Chalk full o' good deeds
Tried to be of some service
To my neighbors' needs.
The lack of love in this world's
Too much to bear
I wash my hands
Of the whole affair.
(couldn't do it.
couldn't do it.
couldn't do it
If I tried 'til I died.)
Only gonna think about little ole me
And first it's gonna seem strange.
But I'll try hard at it day by day
'Til I get used to the change.
Though it may sound selfish
And wicked and cruel,
I'm so tried of playin'
Everybody's fool.
'cause all the good uns die young
From the wear and tear,
I wash my hands
Of the whole affair.
(couldn't do it.
couldn't do it.
couldn't do it
If I tried 'til I died.)

Injun Joe

Without a hurt, the heart is hollow.

Tom Jones

. . .life breaks us all, and afterward many are strong at the broken places.

Ernest Hemingway

The Cross remains constant while the world turns.

John Paul II

If suffering is present in the history of humanity, one understands why His omnipotence was manifested in the omnipotence of humiliation on the Cross. The scandal of the Cross remains the key to the interpretation of the great mystery of suffering, which is so much a part of the history of mankind.

John Paul II

He emptied himself, taking the form of slave, coming in human likeness; then found human in appearance, he humbled himself, becoming obedient to death, even death on a cross.

Phillipians 2:7-8

The condemnation of God by man is not based on the truth, but on arrogance, on an underhanded conspiracy.

John Paul II

If the agony on the Cross had not happened, the truth that God is Love would have been unfounded.

John Paul II

The Death of Christ gives life, because it allows believers to share in His Resurrection. The Resurrection is the revelation of life, which is affirmed as present beyond the boundary of death. . . . "I am the resurrection and the life; whoever believes in me, even if he dies, will live, and everyone who lives and believes in me will never die."

John Paul II

There is only one community and it consists of all peoples.

Nostra Aetate

Suffering and freedom are symbiotic. Following emotion is not freedom but impulse. Following the sex drive is not freedom but bodily reflex. Following whatever is easy is not freedom but conditioned reinforcement. Freedom is choosing the transcendentals in the face of adversity or conflict. One suffers while being free because one's real choices are not impulses, reflexes or Skinnerian reinforcement. Real freedom is choosing the transcendentals and suffering about it otherwise there is no real choosing, which is essential to freedom. Freedom is the hand which gets things done but it must be gloved in suffering if a choice is being made. Freedom and suffering are symbiotic. But there is synergism too: *Joy* occurs when you consciously know that a really free choice is in pursuing the transcendentals in the face of adversity or conflict.

Samuel A. Nigro

MASS IN TIME OF WAR

Over the battlefield a sudden hush
Falls. The skirmish ends. A old rain
Drizzles down indifferently. A rush
From behind the lines toward the shapes of pain,
Toward the huddled bundles spattered with blood
Lying in the old indifferent mud.
Medics with their bandages and dressings
Signed and sealed with red sterile cross
Bring to the wounded dark uncertain blessings,
The wounded, unaware of their own loss,
Ask about their buddies, but in vain.
Out in the alien field a cold rain drenches
The wide-eyed boys lying dead in the trenches.
The chaplain, not unfeeling, makes his way
Among the battered heaps that once were boys
Who'd just begun to learn and love life's joys,
Until the dawning of this dreadful day.
Lips that laughed and loved are struck dumb.
Where one they smiled is all a smear of blood,
The blood that roared and sang spilt in the mud.
The priest, kneeling, anoints each with his thumb
And signs with holy oil each rain washed head
To lift sin's heavy sentence from the dead.

Over the battlefield a pall of night
Descends. Soldiers gather round the fires.
Lie away, alert, awaiting dawn-light,
Remembering old loves, old desires.

The morning watch witnesses the sun's
Silent devastation of the night.
Some men wake, yet others, sleepier ones,
While no one watched, from camp have taken flight.

Over the battlefield a restful hush
Lingers with the morning mist. The priest,
Preparing sacrifice for the deceased,
Sets up his tiny altar near a bush
And hangs the wooden cross among the boughs
Above the altar. Only the morning sparrows
Lend their chant to these sad solemn vows
Of requiem to Christ the Man of Sorrows.

In solitude he hangs on twisted wood
High above the death-dunged battlefield.
For this he spent his life, drained his blood.
For this he let his blood fall like rain,
That man might some finer harvest yield.
And has this sacrifice been all in vain?
Is not this blood enough that we must stain
Our fields to make them run with scarlet mud?

Not only in these rites but in the battle
With boys and bursting shells are you crucified:
Here on an altar of war where, like cattle,
Boys have been led, have struggled, and have died.
The hungry war hawk, vast wings whirring
Hovers over the field. The army is stirring.
Your emptying, O Christ, is it in vain?
For here we seem (on Golgotha again)
To add, with every soldier shot or slain,
To your fierce testament of pain
Our ancient Gift — this sacrifice of Cain.

Br. James M. Deschene
Reprinted with permission
The New Oxford Review, May 1988
1069 Kains Avenue
Berkeley, CA 94706

Christ *is* on earth today; alive on a thousand altars; and He does solve people's problems exactly as He did when He was on earth in the more ordinary sense. That is, He solved the problems of the limited number of people who choose of their own free will to listen to Him.

G.K. Chesterton

Suffering is part of us. Much of life is handling suffering. Jesus shows the way. Suffering is to be handled transcendentally: Matter engaged. Identity as a child of God returning. Truth sought. Oneness maintained. Choices of good made. And ascending by beauty. That is what suffering is all about. It is not so much to be rejected as to be embraced transcendentally when life offers it.

Samuel A. Nigro

The power of Christ's Cross and Resurrection is greater than any evil which man could or should fear. . . . Be not afraid!

John Paul II

God is always on the side of suffering.

John Paul II

Say: ye faint hearted, take courage and fear not: behold our God will come, and will save us.

Isaiah 35:4

Men of Athens, I honour and love you; but I shall obey God rather than you, and while I have life and strength I shall never cease from the practice and teaching of philosophy. . . .I believe that no greater good has ever happened in the state than my service to the God. For I do nothing but go about persuading you all. . .not to take thought for your persons or your properties, but first and chiefly to care about the greatest improvement of the soul.

Socrates

Things enwoven made to blend in oneness with the whole celestial powers who ever take and give transfixing all the world with harmony. . . .

Faust

Angels are the creatures spanning space and time linking perfection. If in the field of spontaneous total integration, more charity comes from considering the angels!

Samuel A. Nigro

The KGB (the brutal Secret Police of the Soviet Union) would fill courtrooms with ringers who were to laugh out loud mockingly at any point made with which they did not agree. So whenever this happens, rest assured that the point has been made and that it is irrefutable.

Michael Coren

To think now and then that there is a man who would give his life to keep a life you love beside you.

Sidney Carton

Love is the heartbeat of the universe, of the entire universe. Mysterious. Mysterious and proud. Torment. Torment's delight. The delight of my heart. This love that is the heartbeat of the universe.

Camille

The man was so dear to him that he could not restrain the feeling in his breast, but in his heart held in the bonds of thought, longing after the dear man flamed against blood. . . .

King Hrothgar

Whoever wishes to be My follower must deny his very self, take up his Cross each day, and follow me.

Luke 9:23

There is a difference between sickness and suffering. Sickness is a condition. Suffering is a vocation; it is redemptive; it is a direct sharing in the sufferings of Jesus. Only chosen souls are called to the ministry and apostolate of suffering.

Anthony M. Pilla

There is an absolute proof that evil neither defines God nor denominates his creatures. The sacrifice of Christ Himself is against all evil and vanquishes all evil. The Cross of Christ is the sin offering of the human race. Mercy Himself lives and dies as "mercy on us." We are called simply to dispense mercy to one another and His generous almsgivers. Let us then dispose of any accusation evil can make against God by confidently saying that while evil obscures God, mercy confirms Him. When a man brings himself to that poverty of spirit where grace actualizes the beatitudes a new man is made. Then the ego resonates with St. Paul, "not I but Christ in me," to heal all pathologies, all dread, where mercy abounds and death is overcome.

Joseph Mauceri

'Tis heaven. . .'tis heaven she sees. . .heaven's God, here lies. She can see heaven and never lift up her eyes. This new guest to her eyesight is given. 'Tis once looked up, 'tis now look down to heaven.

Richard Crashaw about the Virgin Mary with Jesus on her lap

Let's not play Jesus anymore. Let's go back to playing church.

Little boy who found it easier to be the latter than the former

When in doubt, walk up to the high altar, look up at the cross and say: "Jesus died for me and I don't care." Do that three times.

Anthony M. Pilla

All being participates in God's being! From start to finish, the question is: How do we participate?

Samuel A. Nigro

I am the bread of life. He who comes to me will never hunger nor thirst.

John 6:35

My heart is withered because I forgot to eat my bread.

Psalm 102:4

What a great deal of trouble you must have taken to feel like that. . . .

G.K. Chesterton

God often measures his gifts by our desire to receive them and by our co-operation with his grace.

Father Thomas Mahoney

My suffering pales to that of Jesus — my suffering is not so bad — that is one of the things I get out of Holy Communion.

Name Lost

So Jesus told them: "I swear to God, if you don't eat the son of Adam's mortal flesh and drink his blood, you don't possess life. Everyone who feeds on my mortal flesh and drinks my blood possesses real life, and I will resurrect them on the last day. For my mortal flesh is real food, and my blood real drink. Those who feed on my mortal flesh and drink my blood are part of me, and I am part of them. The Father of life sent me, and I have life because of the Father. Just so, anyone who feeds on me will have life because of me. This is the bread that comes down from heaven. Unlike your ancestors who ate [manna] and then died, anyone who feeds on this bread will live forever."

John 6:53-58

Evil is pain and sin, disaster and tragedy. But it is not real; it is the absence of good. Evil only seems to be evil because with it is suffering which is intrinsic to freedom in the universe. True freedom means one must choose a transcendental life, *but* it also means that things can go wrong. . .terribly wrong. Evil is how we willfully respond to that wrong or when we willfully create it. In a perfect world, nothing could go wrong. . .but then there would be no freedom. Suffering is the trade off for freedom. But it really does not matter if with God, if one has chosen a transcendental life.

Samuel A. Nigro

Eucharist — thanksgiving — in the end, comes from above. It is the gift that we cannot fabricate for ourselves. It is to be received. It is freely offered and asks to be freely received. That is where the choice is! We can choose to let the stranger continue his journey and so remain a stranger. But we can also invite him into our inner lives, let him touch every part of our being and then transform our resentments into gratitude. We don't have to do this. In fact, most people don't. But as often as we make that choice, everything, even the most trivial things, become new. Our little lives become great — part of the mysterious work of God's salvation. Once that happens, nothing is accidental, casual, or futile any more. Even the most insignificant event speaks the language of faith, hope, and, above all, love. That's the Eucharistic life, the life in which everything becomes a way of saying "thank you" to him who joined us on the road.

Henri J.M. Nouwen

If then you are the body of Christ and his members, it is your sacrament that reposes on the altar of the Lord. Be what you see, and receive what you are. There you are on the table, and there you are in the chalice.

Saint Augustine

Charity is *deiformity* of the intellect wherein God can be seen to move clearly not as reward but as an intrinsic change of being able to understand and savor the Incarnation.

Samuel A. Nigro

Take him yourselves and crucify him.

John 19:6

"Christ" is Greek for "Messiah." You must know that meaning to understand who Jesus was.

William Marra

The Ten Commandments are strings between people.

Samuel A. Nigro

Sometimes through the universe of matter, God grips us very hard. That grip, though painful, is an indirect contact with his love.

Diogenes Allen

Freedom means that things will go wrong and therefore it further means not that we can do what we want but that we will have to cry.

Name Lost

The alternative to the press and media now is the same as it has been for 2000 years before communication technology ever existed: the Holy Sacrifice of the Mass and ancillary liturgies! The relative newness of the press and media has made us forget that the Mass IS the way, the truth and the light. So communication technology must be recognized for the novelty it is, and, at the same time, the Mass must be brought back to the level of *real* enhancing of and engagement with the world. Liturgists need to remember always that the Mass is not to *compete* with the startling, loud, gross, titillating, entertaining, fraudulent "feel-good", thoughtless excitement of the press and media. The Mass is to be an alternative: solemn, sacred, ponderous, pleasant, placid, piercing to the depths of one's soul; irenically engaged with God by holy matter made more holy by transubstantiation; by total identification with Being as far as possible; by reiteration of deep, ancient, mysterious, truthful secrets of life; by espoused oneness with all desirables known; by liberty defined as a sacrificial choosing of good; and by ascension efforts in uplifting beauty. Liturgies must keep it that way and offer "a break" from the nonsense of the material world except as Incarnated.

Samuel A. Nigro

Let all mortal flesh be silent and stand with fear and trembling and meditate nothing earthly within itself, for the King of Kings and the Lord of Lords, Christ our God comes forward to be sacrificed and to be given for

1000 YEARS OF LATIN MASS *(in part)*

In nomine Patris, et Filii, et Spiritus Sancti.	In the name of the Father, and of the Son, and of the Holy Spirit. Amen.
Introibo ad altare Dei.	I will go unto the altar of God.
Ad Deum, qui laetificat juventutem meam.	To God who giveth joy to my youth.
Judica me, Deus, et discerne causam meam de gente non sancta: ab homine iniquo et doloso erue me.	Judge me, O God, and distinguish my cause from the nation that is not holy; deliver me from the unjust and deceitful man.
Quia tu es Deus, fortitudo mea, quare me repulisti? et quare tristis incedo dum affligit me inimicus?	For thou art God, my strength, why hast Thou cast me off? and why do I go sorrowful whilst the enemy afflicteth me?
Emitte lucem tuam, et veritatem tuam: ipsa me deduxerunt et adduxerunt in montem sanctum tuum et in tabernacula tua.	Send forth Thy Light and Thy truth: they have conducted me, and brought me unto Thy holy hill, and into Thy Tabernacles.
Et introibo ad altare Dei: ad Deum, qui laetificat juventutem meam.	And I will go unto the altar of God: to God who giveth joy to my youth.
Confitebor titi in cithara, Deus. Deus meus: quare tristis es anima mea, et quare conturbas me?	To Thee, O God, my God, I will give praise upon the harp: why art thou sad. O my soul? and why Thou disquiet me?
Spera in Deo, quoniam adhuc confitebor illi: salutare vultus mei, et Deus meus.	Hope in God, for I will still give praise to Him: the salvation of my countenance, and my God.
Gloria Patri, et Filio, et Spiritui Sancto.	Glory be to the Father, and to the Son, and to the Holy Spirit.
Sicut erat in principio, et nunc, et semper, et in saecula saeculorum.	As it was in the beginning, is now, and ever shall be, world with end. Amen.
Introibo ad altare Dei.	I will go unto the altar of God.
Ad Deum, qui laetificat juventutem meam.	To God who giveth joy to my youth.
Adjutorium nostrum in nomine Domini.	Our help is in the name of the Lord.
Qui fecit coelum et terram.	Who hath made heaven and earth.
Confiteor Dei. . .	I confess to Almighty God. . . .
Misereatur tui omnipotens Deus, et dimissis peccatis tuis, perducat te ad vitam aeternam. Amen.	May Almighty God have mercy upon thee, forgive thee thy sins, and bring thee to life everlasting. Amen.

Confiteor Deo omnipotenti, beatae Maria semper Virgini, beato Michaeli Archangelo, beato Joanni Baptistae, santis Apostolis Petro, et Paulo, omnibus Sanctis, et tibi pater, quia peccavi nimis cogitatione, verbo, et opere, mea culpa, mea culpa, mea maxima culpa. Ideo precor beatam Mariam semper Virginem, beatum Michaelem Archangelum, beatum Joannem Baptistam, sanctos Apostolos Petrum et Paulum, omnes Sanctos, et te, pater, orare pro me ad Dominum Deum nostrum.

I confess to Almighty God, to blessed Mary every Virgin, to blessed Michael the Archangel, to blessed John the Baptist, to the holy Apostles Peter and Paul, to all the Saints, and to you, father, that I have sinned exceedingly in thought, word, and deed, through my fault, through my fault, through my most grievous fault. Therefore I beseech blessed Mary every Virgin, blessed Michael the Archangel, blessed John the Baptist, the holy Apostles Peter and Paul and all the Saints, and you, father, to pray to the Lord our God for me.

Misereatur vestri omnipotens Deus, et dimissis peccatis vestris, perducat vos ad vitam aeternam.

May Almighty God have mercy upon you, forgive you your Sins, and bring you to life everlasting.

Deus, tu conversus vivificabis nos.

Thou wilt turn again, O God, and quicken us.

Et plebs tua laetabitur in te.

And Thy people shall rejoice in Thee.

Ostende nobis, Domine, misericordiam tuam.

Show us, O Lord, Thy mercy.

Et salutatre tuum da nobis.

And grant us Thy salvation.

Domine, exaudi orationem meam.

O Lord, hear my prayer.

Et clamor meus ad te veniat.

And let my cry come unto Thee.

Dominus vobiscum.

The Lord be with you.

Et cum spiritu tuo.

And with thy spirit.

Gloria in excelsis Deo: et in terra pax hominibus bonae voluntatis. Laudamus te. Benedicimus te. Adoramus te. Glorificamus te. Gratias agimus tibi propter magnam gloriam tuam. Domine Deus, Rex coelestis, Deus Pater omnipotens. Domine Fili unigenite Jesu Christe. Domine Deus, Agnus Dei, Filius Patris, qui tollis peccata mundi, miserere nobis. Qui tollis peccata mundi, suscipe deprecationem nostram. Qui sedes ad dexteram Patris, miserere nobis. Quoniam tu solus sanctus. Tu solus Dominus. Tu solus altissimus, Jesu Christe, cum Sancto Spiritu, in gloria Dei Patris. Amen.

Glory be to God on high, and on earth peace to men of good will. We praise Thee. We bless Thee. We adore Thee. We glorify Thee. We give Thee thanks for Thy great glory. O Lord God, heavenly King, God the Father Almighty. O Lord Jesus Christ, the Only begotten Son. O Lord God, Lamb of God, Son of the Father, who takest away the sins of the world, have mercy on us. Thou who takest away the sins of the world, receive our prayers. Thou who sittest at the right hand of the Father, have mercy on us. For Thou only art holy. Thou alone art the Lord; Thou only, O Jesus Christ, with the Holy Spirit, art most high in the glory of God the Father. Amen.

Glori tibi, Domine.

Laus tibi, Christe

Orate, fratres, ut meum ac vestrum sacrificium acceptabile fiat apud Deum Patrem omnipotentem.

Suscipiat Dominus sacrificium de manibus tuis ad laudem et gloriam nominis sui ad utilitatem quoque nostram totiusque Ecclesiae suae sanctae.

Per omnia saecula saeculorum.

Sursum corda.

Habemus ad Dominum.

Gratias agamus Domino Deo nostro.

Dignum et justum est.

Sanctus, sanctus, sanctus, Dominus Deus Sabaoth. Pleni sunt coeli et terra gloria tu; Hosanna in excelsis. Benedictus qui venit in nomine Domini. Hosanna in excelsis.

Hoc est enim corpus meum.

Hic est enim calix sanguinis mea, novi et aeterni testimenti: mysterium fidei, qui pro vobis et pro multis effundatur in remissionem pecatorum.

Pater Noster, qui es in coelis, sanctificetur nomen tuum: adveniat regnum tuum, fiat voluntas tua, sicut in coelo, et in terra. Panem nostrum quotidianum da nobis hodie: et dimitte nobis debita nostra, sicut et nos dimittimus debitoribus nostris. Et ne nos inducas in tentationem.

Sed libera nos a malo.

Pax Domini sit semper vobiscum.

Agnus Dei, qui tollis peccata mundi, miserere nobis.

Agnus Dei, qui tollis peccata mundi, dona nobis pacem.

Misereatur vestri omnipotens Deus, et dismissis peccatis vestris, perducat vos ad vitam ae ternam.

Indulgentiam, absolutionem pecatorum vestrorum, tribuat vobis omnipotens et misericors Dominus.

Glory be to Thee, O Lord.

Praise be to Thee, O Christ.

Brethren, pray that my sacrifice and yours may be acceptable to God the Father Almighty.

May the Lord receive the sacrifice from thy hands, to the praise and glory of His name, to our benefit, and to that of His Holy Church.

World without end.

Lift up your hearts.

We have them lifted up unto the Lord.

Let us give thanks to the Lord our God.

It is meet and just.

Holy, holy, holy, Lord God of Sabaoth. Heaven and earth are full of Thy glory. Hosanna in the highest. Blessed is he that cometh in the name of the Lord. Hosanna in the highest.

This is My Body.

This is the Chalice of my blood of the new and eternal covenant: The mystery of Faith, which shall be shed for you and for many unto the forgiveness of sins.

Our Father who art in heaven: hallowed by Thy name; Thy kingdom come; Thy will be done on earth as it is in heaven. Give us this day our daily bread: and forgive us our trespasses as we forgive those who trespass against us. And lead us not into temptation.

But deliver us from evil.

May the peace of the Lord be always with you.

Lamb of God, who takest away the sins of the world, have mercy on us.

Lamb of God, who takest away the sins of the world, grant us peace.

May Almighty God have mercy on you, forgive you your sins and bring you to life everlasting.

May the Almighty and Merciful Lord grant you pardon, absolution and full remission of your sins.

Ecce Agnus Dei: ecce qui tollit peccata mundi.

Domine, non sum dignus, ut intres sub tectum meum: sed tantum dic verbo, et sanabitur anima mea.

Corpus Domini nostri Jesu Christi custodiat animam tuam in vitam aeternam.

Ite, missa est.

Benedicamus Domino.

Deo Gratias.

Requiescant in pace.

Benedicat vos omnipotens Deus, Pater, et Filius, et Spiritus Santus.

O Salutaris Hostia!
quae coeli pandis ostium:
Bella premunt Hostilia,
Da robur, fer auxilium.
Uni trinoque Domino
sit sempiterna gloria;
Qui vitam sine termino,
Nobis donet in patria.

Tantum ergo Sacramentum
Veneremur cernui:
Et antiquum documentrum,
Novo cedat ritui:
Praestet fides supplementum,
Sensuum defectui.
Genitori, Genitoque,
Laus et jubilatio,
Salus, honor, virtus quoque,
Sit et benedictio:
Procedenti ab utroque,
Compar sit laudatio.

Panem de coelo praestitisti eis.

Omne delectamentum in se habentem.

Behold the Lamb of God who takes away the sins of the world.

Lord, I am not worthy that Thou shouldst come under my roof; but only say the word, and my soul will be healed.

May the Body of our Lord Christ preserve your soul unto life everlasting.

Go, you are sent forth.

Let us bless the Lord.

Thanks be to God.

May they rest in peace.

May Almighty God bless you, the Father, the Son, and the Holy Spirit.

O Saving Victim, open wide
The gate of heaven to man below.
Our foes press on from every side;
Thine aid supply, Thy strength bestow.
To Thy great name be endless praise,
Immortal Godhead, one in three!
O grant us endless length of days.
In our true native land with thee.

Down in adoration falling,
Lo! the Sacred Host we hail;
Lo! o'er ancient forms departing
Newer rites of grace prevail;
Faith for all defects supplying
Where the feeble senses fail.
To the everlasting Father,
And the son who reigns on high,
With the Holy Spirit proceeding
Forth from each eternally,
Be salvation, honor, blessing,
Might and endless majesty!

Thou didst give them bread from heaven.

Containing in itself all sweetness.

food for the faithful. And the bands of angels go before him with every Power and Dominion, the many-eyed Cherubim, and the six-winged Seraphim covering their faces and crying aloud the hymn "Alleluia, Alleluia, Alleluia."

Lord, I would have a lake of the finest ale!

I would welcome the poor to my feast,
For they are God's children.
I would welcome the sick to my feast,
For they are God's joy.
Let the poor sit with Jesus at the highest place,
And let the sick dance with the angels,
God bless the poor,
God bless the sick,
And bless our human race.
God bless our food,
God bless our drink.
All homes, O God, embrace.

— St. Brigid of Kildare

The love of God is not a mild benevolence but a consuming fire.

— Bede Griffiths

If everything else could disappear and only this could remain, this one experience wrapped and beholden in inward joy so that all of life became like that single moment. Would that not mean that we have entered into the joy of the Lord? Listen. Pray fervently. Pray often. Pray truly. Pray with the eyes of your soul properly focused on the right thing which is the presence of a high priest. Pray with your heart hoping and cherishing eternal life not only for yourself but those dear to you and for the whole Church and for the whole world, and your life will change. And that most precious of all human experiences will gradually begin to grow in your life. That even in this valley of tears, in this sad world, you will know that He is with you. "I will be with you until the end of the world." The realization of that fact is what Christian prayer is about. Amen.

— St. AugustineDivine Liturgy of St. James

Where are the weak to find safety and rest but in the Savior's wounds?

St. Bernard of Clairvaux

When you draw near to the awe-inspiring Chalice, so approach as if you were going to drink from the side of Christ.

St. John Chrysostom

Remove from yourself, therefore, every bit of self love and egoism, and enter within the Wounds of Christ crucified, where there is perfect and true security.

St. Catherine of Siena

"Let his blood be on us and on our children. . . ." Yes! That was the mission of Jesus. . . . His Sacrifice requires our sacrifice. The Eucharist makes it so.

Samuel A. Nigro

Whenever you see a poor, wooden Cross alone, uncared-for, worthless. . . and without a Corpus, don't forget that that Cross is your Cross — the everyday hidden Cross, unattractive and unconsoling — the Cross that is waiting for the Corpus it lacks: and that Corpus must be you.

Msgr. Escriva

Some believe that the poor are poor because the rich are rich. But the poor are poor usually because they do not know how to be rich.

James Schall

Loneliness, then, is a sign that we are never satisfied with any earthly love or work, a sign of the dignity of our creation.

James Schall

In the temporal order, a *field* is a matrix existing throughout space and time. So is Holy Eucharist. Make the most of it.

CHAPTER 6:

CONFIRMATION

In the physical order, a quantum is the indivisible unit of receiving or giving energy. Your human beingness is a quantum.

In the spiritual order, *Confirmation* is a *quantum* of *identity*, given and received, as a unique individual and as a member of the human race. By "assisting emotions" *prudence* is conveyed by which one sees and recognizes the will of God in all things and an awareness of the interdependence of all virtues in life.

"My God, my God, why hast thee forsaken me?"

Confirmation makes you a quantum — a prudent portraying of your total identity.

Live Confirmation — a reserving of one's energies to God's will, whatever it may be, and trying to carry it out.

To be in the Holy Spirit.
To enter the World of Relating and to participate in the Incarnation.

In physics, a *quantum* is the indivisible unit of receiving or giving energy. So is Confirmation.

Confirmation is a Sacrament through which we receive the Holy Spirit to make us strong and perfect Christians and soldiers of Jesus Christ. Confirmation is a *quantum*.

Confirmation is a pattern of "assisting emotions" as coinciding with *quantum*, i.e. energy units being given and received in the physical world. The resulting human principle is *identity* leading to the activity of *prudence* wherein one's own identity is willed to energize all interdependently as well as in concert with God.

Affect Assistance. . .

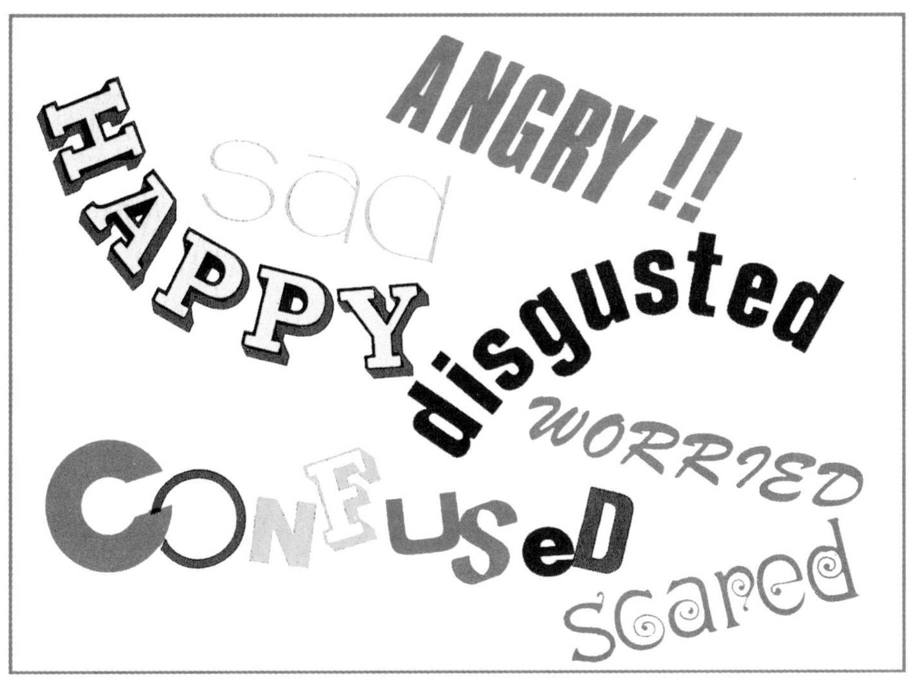

. . . One way to be a human being. Animals do not verbalize feelings or emotions but merely act out instead. A human being, however, expresses the affects:

> I am angry. You are angry. I am worried. You are worried. I am scared. You are scared. I am sad. You are sad. I am disgusted. You are disgusted. I am confused. You are confused. I am happy. You are happy.

By the calm expression of affects, unconditional help is given to oneself and to others in mutual self-understanding, in tactic-less interaction, and in self-aware interpersonal commitment to truth. Therefore, help yourself (and help me) with our feelings. To know and to express them is to create humanbeingness and is *to care.*

AFFECT ASSISTANCE

This is to underscore the need to label the emotions evident to us. Labeling emotions is therapeutic. The major emotions to be identified are those of: angry, scared, sad, worried, disgusted, and confused.

In addition, there is the affect of happiness. Nothing is wrong with happiness except when it becomes excitement.

Affect assistance is extremely appropriate for excitement levels. When you see and feel the excitement, one must move to those excited and talk about "the increasing excitement" with the clear message: "I feel tension building — let us control the excitement." Something like this may diminish the excitement so the happiness is not spoiled.

If left alone, excitement must end by aggressive acting-out, which is the natural evolving of excitement unless consciously talked down. This is especially so with anger, but all the affects run the same course: building of tension — excess excitement — disruptive behavior — end of happiness.

* * * * *

When Jesus said "to love others as yourself," He obviously implies that you are to love yourself also.

Samuel A. Nigro

I think I shall not hang myself today.

G.K. Chesterton's Morning Prayer

Go where life takes you but never stop working or praying the whole time.

Evelyn Nigro

Unhappiness is the ultimate form of self-indulgence.

Tom Robbins

Life is like riding a bicycle. You don't fall off unless you stop pedaling.

Claude Pepper

I love you, not only for what you are, but for what I am when I am with you.

Roy Croft

In the language of love there are only proposals never commands. Let us restrict commandments to things. We have no rights over each other.

Donald DeMarco

Are you afraid to be fully human? If you confine yourself to that which distinguishes you and "your kind" from others, you are being less fully human than you need to be and less fully human than the world needs you to be. Indeed, to be caught up only in "your kind" may lead you to be *inhuman*.

Samuel A. Nigro

Always leave 'em laughing, smiling, and still wanting you around. . . .

Charles C. Nigro

Anyone can become angry — that is easy. But to be angry with the right person, to the right degree, at the right time, for the right purpose, and in the right way — that is not easy.

Aristotle

> Of equal difficulty if not more is the ability to accept reasoned, angry criticism graciously without needing to retaliate (how dare you. . .), to mirror (well, you did. . .) or to make excuses (explanations are acceptable).

It doesn't hurt to be optimistic. You can always cry later.

Lucinar Santos de Lima

Be awful nice to 'em goin' up, because you're gonna meet 'em all comin' down.

Jimmy Durante

Being bored is all in your head. The world will not come and entertain you. Find something good to do.

Evelyn Nigro

TV precludes any type of friendship except the empty greeting, "Hi, how are you? Have you seen the last program?". . .there is the kind of loneliness begotten by machines. . .loneliness is stalking the land.

Catherine de Hueck Doherty

I owe much to my friends; but, all things considered, it strikes me that I owe even more to my enemies. The real person springs to life under a sting even better than under a caress.

Andre Gide

The difference between a conviction and a prejudice is that you can explain a conviction without getting angry.

Anonymous

Extending your hand is extending yourself.

Rod McEwen

One man practicing sportsmanship is far better than 50 preaching it.

Knute K. Rockne

No right-minded man forsakes truth for falsehood.

Saint Justin Martyr at his
beheading, Circa 165 A.D.

The best thing for being sad is to learn something. That is the only thing that never fails.

T.H. White

Wall bangers should use their heads.

Samuel A. Nigro

A wise man is one who savors all things as they really are.

Bernard of Clairvaux

Good morality is good medicine.

John Cardinal O'Connor

Only boring people say things are boring.

Samuel A. Nigro

Is anybody happier because you passed his way?
Does anyone remember that you spoke to him today?
Can you say tonight, in parting with the day that's slipping fast,
That you helped a single person of the many that you passed?
Is a single heart rejoicing over what you did or said?
Does the man whose hopes were fading now with courage look ahead?
Did you leave a trail of kindness, or a scar of discontent?
As you close your eyes in slumber, do you think that God will say
"You have earned one more tomorrow by the work you did today?"

Anonymous

With good prevention, you never know what disasters you are missing.

Samuel A. Nigro

Almost anything you do will be insignificant, but it is very important that you do it.

Mohandas K. Gandhi

Of all music, that which most pleases the ear is applause. But it has no score. It ends and is carried off by the wind. Nothing remains.

Enrique Solari

The real sword has no "s."

Samuel A. Nigro

Happiness, I have discovered, is nearly always a rebound from hard work.

David Grayson

Be angry and sin not; do not let the sun go down upon your anger.

Ephesians 4:26

Be not quickly angry, for anger rests in the bosom of a fool.

Ecclesiastes 7:10

Be a peacemaker, not a troublemaker.

Samuel A. Nigro

Nations do not mistrust one another because they have weapons; they have weapons because they mistrust one another.

Ronald Reagan

Never put off till tomorrow what you can do today!

Florence Hill

I imagine one of the reasons people cling to their hates so stubbornly is because they sense, once hate is gone, they will be forced to deal with pain.

James Baldwin

How we are known by God is our Being. How we know God is our virtue.

Samuel A. Nigro

A dog is a dog except when he is facing you. Then he is Mr. Dog.

Haitian Farmer

Love doesn't just sit there, like a stone; it has to be made, like bread, remade all the time, made new.

Ursula K. LeGuin

Everybody is somebody.

J. Morgan Puett

You can always tell losers because they talk about what was on television or in the movies instead of something real.

Samuel A. Nigro

He is a dirty, stinking, lousy, filthy, worthless polecat.

The Lone Ranger

Be your own best friend.

Anonymous

He who regards himself does not shine.

Lao-Tse

The superior man thinks always of virtue; the common man thinks of comfort.

Confucius

Confirmation is a Sacrament through which we receive the Holy Spirit to make us strong and perfect Christians and soldiers of Jesus Christ.

Baltimore Catechism

To act and take no account of it — that is profound virtue.

Lao-Tse

When it comes to staying young, a mind-lift beats a face-lift any day.

Marty Bucella

In God's name, I beg of you to think.

Demosthenes

When regard for truth has been broken down or even slightly weakened, all things will remain doubtful.

St. Augustine

In our doing and acting everything depends on this, that we comprehend objects clearly and treat them according to their nature.

Goethe

Never look down at someone unless you are bending over to help them up.

Anonymous

Virtue is energy of the soul employed for the common good.

Russell Kirk

You don't stop laughing because you grow old; you grow old because you stop laughing.

Michael Pritchard

I get satisfaction of three kinds. One is creating something, one is being paid for it, and one is the feeling that I haven't just been sitting on my ass all afternoon.

William F. Buckley, Jr.

You never know the love of the parent until we become parents ourselves.

Henry Ward Beecher

The only argument against losing faith is that you also lose hope — and generally charity.

G.K. Chesterton

Sorrow and pessimism are indeed, in a sense, opposite things, sorrow is founded on the value of something, and pessimism upon the value of nothing.

G.K. Chesterton

If you want your paperwork to disappear, only touch a piece of paper once; and if you want your problems to disappear, only talk about them once.

Samuel A. Nigro

Work, but success never happens in your own time!

Samuel A. Nigro

Every problem has a simple solution. Unfortunately, the simple solution is always wrong.

Winston Churchill

Problem solvers have more fun.

Samuel A. Nigro

Despair does not lie in being weary of suffering, but in being weary of joy.

G.K. Chesterton

If a man cannot make a fool of himself, we may be quite certain that the effort is superfluous.

G.K. Chesterton

The pagan determined with admirable sense to enjoy himself. But by the end of his civilization, he had discovered that a man cannot enjoy himself and continue to enjoy anything else.

G.K. Chesterton

Stand fast, and hold the traditions which you have learned, whether by word or by our Epistle.

2 Thessalonians 2:15

Go, therefore, making disciples of all nations.

Matthew 28:19

Alcohol and street drugs are abortion machines which grind you up into nothing.

Samuel A. Nigro

Hope would not be hope at all if its object were in view; how could man still hope for something which he sees?

Romans 8:24

I'm gonna take dis club and knock yoah head clean off.

Brer Bar

If all the world wre made up of people like you and your family, would it be a better place?

Name Lost

If you can't bear the cross, then you can't wear the crown.

Anonymous

Ideas rule the world and its events. A revolution is a passage of an idea from theory to practice. Whatever men say, material interests never have caused and never will cause a revolution.

Giuseppe Mazzini

First and foremost, the most important aspect of life is the salvation of your immortal soul.

Jesuits everywhere

I adjure Thee by the living God, that Thou tell us if Thou be the Christ, the Son of God. . ."Thou hast said it."

Matthew 26:63

When the Apostles who were in Jerusalem had heard that Samaria had received the word of God, they sent unto them Peter and John, who, when they were come, prayed for them that they might receive the Holy Spirit; for He was not yet come upon any of them, but they were only baptized in the name of the Lord Jesus. Then they laid their hands on them, and they received the Holy Spirit.

Acts 8:14-17

If you think you've succeeded, then you have quit.

Samuel A. Nigro

Pray like all depends on God. Work like all depends on yourself.

St. Augustine

Freedom does not mean you can do what you want to do. It means you passively accept the consequences of your behavior. Only when freedom is coupled with obedience to God does happiness occur.

Samuel A. Nigro

One should either write ruthlessly what one believes or shut up.

Arthur Koestler

An evil law is no law.

St. Thomas Aquinas

Those to whom evil is done
Do evil in return.

W.H. Auden

But I say unto you which hear, Love your enemies, do good to them which hate you.

Luke 6:22

. . .test everything; hold fast what is good.

1 Thessalonians 5:21

Do not speak to victory. Speak to people.

Name Lost

As the Father has sent Me, now also I send you. . .

John 20:21

And he who does not take up his cross and follow me, is not worthy of me. He who finds his life will lose it, and he who loses his life for my sake, will find it.

Matthew 10:38-39

We are the Body of Christ. We at least are the hands and feet of God. We gotta do some good for everybody.

Wally Hyclak

The sense of indestructibility and know-it-all-ness are a dangerous combination in teenagers.

Samuel A. Nigro

Those who cannot remember the past are doomed to repeat it.

Santayana

Those who remember the past too well *are* repeating it.

Samuel A. Nigro

Master, master! We are about to die!. . .
Where is your faith?

Luke 8:24-25

Pay to the Emperor what belongs to him, and pay to God what belongs to God.

Matthew 22:21

Governments are beasts that hustle and shake down the people. Therefore, you must pretend to be for the government by going through the motions of keeping civil obligations. Remember, however, that this is an act, an imposture, in order to get what you can to enhance your family. Under no circumstances should traditional family people do anything that actually injures their family. Sacrifice for the family. Let non-family people sacrifice for the government.

Samuel A. Nigro

He who loves the world as he loves his own body can be entrusted with the world.

Lao-Tse

Love your enemies, do good to those who hate you, bless those who curse you, and pray for those who mistreat you.

Luke 6:27-28

If anyone wants to come with me, he must forget himself, carry his cross, and follow me.

Matthew 16:24

You cannot call every bastard, a bastard. Some bastards cannot bear it.

James Schall

Study like your life depends on it because it does.

Name Lost

No heart, no mind.

Charles C. Nigro

When boredom no longer bothers you, you are truly mature and have learned to savor Life.

Samuel A. Nigro

A genuine hero is a person who, upon being pressured to do what is wrong, tells a peer group to "go to hell."

Samuel A. Nigro

Listen, do not take your lives because men of good will are with you. In some corner, in your honor, and in your memory, there will always be the note of a violin, the note of compassion of those who will defend you. Look, you are not an animal. Do not take your life. Liberty will never disappear from the face of the earth.

Armando Valladares

". . .only by a maximum exertion of will is it possible to retain one's. . .scale of values. . . . But in doing so, you must not, under any circumstances, allow yourself to hate. Not because your tormentors have not earned it. But if you allow hatred to root, it will flourish and spread during your years in the camps. . .and ultimately corrode and warp your soul. You will no longer be yourself, your identity will be destroyed, all that will remain will be a hysterical maddened and bedeviled husk of the human being that once was. And this is what will come before God should such a creature die while still behind bars. And this is just what "they" want.

Irena Ratushinskaya

I don't need to go to the zoo — I just turn on the television set.

Anonymous

Being a man is practicing your materialness (matter), your truth and your goodness. That is what being a man is. Being a woman is practicing your identity (form), your oneness, and your beauty. That is what being a woman is.

Samuel A. Nigro

The biggest soap opera in the world is the evening news about politicians and journalists.

Anonymous

Feelings alone are irrelevant unless:
1) Acted out by a thoughtless capitulation to them;
2) Neutralized by reasoned judgment;
3) Or positively empowered by the will seeking to improve the world by improving oneself.

Samuel A. Nigro

Enjoy life when it is good, but watch where you are stepping — there is always a huge pile of crap around the corner.

Name Lost

Men are always looking for sex. It is up to women, all women, to tell them: "No one but your wife."

Anonymous

Mental stability is the ability of getting mad without being mad.

Name Lost

Discipline is not order.

G.K. Chesterton

A Natural Law principle evident is that no animal species reaches fulfillment unless the females remain true to their nature leading males to do the same.

Samuel A. Nigro

The persistent emotional sexuality of all male creatures requires, in nature, that the females exert a control, and if such does not occur, then nothing, absolutely nothing works well. Perhaps this is the message of Adam and Eve in the Garden of Eden: If the female does not say "no," paradise is lost.

Samuel A. Nigro

Getting along by going along never works.

Name Lost

A little neglect may breed mischief. . .
For want of a nail the shoe was lost;
for want of a shoe the horse was lost;
for want of a horse the rider was lost;
and for want of a rider the kingdom was lost.

Benjamin Franklin

Let me be swift to hear, but slow to speak and slow to anger.

James 1:19

H.A.L.T.:
Don't get too Hungry
Don't get too Angry
Don't get too Lonely
Don't get too Tired

From mini-program of Alcoholics Anonymous

Fake it 'til you make it. . . . Choose to be happy. Period.

AlAnon Principle

Yearning for union with Christ is called Oneing by St. Julian of Norwich. Oneing is three gifts: laughing Satan out of our lives; seeing ourselves as the prize of his passion; and recognizing eternity is the Ultimate Oneing.

Calvin Miller

You shouldn't believe everything you read.

Stephen Hawking

One has to be grown up enough to realize that life is not fair. You just have to do the best you can in the situation you are in.

Stephen Hawking

One must always choose sides.

G.K. Chesterton

The covers of this book are too far apart.

Ambrose Bierce

May heaven punish the malefactor who invented that deadly, dull thing, a good time.

Ambrose Bierce

Much may be made of a Scotchman if he be caught young.

Samuel Johnson

You feed off fear as if it's a high-energy candy bar. It keeps you focused and alert.

American Test Pilot Chuck Yeager

Win one for the sonofabitch.

Florence King

Everybody's friend is everybody's fool.

Old Maxim

I sign thee with the sign of the Cross and I confirm thee with the chrism of salvation in the name of the Father, the Son, and the Holy Spirit, Amen.

Form of Confirmation

My kids are not going to date until they are married.

Dennis J. O'Hare, M.D.

I am not asking you to believe anything, all that I am asking you to do is *assume* that there is a God, and that He'll help you if you ask Him. You just do this from now on. It doesn't hurt you any. When the day comes that you leave this world, if there is a God you will find out. And if there isn't, you'll never know the difference, so how can you lose?

Sister Ignatia Gaven

First the man takes a drink,
Then the drink takes a drink,
Then a drink takes the man.

Japanese adage

The modern woman's new submissiveness is often disguised, even to herself, by the language of liberation. She's bold, she's brave, she's flouting convention, sexually "liberated" enough to do exactly what her man wants, no questions asked.

Maggie Gallagher

Almost nowhere in the anthropological records is found evidence of Freudian penis envy (except among other men), but womb envy is ubiquitous. It confirms female sexual superiority as a basic reality of human life, universally apparent but feverishly denied, and aggressively countervailed in action — by posturing men in all societies.

George Gilder

To believe in God means to do His will.

St. Irenaeus, Circa 180 A.D.

This is the definition of sin: The misuse of powers given us by God for doing good, a use contrary to God's commandments. Virtue is the use of the same powers based on a good conscience in accordance with God's commands.

St. Basil the Great, Circa 350 A.D.

Power is the unfree universal slaver. . . an idol for idiots. . . an unnatural competitor for Nature's flow. . . . It is a false god . . . Promethean power and control: it is anti-transcendental.

Samuel A. Nigro

There is no sin nor wrong that gives a man such a foretaste of hell in this life as anger and impatience.

St. Catherine of Siena, 1380 A.D.

Charity is not able to sin.

St. Angela Merici 1540 A.D.

To promote only your own kind is a denial of the humanity of yourself. Be a Catholic — "one" everywhere. . .a full human being.

Samuel A. Nigro

All life is a karate cada to be performed with joyful Italian elan. To mess it up just ask "how do you feel about it?"

Name Lost

Frivolity is, in a sense, far more sacred than seriousness.

G.K. Chesterton

Most creatures' bodies are not made for indiscriminate sex, particularly at the level of mammals. Bodies are made for reproduction in a unitive way. To make your body available for sexual purposes without reproduction and commitment is not only stupid but dangerous.

Samuel A. Nigro

A young man should read five hours a day, and so may acquire a great deal of knowledge.

Samuel Johnson

Discipline is remembering what you want.

David Campbell

Where your treasure is, there is your heart also.

Matthew 6:21

Character obliges us to do more than seek the pleasant and avoid the unpleasant; it obliges us to do what is meaningful, what is right.

Donald DeMarco

Feelings are the somatic resonance to love, that is, the counterpart on the physical side to what lies essentially in our spiritual soul.

Fr. William G. Most

Love is to will or wish good to the other for the other's sake. This lies in our spiritual will, not in our feelings.

Fr. William G. Most

Winning means you cannot lose
Because everyone wins:
By the maximum effort (courageously!),
By expecting success (in composure!),
By respecting one another (with dignity!),
By coping with the elements (resourcefully!),
By learning (with class!),
By being pointed for (quality shows!),
And by trying to be the best. . .

Samuel A. Nigro on sports

Argument ceases to be civil when it is dominated by passion and prejudice; when its vocabulary becomes solipsist, premised on the theory that my insight is mine alone and cannot be shared; . . .when things like this happen, men cannot be locked together in argument. Conversation becomes merely quarrelsome or querulous. Civility dies with the death of dialogue.

John Courtney Murray, S.J.

When a true genius appears in the world, you may know him by this sign, that the dunces are all in confederacy against him.

Jonathan Swift

You learn to grow by getting your ego hurt.

Mike Krzyzewski

What, Sir? You would make a ship sail against the wind and currents by building a bonfire under her deck? I pray you, excuse me. I have no time to listen to such nonsense.

Napoleon Bonaparte to Robert Fulton,
American Inventor

. . .whosoever, aspiring, struggles on, for him there is salvation.

Goethe

Do not hate. Loathe!

Name Lost

(The founder of Christianity) was some feeble individual. ..some puny wretch.

Marquis de Sade

There is no adequate defense except stupidity against the impact of a new idea.

Percy W. Bridgeman

I come from the town of Stupidity; it lieth four degrees beyond the city of Destruction.

Bunyan

And whoever begins by being a dupe ends in being a scoundrel.

Voltaire

"So be it!"
"Praise Him"

Polish Greeting

The difference between making the world a better place and demanding the world as you want it, is the difference between being a good guy and a selfish son-of-a-bitch.

Samuel A. Nigro

If you are not aware of and projecting your transcendentals, you are not free but are controlled by forces other than yourself.

Anonymous

The underlying meaning of "earning a living" — earning one's *life* — is at the heart of human happiness.

Charles Murray

Whenever economic policy is driven by envy, ruin results.

Robert's Law

SUCCESS: To laugh often and much; to win the respect of intelligent people and affection of children; to win the appreciation of honest critics and endure the betrayal of false friends; to appreciate beauty, to find the best in others, to leave the world a bit better, whether by a healthy child, a garden patch or a redeemed social condition; to know even one life has breathed easier because you have lived. This is to have succeeded.

Ralph Waldo Emerson

Nothing is so beautiful, nothing is so consistently fresh and surprising, so full of sweet and perpetual ecstasy as the good. No desert is so dreary, monotonous and boring as evil. But with fantasy, it's the other way 'round. Fictional good is boring and flat, while fictional evil is varied, intriguing, attractive and full of charm.

Simone Weill

Only a madman could maintain that the distinction between honorable and dishonorable, between virtue and vice, is only a matter of opinion.

Cicero

Feelings are liars. Feelings do not tell the truth. Do not believe or act on your feelings. Use your reason.

Samuel A. Nigro

Wealth from gambling quickly disappears; wealth from hard work quickly grows.

Proverbs 13:11

There are those who maintain that, in this old world of ours, everybody gets about the same break in life, and that may be true. I have observed, for example, that everybody gets about the same amount of ice. The rich get it in the summertime and the poor get it in the winter.

Bat Masterson, American Gunfighter

Melody is for the mind; harmony is for the heart; and rhythm is for the rump.

Samuel A. Nigro on music

The world is a comedy for those who think and a tragedy for those who feel.

Horace Walpole

Lord, Jesus, Carpenter of Nazareth, you are a worker as I am.

Worker's Prayer of the Association of Catholic Trade Unions

You are the future of family life.
You are the future of the joy of loving.
You are the future of making your life
something beautiful for God. . .
A pure love.
That you love a girl
or that you love a boy
is beautiful
But don't spoil it
don't destroy it.
Keep it pure.
Keep your heart virgin.
Keep your love virgin,
so that on the day of your
marriage,
you can give something
beautiful to each other. . .
the joy of pure love.

Mother Teresa of Calcutta to young people

I am not supposed to think because school is out.

12-year-old boy

High standards only discriminate against those who do not meet them.

Gayle Yiotis

There is no substitute for virtue.

Leo Strauss

Sex Liberation? That is pure myth, social poison, as about as unnatural as one can get for creatures on this planet.

Phil, the poker player

Unnatural, irrational, excessive excitement, once it is over, leads to malaise which then leads to spiritual poverty because there is an incapacity to see beyond the superficial unnatural, irrational excitement.

Name Lost

Humor is our best friend. . .
Temper is our worst enemy.

Alcoholics Anonymous

Do your best — God will do the rest.

Alcoholics Anonymous

Take the good and leave the rest behind.

Alcoholics Anonymous

One day at a time. . .

Alcoholics Anonymous

Good guys want the gals to say, "NO." They will test — and probably will not turn down if you say "yes," but then they will categorize you as a "quick piece of meat" rather than as a special person who could be part of a special relationship like a permanent commitment, like marriage. Good guys want you to say "no."

Anonymous

. . .being happy is not so important as having a jolly time. Philosophers are happy, saints have a jolly time. The important thing in life is not to keep a steady system of pleasure and composure (which can be done quite well by hardening one's heart or thickening one's head) but to keep alive in one's self the immortal power of astonishment and laughter, and a kind of young reverence.

G.K. Chesterton

Speaking truth to power implies a submission to truth represented in a higher power and nonsubmission to nontruth as represented in statements from other powers.

Michael H. Crosby

You have to believe in happiness or happiness never comes.

Douglas Malloch

If your project doesn't work, look for the part you didn't think was important.

Arthur Bloch

Better a friendly refusal than an unwilling promise.

German Proverb

Never cut a tree down in wintertime. Never make a negative decision in the low time.

Robert H. Schuller

Work. There is nothing else.

Albert Einstein

Do not hold the delusion that your advancement is accomplished by crushing others.

Marcus Tullis Cicero

Do not expect justice where might is right.

Phaedrus

According to vivid video and movie portrayals, the mind has the ability to do fantastic things with special extrasensory mind-over-matter powers. This is neither joke nor imagination. This is the contemporary way of recognizing that Heaven exists. But to acquire these powers, you have to lead a good life according to Natural Law and then die in the state of Grace.

Samuel A. Nigro

When you are behind in a foot-race, the only way to get ahead is to run faster then the man in front of you. . .stay up and burn the midnight oil.

Martin Luther King, Jr.

Earth! You seem to look for something at my hands,
Say, old top-knot, what do you want?

Walt Whitman

Does your belief system help you to think or to hate? To know truth or to buy something? To be political or to be human?

Name Lost

If all the people in the world were like you, would it be a better place?

Anonymous

We're all the same. . . we're all the same even though we're different! You are only different if you don't know that!

Charles C. Nigro pounding the dinner table
during a discussion of race and religion

Hatred and bitterness are *the* most polluting, energy-wasting events in the world — hate and bitterness require a tremendous amount of energy without anything positive produced.

Name Lost

If you cheated and won, then you really did not win — you only *thought* you won.

John Renner

A generation is now growing old, which never had anything to say for itself except that it was young. It was. . .a generation that believed in progress and nothing else. It was simply that the new thing was always better than the old thing; that the young man is always right and the old man wrong. And now that they are old men themselves, they have naturally nothing whatever to say or do. Their only business in life was to be the rising generation knocking at the door. Now that they have got into the house, and have been accorded the seat of honor by the hearth, they have completely forgotten why they wanted to come in. The aged younger generation never knew why it knocked at the door; and the truth is that it only knocked at the door because it was shut. It had nothing to say; it had no message; it had no convictions to impart to anybody. Now that it has grown old in its turn, it cannot influence its children. . .simply because it has nothing to tell them.

G.K. Chesterton

Today's women are incredible. I can get a hand job, a blow job, or a quick screw from any of them. It's about as meaningful for our relationship as taking a leak.

25-year-old male patient, 1990

If I do not perform the works of my Father, do not believe. But if I do perform them, and if you are not willing to believe me, believe the works, and you may know and believe that the Father is in me and I in the Father.

John 10:37-38

The so-called "sex revolution" is nothing more than the recognition that a simple body reflex can become a series of lifestyles. A body reflex has been found to be able to be stimulated and exaggerated because of a good spasm-like feeling similar to the ejaculation reflex in males. This has been called "orgasm." Thus, the sex revolution is nothing more than the orgasm generation abusing the human body by its infatuation and addiction to what in nature is nothing more than the male ejaculation reflex.

Samuel A. Nigro

If you give a man a bad name, you may as well hang him.

Betty Steele's mother

There is not one happy person on the face of this earth who has not learned to serve others.

Albert Schweitzer

We have seen the enemy — and she is *us*.

Maureen Sabia on professional feminists

If orgasm is the end-all, nothing else matters but "did it happen." But. . . then what? What is the significance of purposeless sperm? What is more meaningless than sperm as pollutant unless it is little spasms by pseudo-ejaculating, penisless women?

Samuel A. Nigro

Those crazy women who go around all disheveled and hate men? They're crazy, crazy. But how can one accept such crazy women who think it's a misfortune to get pregnant and a disaster to bring children into the world? And when its the greatest privilege we women have over men!

Golda Meier

Laudably, feminists are quite forthright about their wanting POWER. But in the final analysis, theirs is a shrieking self-contradictory demand bereft of power because they essentially want power GIVEN to them crying "inequality" to get others, men especially, to not use power to retain the power naturally received and which is supposed to be wanted by women only. According to this formulation, men are supposed to abandon power to women so women can have the power as perceived instead of the men. Well, if POWER is the goal, men would be stupid to acquiesce to this sort of thinking and contest. This sort of "power orientation" is essentially untrue, unnecessary and an internecine phenomenon which should only be embraced in order to defeat it.

Samuel A. Nigro

If male-female relationships are simply a matter of power, then the only way that women can "win" is by men not using the power at their disposal.

Name Lost

You cannot plough a field by turning it over in your mind.

Anonymous

To be or not to be.

Shakespeare

Do be or do not be.

Nietzsche

Do be do be doo.

Sinatra

Never show up for an interview in bare feet.

W.C. Fields

Whatever you think, be sure it is what you think; whatever you want, be sure that it is what you want; whatever you feel, be sure that it is what you feel. It is bad enough to think and want the things that your elders want you to think and want, but it is still worse to think and want just like all your contemporaries.

T.S. Eliott

Out of clutter find simplicity. From discord make harmony. In the middle of difficulty lies opportunity.

Albert Einstein's three rules of work

In the modern world it is no longer a question of liberty from kings and captains and inquisitors. It is a question of liberty from catchwords and headlines and hypnotic repetitions and all the plutocratic platitudes imposed on us by advertisement and journalism.

G.K. Chesterton

Do what you gotta do as if you wanna do, because if you don't wanna do what you gotta do, then you gotta do what you don't wanna do.

Samuel A. Nigro

Conscience is a student, not a teacher.

Pope Pius XII

I am not going to leave you much money — people will take it all from you anyway. But I will leave you a good education — no one can take that away from you.

Charles C. Nigro

An act becomes a habit, which becomes a character, which becomes a destiny.

Aristotle

Life is short; bilge is long; hell no, we won't read it.

Windi Carnes on Contemporary "Writings"

When you are in a minority, talk; when you are in a majority, vote.

Roger Sherman

Follow the first law of holes: If you are in one, stop digging.

Dennis Healey

The first thing to do in life is to do with purpose what one proposes to do.

Pablo Casals

Do not wait to strike until the iron is hot; but make it hot by striking.

William D. Sprague

Watch out for emergencies. They are your big chance!

Fritz Rianer

If you fail to plan, you are planning to fail.

Anonymous

Go out into the world, find work that you love, learn from your mistakes, and work hard to make a difference.

Maurice R. Greenberg

The secret of life is not to do what you like, but to like what you do.

American Proverb

If it makes you happy to be unhappy, then be unhappy.

Anonymous

There is no man who is happy in every way.

Euripides

Fear the goat from the front, the horse from the rear, and the man from all sides.

Russian Proverb

There are those who dislike playing the fool, preferring to act the part in a more serious spirit.

G.K. Chesterton

Never feel self-pity, the most destructive emotion there is. How awful to be caught up in the terrible squirrel cage of self.

Millicent Fenwick

When all else fails, read the instructions.

Arthur Block

Make money your god and it will plague you like the devil.

Henry Fielding

Look up and not down; look out and not in; look forward and not back, and lend a hand.

Edward Everett Hale

Cantate, cantate! (Sing, sing!)

Arturo Toscanini

When a piece gets difficult, make faces.

Arthur Schnabel

Society doesn't applaud peoples looking bad. Looking bad means we feel bad about ourselves.

Charles Hix

You should aim to be independent of any one vote, of any one fashion, of any one century. Right: Go Catholic.

Baltasar Gracian

Be grateful for luck. Pay the thunder no mind — listen to the birds. And don't hate nobody.

Eubie Blake

The happiness of your life depends upon the quality of your thoughts: therefore, guard accordingly.

Marcus Antonious

The human mind is like a magnifying glass: It exaggerates. A simple rule of thumb: Whatever you're looking for is not as big a deal as you think it is.

Daniel Meacham

To achieve great things we must live as though we were never going to die.

Vauvenargues

Yes! Christianity of course. Believe in dreams. Never believe in hurts. You can't let the grief and the hurts and the breaking experience of life control your future decisions.

Robert H. Schuller

Nature, to be commanded, must be obeyed.

Sir Francis Bacon

People are more easily led than driven.

Jewish Proverb

Human history becomes more and more a race between education and catastrophe.

H.G. Wells

Some people go through their lives like the simple workmen who "make bricks," while others, doing the very same tasks, "build cathedrals."

Samuel A. Nigro

War, Famine, Pestilence and Death have long been known as the Four Horsemen of the Apocalypse. Few are aware of the Four Horsewomen of the Apocalypse: Noise, Promiscuity, Pollution and Power. Both quartets, however, are interchangeably mare or nag.

Samuel A. Nigro

. . .bear witness to the Church of the Gospel by feeding the hungry, sheltering the homeless, and clothing the naked, without a whole lot of gad. . .

Barbara Grizzuti Harrison

Natural Law is never spent; therein is life, love and all truth.

Samuel A. Nigro

The story may not be true — who cares? Any story, once told, has a certain kind of truth.

Barbara Grizzuti Harrison

Man left to himself is a victim of moods.

G.K. Chesterton

Insanity is the placing of the will before the intellect.

Frank A. Petta

The sex revolution is nothing more than the misappropriation of the ejaculation (orgasm) reflex from sperm emission consistent with procreation to an end in and of itself by any means available. This is a bizarre magnification of a simple body reflex beyond offspring, family and environment. Resultant is the waste of an extraordinary part of one's life seeking old or new ways to ejaculate, perseverating like the brain-damaged, preoccupied like addicts, never failing to conjure up another useless but exciting permutation of ejaculation possibilities. At best, this is "advertising"; at worst, it is a plague. In the final analysis, ejaculation (orgasm) as end-all is the grotesque denial of one's linkage to the animal kingdom, of one's obligation to comply with planetary norms, and of one's responsibility to the environment. Indeed, jaculasis or ejaculation reflex people (ERPs) are the very worst examples of human disdain for the environment because their adoration of the ejaculation reflex is a personal rejection of one's own self as a normal animal on the planet. Thus one becomes a pollutant oneself. It is to live irreverence.

Samuel A. Nigro

For centuries, men have been trying to figure out how to get women to submit to them sexually without expectations. Thanks to contraception and Planned Parenthood, it has finally been accomplished in the 1990's.

Samuel A. Nigro

Chastity is the only solution that is 100% effective, costs nothing, has no harmful side effects, and puts you in control of your own life. . . . Why aren't more people promoting chastity as a solution for teen pregnancy, sexually transmitted diseases, and abortion? (Because) chastity does not make money. No one can sell it, put it in pill form, or make it into a spray repellant to be used before going out on a date.

Molly Kelly

Because the press and media can influence you and me, they revel in a perverse state of self-importance. They inflate an act — whatever it may be — so they can savor how they influenced us. And whatever it is, this is not communication.

Samuel A. Nigro

Of all the fairy tales ever in the universe, none are less true than anything in the press and media and none are more true than Roman Catholicism.

Samuel A. Nigro

One and one is two, two and two is four; and five will get you ten if you know how to make it work.

Mae West

Duties change, but truth never.

John Henry Newman

There is nothing I wouldn't do for ____, and there's nothing ____ wouldn't do for me, so we go through life doing nothing for each other.

Mark Shields

We need not dispute, we need not prove, we need but define.

John Henry Newman

The presence of such members (homosexuals) adversely affects the ability of the Armed Forces to maintain discipline, good order and morale.

United States Defense Department

Hate hurts the hater more than the hated. Hate is from the fear of recognizing that one's nothingness may be discovered. Hate is an amalgamation of pride, envy and self-pity.

Name Lost

How canst thou endure without being mad?

Ahab

The most consistent correlation of "success" by whatever definition is with the size of one's vocabulary.

Samuel A. Nigro

The gentlemen is a liar and a scoundrel. I use the words in no personal sense.

G.K. Chesterton

Just as flirting is a profanation of holy love, so sulking is a profanation of holy hatred.

G.K. Chesterton

Contemporary entertainment is designed to trick women into submitting to sexual activity without realizing that they are submitting.

Samuel A. Nigro

God will not help with that you can do yourself.

Name Lost

Everybody starts out Saul and ends up Paul.

Ralph Ellison

Go to bed early, get up early; this is wise.

Mark Twain

Do not carry a spirit of contradiction, for it is to be freighted with stupidity and with peevishness, and your intelligence should plot against it; though it may well be the mark of mental genius to see objection, a wrangler about everything cannot escape being marked a fool, for he makes guerrilla warfare of quiet conversation.

Baltasar Gracian

Do not consider a thing as proof because you find it written in a book; for just as a liar will deceive with his tongue, he will not be deterred from doing the same thing with his pen. They are utter fools who accept a thing as convincing proof simply because it is in writing.

Moses Maimonides

Cultivate the habit of early rising. It is unwise to keep the head long on a level with the feet.

Henry David Thoreau

Never advertise what you don't have for sale.

Mother's advice to daughters

Never praise a woman for having masculine traits.

English Proverb

Rule of survival: Pack your own parachute.

T.L. Hakala

If you don't get the better of yourself, someone else will.

Anonymous

Remember, my son, if you ever need a helping hand, you'll find one at the end of your arm.

The father of Sam Levenson

Anybody who has been seriously engaged in scientific work of any kind realizes that over the entrance to the gates of the temple of science are written the words: *Ye must have faith.* It is a quality which the scientist cannot dispense with.

Max Planck

When the character of a man is unclear to you, look at his friends.

Japanese Proverb

Fake feeling good. You're going to have to learn to fake cheerfulness. Believe it or not, that effort will pay off: you will actually start feeling happier.

Jean Bach

You have to help a child understand the role of money. You want to establish that money doesn't grow on trees.

James Comer

If you want a thing done well, do it yourself.

Napoleon I

If you want to "get in touch with your feelings" fine — talk to yourself, we all do. But if you want to communicate with another thinking human being, get in touch with your thoughts. Put them in order, give them a purpose, use them to persuade, to instruct, to discover, to seduce. The secret way to do this is to write it down, and then cut out the confusing parts.

William Safir

Don't watch the clock; do what it does. Keep going.

Sam Levenson

Do your job and demand your compensation — but in that order.

Cary Grant

Way of the world or way of the Lord?
TV or not TV? These are the questions.

Name Lost

False pride is pride in anything other than what you are doing right now.

Samuel A. Nigro

. . .all the claims so glibly made about societies ruled by women are nonsense. We have no reason to believe that they ever existed. . . . Men have always been the leaders in public affairs and the final authorities at home.

Margaret Mead

Virtue — even attempted virtue — brings light; indulgence brings fog.

C.S. Lewis

Where promiscuity prevails, there will therefore always be more often the victims than the culprits.

C.S. Lewis

Never bring shame on your family, never tell a lie, and never brag about what you do.

Toil Okazaki

Violence may be wrong, but it can be used at times. After all, St. Peter drew the sword while Judas used a kiss.

G.K. Chesterton

Beware of the danger signals that flag problems: Silence, secretiveness, or sudden outbursts.

Sylvia Porter

Put first things first and we get second things thrown in: put second things first and we lose *both* first and second things.

C.S. Lewis

I prefer to combat the "I'm special" feeling, not by the thought "I'm no more special than anyone else," but by the feeling "Everyone is as special as me."

C.S. Lewis

Standing in the middle of the road is very dangerous; you get knocked down by the traffic from both sides.

Margaret Thatcher

If thou has commenced a good action, leave it not incomplete.

The Talmud

Anything half done, or half known, is, in my mind, neither done or known at all.

Lord Chesterfield

Think — or be damned!

Bryan Penton

If you want to kill time, why not try working it to death.

Sam Levenson

Trust in Allah, but tie up your camel.

Turkish Proverb

Establish the eternal truth that acquiescence under insult is not the way to escape war.

Thomas Jefferson

Of course (healthy) patriotism. . .is not in the least aggressive. It asks only to be let alone. It becomes militant only to protect what it loves.

C.S. Lewis

To make good you must have some talent other than determination.

William Feather

If those people had read or gone to school instead of watching soaps and television, they would have accomplished something instead of nothing.

Betty Howard

Humanity has a natural affinity with the animal kingdom and with the earth. Humans are not aliens upon this planet. It just seems that way when we violate our roots by anti-life actions against the environment and by anti-animal actions in regards to natural sexuality. Indeed, none of the animals treat sexuality the way humans do, just as none of the animals treat the environment the way humans do. Natural Law places humanity at one with our animal origins and with our roots in the planet.

Samuel A. Nigro

Be led by reason.

Greek Proverb

If you knew everything you thought you knew, why aren't you teaching the class.

Charles C. Nigro to his teenage son about school

Why don't you talk about it!

A child psychiatrist's exhortation to two fighting 2-year-old boys

True liberty is not liberty to do what we wish, but liberty to do what we ought.

Lord Acton

All right, kids, GROW UP!

Sister Mary Francetta and all the Sisters of Charity

The only time you get bored is when you are not learning something.

Samuel A. Nigro

The man who says there are no sexes or no nations fares simply and precisely like the man who says there are no chairs and tables. He falls over them.

G.K. Chesterton

Dig a well before you are thirsty.

Chinese Proverb

The press and media do not appeal to the mind; they appeal to emotions.

Anonymous

You can observe a lot just by watching.

Yogi Berra

The denial of identity is the very signature of Satan.

G.K. Chesterton

The world of media is full of easy answers, wash-and-wear philosophies, instant ecstasies, what-me-worry Epiphanies. Probably readers want a little more.

Umberto Eco

When people waste their time on nonsense, they can only get mad when challenged.

Samuel A. Nigro

If you get in trouble with the authorities, police, teachers, whoever, you are on your own, buddy. . . . Don't call me.

Charles C. Nigro to his 14-year-old son

An exaggeration is a truth that has lost its temper.

Kahill Gibran

Cast the net on the right side of the boat and you will find some.

John 21:6

Truly, truly, I say to you, when you were young, you girded yourself and walked where you would; but when you are old, you will stretch out your hands and another will gird you and carry you where you do not wish to go. . . . Follow me.

John 21:18

Render to Caesar the things that are Caesar's, and to God the things that are God's.

Mark 12:17

When we speak about virtue, we speak about Christ.

St. Ambrose

Virtue is it! Virtue perfects.

Name Lost

The only substance of feelings is that which you give them. Therefore, you can control the impact of feelings.

Samuel A. Nigro

Feelings are important nothings. They cannot have the impact of being hit by a brick. To give feelings the power of reality is self-destructive.

Samuel A. Nigro

To really feel good, find something to do greater than yourself and keep doing it.

Name Lost

Why should you learn this stuff in school? Because somebody you are going to be on a quiz show and you'll answer the question, winning one million dollars.

Samuel A. Nigro

Are you going to build a cathedral today? Or make a brick?

Sister Florence Marie

People generally quarrel because they cannot argue.

G.K. Chesterton

We can all disagree without being disagreeable.

U.S. Congressional motto

If you drink, don't drive. Don't even putt.

Dean Martin

It is only for God (the bestower and creator of forms), and perhaps also for angels or pure intelligence at once to recognize supremely universal forms at the first glance of contemplation.

Sir Francis Bacon maintaining that human thought proceeds gradually from particular to universal.

Nothing lasts on earth but your family, good books, and virtue.

Samuel A. Nigro

Short term feel-goods make for long term misery.

Anonymous

It is not always a disadvantage to have disadvantages.

G.K. Chesterton

It is not bigotry to be certain we are right; but it is bigotry to be unable to imagine how we might possibly have gone wrong.

G.K. Chesterton

Every child must experience *appropriate* anger about an act that was wrong — an anger that does not crush or injure but that hurts-out-of-concern merely for the wrongness of the act. This is how the conscience is formed.

Samuel A. Nigro

Nature has tended to endow human males with a greater muscle mass. Because of this expectation on the part of the brain in the developing years, boys tend to be more vigorous, assertive and aggressive than girls.

Name Lost

Nobody hands you anything on a silver platter — you have to work for it.

Evelyn Nigro

Your life project is your own way of being — it should be a work of art in which you affirm your being using transcendentals in a process of living the Sacraments, just as a self-portrait is made by an artist using paints in a process of living his abilities.

Name Lost

Of all that might be omitted in thinking, the worst was to omit your own being.

Saul Bellow

Winning isn't everything; wanting to win is.

Vincent Lombardi

Far better it is to dare mighty things, to win great triumphs, even though checkered by failure, than to rank with those poor spirits who neither enjoy much or suffer much, because they live in the gray twilight that know neither victory nor defeat.

Theodore Roosevelt

If you want your dreams to come true, don't sleep.

Yiddish Proverb

If you want joy out of life, learn the transcendentals and project them.

Name Lost

Of course, I trust you. . .it is the world that I do not trust. . .so you cannot date one-on-one. . .you can only go out with a group of your friends.

Mother to her 15-year-old daughter

Pornography is the Big Mac of sex. It titillates and teases. It may even seem to satisfy for the moment. But the more you get, the sicker you become, and eventually you forget what real food or real women (with real names) are like.

Thomas Fleming

Problems are only opportunities in work clothes.

Henry J. Kaiser

Make yourself into a sheep, and you'll meet a wolf nearby.

Russian Proverb

All teenagers go through a *Romeo and Juliet* stage where everything goes wrong by their own stupidity and if unlucky, they end up dead.

Name Lost

The world suffers if women are not focused on identity, oneness and beauty; the world suffers also if men are not focused on matter, truth and goodness.

Samuel A. Nigro

. . .which of you being anxious can add a cubit to his span?

Luke 12:22-25

Never be entirely idle; but either be reading, or writing, or praying, or meditating, or endeavoring something for the public good.

Thomas a Kempis

Television negates depth; it superficializes everything so that one is diluted to nothing, i.e. the personal equivalent of a vacuum in astronomy. At the opposite extreme is psychoanalysis which accentuates self-depth so that one is constricted to nothing, i.e. the personal equivalent of a "black hole" in astronomy. One can embrace the universe with neither television nor psychoanalysis. Both are a form of withdrawal from active free participation in the world.

Samuel A. Nigro

Before undergoing a surgical operation, arrange your temporal affairs. You may live.

Ambrose Bierce

Make not thy stomach an apothecary's shop.

English Proverb

And that means drugs.

Trust your hopes, not your fears.

David Mahoney

Treat your superior as a father, your equal as a brother, and your inferior as a son.

Persian Proverb

If sexual activity is separated from reproduction, it becomes then a matter of orgasm. If sexual activity becomes a matter of orgasm, then it becomes separated from gender. If sexual activity becomes degenderized, then it becomes separated from humanity. If sexual activity becomes dehumanized, then it becomes a matter for subhuman animals and inanimate objects. If sexual activity becomes a matter for subhuman animals and inanimate objects, it has been totally denaturalized from Life on the planet. Humanity, thusly, treats sexual activity consistent with its violating almost all other Natural Laws of the planet, from pollution to the disrespect for natural life, from oil spills to nonreproductive sexual activity. Not even subhuman animals behave this way. And, the sole promoter of genuine sex (not separated from reproduction) in Nature in the full realm of humanity is: the Roman Catholic Church.

Samuel A. Nigro

Now the works of the flesh are plain: fornication, impurity, licentiousness, idolatry, sorcery, enmity, strife, jealousy, anger, selfishness, dissension, factions, envy, murder, drunkenness, carousing, and the like. I warn you, as I warned you before, that those who do such things shall not inherit the kingdom of God. But the fruit of the Spirit is love, joy, peace, patience, kindness, goodness, self-control; against such there is no law. And those who belong to Christ Jesus have crucified their flesh with its passions and desires.

Galatians 5:19-24

The primary impulse of each is to maintain and aggrandize himself. The secondary impulse is to go out of the self, to correct its provincialism and heal its loneliness. In love, in virtue, in the pursuit of knowledge, and in the reception of the arts, we are doing this. Obviously this process can be described either as an enlargement or as a tempory annihilation of the self. But that is an old paradox: He that loseth his life shall save it.

C.S. Lewis

The press is lazy, ideological, politicized, stupid, mean, and vindictive. It is comprised of a bunch of public relations puppeteers who have strung our politicians. Thus the government has actually been overthrown by the press, and the people have been deprived of the First Amendment which has been stolen by a bunch of thugs known as editors and journalists who, pretending objectivity, never fail to impose their own personal inclinations.

Samuel A. Nigro

One must first give battle to be able to proclaim victory; he who begins nothing, finishes nothing. . . . Those who do not recognize opportunity when it comes, find misfortune when they do not look for it.

Isabel of Spain: The Catholic Queen,
The Greatest Women Ruler in History

Is there Joy in it?

Name Lost

Beware of the twelve confusions:

1. Of dissent for intolerance.
2. Of independence for error.
3. Of minority correctness for inferiority special pleading.
4. Of precise justice for cruelty.
5. Of tradition for unfashionability.
6. Of morality for arbitrariness.
7. Of leadership for consensus.

8. Of forthrightness for obstructionism.
9. Of real civilization for the inability to read.
10. Of truth for a fake press proclaiming to be free.
11. Of salvation for cannibalism.
12. Of goodness for evil-claiming-to-be-nice.

Name Lost

Loquere igitur; inquit, adolescens, ut te videam. — well, then, my lad, speak, so that I can see you.

Socrates

First deserve, and then desire.

English Proverb

I have six honest serving men; they taught me all I knew. Their names are How and Why and Where, and When and What and Who.

Rudyard Kipling

Overturning the chess board is not a chess move.

Andre Malraux

An effective way to get the troubles out of your mind is to write them on a sheet of paper — a problem things-to-do list. Then let the list both remember and fret for you.

Samuel A. Nigro

Lust is like mud. Its opposite is like clear water, or clean air. It is called purity of heart.

Peter Kreeft

A man with a violin case under his arm stood in Times Square looking lost. He asked a policeman, "How can I get to Carnegie Hall?" The policeman answered, "Practice, man, practice." There is no short cut to sanctity either. Or happiness, or salvation.

Peter Kreeft

For what will it profit a man if he gains the whole world, and loses his own soul?

Mark 8:36

Talk is cheap and it doesn't mean a damn thing.

Charles C. Nigro

The gluteus maximus should not control the eyes.

Samuel A. Nigro

A foul mouth is always linked to an empty mind.

D.J. O'Hare

Humans are the only creatures in the entire animal kingdom for which sex is used for something other than procreation — talk about being out of touch with Nature and the Planet!

Samuel A. Nigro

Nothing worthwhile is easy. . .you have to work for it.

Evelyn Nigro

Everything is easy if you know how.

Charles Nigro

Go where life takes you. Do not second guess.

Evelyn Nigro

They will steal your money and all your belongings, but no one can take your education from you — so if I leave you anything, it will be an education.

Charles C. Nigro

If you cannot do anything about it, then you can cry — otherwise you should be laughing or singing.

Evelyn Nigro

Hey, listen, you have to work at having fun too!

Evelyn Nigro

Nothing is so strong as gentleness. Nothing is so gentle as real strength.

St. Francis of Assisi

Easy sex is a denaturalized pattern. . . . For humans, like so many other unreflective activities, easy sex is against all animal life and the Planet itself.

Name Lost

Sex preoccupation in a society is an environmental disease. That you are not preoccupied with orgasm all the time does not mean that something is wrong with you. That you are not preoccupied with heterosexual orgasm does not mean that you are homosexual. Ejaculation reflex people (ERPs) think otherwise and they are not only wrong but sick. Sex preoccupation or sex as recreation is an environmental disease because it is out of synchrony with procreation and unition. Sex as recreation is the simple adoration of a bodily reflex. Period. It is an environmental disease.

Samuel A. Nigro

A man is a slave to anything he cannot part with that is less than himself.

George MacDonald

He that is angry without cause shall be in danger, but he that is angry with shall not.

St. John Chrysostum

Brainwashing is not propaganda; brain-dirtying is propaganda.

Peter Kreeft

Sow a thought, reap an act.
Sow an act, reap a habit.
Sow a habit, reap a character.
Sow a character, reap a destiny.

Samuel Smiles

All that we are is dependent on our thoughts. It begins with our thoughts, it continues with our thoughts, it ends with our thoughts.

Buddha

Passions (feelings) are like horses; reason is like a rider.

Peter Kreeft

Do not seek flattery — nor give it — if you are focusing on your Transcendentals, you really do not have to care.

Name Lost

Man has free-will: otherwise counsels, exhortations, commands, prohibitions, rewards and punishments will be in vain.

St. Thomas Aquinas

Virginity is not only symbolic of innocence and purity, but it is Transcendentally (specifically *immanentally*) supreme with unintruded essence, unfragmented oneness, and undeterred ascendancy. Virginity means that one has full control of one's own material being.

Samuel A. Nigro

True law is right reason in agreement with Nature.

Cicero

It is against reason to be burdensome to others, showing no amusement and acting as a wet blanket. Those without a sense of fun, who never say anything ridiculous, and are cantankerous with those who do, these are vicious and are called grumpy and rude.

St. Thomas Aquinas

There are natural reasons why people can get along together. They are evident in deliberative balanced discourse which apply rules of reason acceptable to all parties. It is the universal acceptance of these rules of reason observed during dialogue that provide the vanguard of judging, enabling the acquisition of truth and the seeking of good, fundamental to which is the deliverance from gullibility.

Samuel A. Nigro

Happiness (*eudaimonia* in Greek, *felicitas* in Latin) means not merely subjective contentment, or a rest of desire, but also real blessedness, a state of possessing the objective good for man. It is contentment, but contentment in the true good.

Peter Kreeft

Man is created to praise, reverence, and serve God our Lord and by this means to save his soul.

And the other things on the face of the earth are created for man and that they may help him in prosecuting the end for which he is created.

From this it follows that man is to use them as much as to help him on to his end, and ought to rid himself of them so far as they hinder him as to it.

For this it is necessary to make ourselves indifferent to all created things and all that is allowed to the choice of our free will and is not prohibited to it; so that, on our part, we want not health rather than sickness; riches rather than poverty; honor rather than dishonor; long rather than short life; and so in all the rest, desiring and choosing only what is most conducive for us to the end for which we are created.

Beginning of the Ignatian Credo

It is better to love God than to know God, but it is better to know material things than to love them.

Peter Kreeft, paraphrasing St. Thomas Aquinas

Always try to please Jesus.

St. Therese of Lisieux

Virtue means energetic manliness.

Russell Kirk

The importance of genuine women being genuinely female is symbolized as ideal by the Blessed Virgin Mary, as to be admired by Beatrice for Dante, and as gone wrong by the story of Eve. The impact of a genuine woman being genuinely female is absolutely irreplaceable.

Name Lost

Just do good and avoid evil; time is on your side.

Samuel A. Nigro

. . .the new life begins. . .

Dante on first seeing Beatrice

All men by nature desire to know.

Aristotle

"Selling one's soul" is merely the investing of oneself in one's own body (*res*) to the slighting of the other transcendentals, i.e. by investing so much in the material self, one's spiritual components are forgotten.

Samuel A. Nigro

I can act stupid without getting drunk. . . . So why drink?

Samuel A. Nigro

Homosexuality in nature does not exist as a consistent stable social phenomenon. However, humans, having the mental capacity and need to rationalize all behaviors, create an epiphenomenon called "homosexuality" which is actually a masquerade behind which is nothing more than orgasm addiction for any stimulation other than natural sexual intercourse.

Samuel A. Nigro

An excellent plumber is infinitely more admirable than an incompetent philosopher. The society which scorns excellence in plumbing because it regards that as a humble activity and tolerates shoddiness in philosophy because it regards that as an exalted activity will have neither good plumbing nor good philosophy; neither its pipes nor its theories will hold water.

John William Gardner — Former Secretary,
U.S. Dept. of Health, Education & Welfare

No matter how well intentioned, nothing can be corrected or "made right" by telling lies.

Samuel A. Nigro

The rule of reason is the most basic guide for mankind.

St. Thomas Aquinas

Labor the more that by good works you may make sure your calling and elections sure.

2 Peter 1:10

Anxiety is not the same as failure.

Name Lost

The most effective method of defying all the unrealistic emotional craziness offered as reality is to be aware and project one's Transcendentals. They truly set one free and will create the new man: male or female.

Anonymous

Haste makes waste.

Simple, true, unimprovable, and not to be forgotten

Acts of the sensitive appetite, inasmuch as they have annexed to them some bodily change, are called passions; whereas acts of the will are not so called. Love, therefore, and joy and delight are passions; insofar as they denote acts of the sensitive appetite. But insofar as they denote acts of the intellective appetite, they are not passions. It is in this latter sense that they are in God.

St. Thomas Aquinas

Prayer does not change God, but it changes things and people. The reason to pray is not to change God's will, but to fulfill it. It is the same reason as the reason to work.

Peter Kreeft

A man should pride himself more on serving well than on commanding well.

Plato

Mediocre people are always at their best.

Old adage

Music sings what our words would like to say, but can't.

Alice von Hildebrand

Catholic guilt is better than Protestant superficiality or non-Catholic stupidity.

Michael D. Nigro

Arm yourself and be ye men of valor, for it better to perish in battle than look upon these insults to our home and to our altar.

Joshua 1:14

Modesty is the virtue which guards the intimate sphere of your sexuality and ensures that it won't be desecrated.

Alice von Hildebrand

Your body is only 1/7 of your soul — and each of the other six parts deserve as much attention and activity as your body.

Samuel A. Nigro

Genuine guilt is about intellectual misapprehending.

Name Lost

Television and movies are ways of vicarious living, mainly lies and thus most are a waste of time.

Anonymous

The proper study of mankind is everything.

C.S. Lewis

Feelings violate integrity unless they are dealt with by right reason.

Samuel A. Nigro

The two most ridiculous activities I have ever been engaged in have been war and sex.

Malcolm Muggeridge

I am willing to appear on T.V., but not to own one.

Malcolm Muggeridge

No one is more homeless than those living on unnatural sex.

Name Lost

A gentlemen is tender towards the bashful, gentle towards the distant, and merciful towards the absurd.

Cardinal Newman

There have always been two types of free people in the world: those who are genuinely free and in touch with Nature and those who listen to people who pretend to know but do not know. This is particularly so today with the press and media. In order to be genuinely free, you must know how to be focused intently on Truth that is at One with Nature. This means you can listen to what the press and media have to say, but you must not believe it until you have confirmed it independently in detail. Only then can you genuinely be free because that which is untrue or that which is unNatural will make you a slave.

Samuel A. Nigro

Whatever — make an effort! With all you got — like the world will end if you do not succeed. Make an effort.

Sister Agnes Virginia

Be you perfect as also your heavenly Father is perfect.

Matthew 5:48

About homosexuality: when someone says it is normal, I cannot agree without violence to what I know in my own experience. However, when someone says it is a disorder and the individuals with it want to be treated normally, then I can understand and can help.

Samuel A. Nigro

Don't lose looking bad.

Mrs. Vince Lombardi

All which is not you, you should have to worry about — it is the other guy — always look out for the other guy.

Charles C. Nigro

If everybody in class jumped off a cliff, would you do it too?

Sister Florence Marie

The public does not know what to believe until it is *told* what to believe.

Ed Simmons, Jr. on television and movies

When the archer shoots for nothing, he has all his skill. When he shoots for a brass bubble, he is already nervous. When he shoots for a prize of gold, he goes blind! He's out of his mind! He sees two targets! His skill has not changed but the prize divides him. He cares. He thinks more of winning than of shooting. And the need to win drains him of power. . . .

Quang Tse about 2500 B.C.

My mother really wants me to be a priest, but my father has warned me against taking a job where I have to wear a dress to work.

Ed Stivender, 5th grader

Oh, yeah, well, never get a job where you have to wear a hat to work.

Diane Tasca, 5th grader

DEFY EVIL!

Anonymous

I have six bottomless-pitted feminists to serve; they take all that is mine. Their names are Harangue and Weasel and Wretch, and Want and Whimper and Whine.

Apologies to Rudyard Kipling

My people are destroyed for lack of knowledge. . . .

Hosea 4:6

You can always tell a Harvard man, but you can't tell him much.

Name Lost

When one can no longer dislike what one dislikes. . .but when all must like alike, that is real tyranny and Defiance is called for.

Samuel A. Nigro

. . .true progress consists in looking for the place where we can stop.

G.K. Chesterton

The pursuit of happiness is. . .learning how to experience our experience. . . learning how to enjoy our enjoyment.

G.K. Chesterton

If you wish to love your enemy fight him. If, however, you wish to hate him with really hellish hatred, surrender to him.

G.K. Chesterton

Politeness is an armed guard, stern and splendid and vigilant, watching over all the ways of men; in other words, politeness is a policeman.

G.K. Chesterton

The world will not entertain you, so make your own fun. It won't feed you either, so work. And it won't love you, so stay right with God.

Evelyn Nigro

Virtue renders feelings to be irrelevant. When feelings strike, find a Transcendental to do.

Anonymous

The more we anticipate a pleasure, the more we lose our grasp.

Thomas Fleming

Sincerity merely means actuality. It only means that a man's opinion undoubtedly is his opinion.

G.K. Chesterton

If you give in to your feelings, you will be enslaved by them.

Sister Honorius

Disturb us, Lord, when
We are too well pleased with ourselves,
When our dreams have come true
Because we dreamed too little

When we arrived safely
Because we sailed too close to shore.
Disturb us, Lord, when
With the abundance of things we possess
We have lost our thirst
For the abundance of life;
We have ceased to dream of eternity.
And in our efforts to build a new earth,
We have allowed our vision
Of the new Heaven to dim.

Disturb us, Lord, to dare more boldly,
To venture on wider seas
Where storms will show you mastery;
Where losing sight of land,
We shall find the stars.

We ask you to push back
The horizons of our hopes;
And to push us in the future
In strength, courage, hope and love.

Sir Francis Drake

MASTURBATION

Masturbation as a phenomenon acquires exaggerated significance for those against it and, in mirror image, for those for it. For individuals, masturbation looms large also because of its simplicity (for males at least) and its frequency. Indeed, how can masturbation be "wrong?"

Well, once again, the psychosocial detriments are found upon analysis to coincide with the Church's moral wisdom.

Psychologically, masturbation (and any equivalent, i.e. oral or anal sex) often has a more satisfying intensity even than sexual intercourse. This very satisfaction has significance in the totality of human beingness, because a person is tricked into believing that one can be satisfied by self or by what is incomplete in or overtly counter to genuine nature accurately appreciated.

To grasp the totality of being and be committed to the transcendentals of truth, beauty, and goodness et cetera is to demand global environmentalism, and, if consistent, is also to demand its *sine qua non*: individual virtue, which does not allow personal selfish unsanitary and dangerous activities any more than international businesses are allowed to foul up the environment. Only Natural Law serves the purpose of total faithfulness to the universe, and it cannot be applied willy-nilly.

For example, an environmentally-oriented and thereby Natural Law enthusiast would, if logically consistent, object to that which is unsanitary and downright dangerous (from oil spills on the community level to anal sex on the individual level).

Such is the moral "high ground" when it comes to masturbation and its equivalents.

At the personal "low ground," however, masturbation is so common. . .it is so pleasurable. . .it is so easy. . .so uncomplicated. . .so benign! And it does not foul the environment! (All these composing the most common promotions *for* masturbation.)

Well, perhaps it is not as private as one thinks — anymore than not dealing "properly" with trash by separating that which can be recycled from the rest. "Privacy" in the psychological spiritual sense may be more widely impacting than the claims that one's secret feelings, fantasies, and non-public simple activities affect no one else.

On three grounds, psychologically at the personal level, masturbation can be recognized as something to be avoided:

1. It is habit forming;
2. It is distracting and interfering with higher functions;
3. It is counterproductive to a fulfilling relationship.

Considering addiction aspects, there can be little argument about masturbation's (1) habit-forming and (2) distraction-interference detriments. Masturbation, like any addiction, can have profound, far-reaching implications easily discernible by the briefest introspection. Actually, addiction theories in regard to sexual patterns are as valid for masturbation as for anal sex, oral sex, violent sex, homosex as well as chemical addictions (alcohol, cocaine).

Masturbation as an addiction phenomenon has all the negatives of any other addiction. Deserving emphasis especially is its strong tendency to dull enthusiasm for objectivity, replacing the objective by the subjective self. Truly, masturbation is the subjective plundering of objective good, and the mind's chemistry becomes prone to decondition, coarsen, and cheapen objective truth, beauty, and goodness for a simple, common, intense "feel good" spurious benignity, devoid of external positivity except in fantasy which emphatically is not real.

Now, for (3) that masturbation is counterproductive to a fulfilling relationship, helpful is the extreme example of when one masturbates so that one's spouse is rendered either uninteresting or unnecessary — this occurrence usually because of an unresolved fear of the spouse or inability to cope with one's loneliness in a social way. Clearly, masturbation is counterproductive for one's marriage in these circumstances. It *removes desire* and need for the other. It detracts from seeking unitive wholesome maleness/wholesome femaleness together. Indeed, if you want to mess up your interest in your spouse by rendering him or her redundant, then masturbate. If you want to cultivate desire and save your marriage, do not masturbate, but seek each other out by practices which are not lessened by this so-called "benign" self-interest of masturbation.

Such an example holds true for the imperfect other alternatives to sexual intercourse which are essentially "masturbation by other means" (oral, anal, et cetera sex).

People are *used* rather than related to.

While the subjective pleasures are undeniable in terms of (1) the power felt when creating such ecstasy in another and (2) the orgasmic relief itself, this act becomes either an act of a human (subjective biological relief plus a social use of another) or a *human act* (objective moral good with self-fulfillment plus spiritual loving with self-satisfying trust independent of orgasm the latter becoming actually not that important).

That is, the genuineness of one's mutual commitment is linked to the oneness achieved in a mutually fulfilling sharing that which intrinsically entails the naturalness of the action in the highest sense of truth, beauty, and goodness. There exists a nagging quality of mechanicalness, of exploitation, of undignity, of disintegrity, of non-unity, and lack of cohesive identity with one's partner when sexual activity is characterized by masturbation or its equivalents than when by mutual sharing through natural sexual intercourse.

Masturbation is an ultimate test of moral choice, self-discipline, and integrity. To some extent, only you and God know your decisions. But your identity and your image will be known to yourself as integrated in nature's future mode or in a stagnating me-only mode which is known, in spite of many defenses to the contrary, as a violation of your worthy and full participation in life processes.

Masturbation is a defect even if it is pleasurable, common, routine, satisfying, or whatever. As a defect, it diminishes you, all the fantasized "positives" notwithstanding. Masturbation on deeper analysis is an incontrovertible defect as we are incontrovertibly all sinners. However, reality and you are better served by not calling it either normal or good.

Such is a basic defect of original sin: We must insist that what wrongs we do are "right." This applies nowhere intensely as in regard to masturbation (closely followed by abortion and television/movies).

Masturbation's effects on the "other" cannot be overlooked either. For the spouse of a masturbator, it leaves a sense of failure and/or emptiness. That is, there exists an increasing distance between you and your loved one when one of you prefers masturbation to the life-compatible sexual union.

Missing is the marital bonding of "I-am-yours-you-are-mine-we-are-one."

Further missing is the pleasure of mutual desirability, i.e. the profound unitive dimension of two people intensely responding to each other by exhilarating participation in nature's procreative process: Awesome in its life-giving power; holy in its hope; faithful in its truth; loving in its beauty; amusing in its geometry; appeasing the brutal beastliness; intellectually known as good; and confident in the origin of mutual virginity and total commitment giving genuine form to the substance of the marriage — this is never possible for sexual activity outside of marriage or by masturbation in any of its forms.

If the relationship is merely animal. . .okay, but if there is to be a human meeting of minds with uplifting of the person(s), there is little room for anything other than an awareness of the beingness of both parties complying with the natural procreative process of nature which hints at the sensations of Heavenly bliss.

In summary, as an ephemeral developmental-experimental state, masturbation deserves reluctant acceptance but only as a biological exigency rather than a gluttonous self-induced regurgitative-like distortion of normal appetite akin to "eat and vomit," "eat and vomit," "eat and vomit" of ancient Roman orgies.

Similarly, the habit-forming danger existing in the biological-exigency excuse for masturbation, needs preventing because masturbation may become a preferred way of sexual experience of surprising power later, even when one is married.

Fundamentally, masturbation is a negative experience, psychologically disserving the individual and community because it is as against Natural Law as is industrial pollution.

Indeed, if nature is sacred in the broad community sense and demands environmental respect, then nature is sacred in the interpersonal and intrapersonal dimensions also. Natural Law calls for virtue which spans from the broadly environmental to the intensely personal. Such self-discipline cannot be easily garnered for broad issues if it is not expected at the personal level.

The macro- and micro- dimensions of the Roman Catholic Church's Natural and Revealed Laws always are consistent with the Church's moral teachings. This is no less true in all dimensions of human sexuality.

Samuel A. Nigro

ADDENDUM: JACULASIS

(From the Latin *jacul* — "to throw" from which "ejaculation" is derived.)

Jaculasis is a psychosocial disordered state of involuntary emotional repetition-compulsion of ejaculation attempts voluntarily professed to be essential to one's identity.

More specifically, jaculasis is the disorder of unnatural seeking of orgasm which is nothing more than mere neurophysiologic reflex spasms with a feel-good, breath-taking, eye-opening, head-shaking, whole-body exercise charge-up of about ninety seconds duration, who counts. Still, orgasm has no cosmic significance. This kind of reflex also is no big bodily deal either and can be artificially induced in other ways as vomiting in bulemics, gagging in oral sex, and anal stretching in homosexuals' "fisting." Bodies can be tricked into all sorts of spurious "feel-good" states none of which have any significance except as selfishness, social pollution, and simple physical reflex. Because of all this, it rarely if ever is the source of clinically significant distress.

The creation and focusing on a reflex like this is a selfish and self-constricting isolation of a part of the human from his entirety, a violation of one's unity as a total social human being. Such orgasm emphasis fragments humans from themselves, the species itself, the entire animal kingdom and all nature. And *that* is what is wrong with masturbation and its equivalence for *individuals*. But jaculasis applies all this as a social phenomenon to encompass the entire erection-ejaculation-orgasm culture of masturbation, feminism, homosexuality, pornography in all its forms, and the unreal and perverse fantasy, vicarious living and selfish bodily reflex styles of nonbeing presented by press, media and cult overemphasis on sexual feelings, untruths, errors and advertising promotions.

When jaculasis is rampant, created is a dissocial phenomenon. Any society which accepts and promotes masturbation (as jaculasis) is constricting itself to a selfish and perverse track which is anti-evolutionary if not anti-developmental. Indeed, if one accepts masturbation, there is no reason not to do it in whatever way it can be intensified. And that is what happens.

The case can be made that jaculasis (masturbation *uber alles*) especially predisposes and increases the frequency of homosexuality (and now you know why gays, lesbians and feminists are so enthusiastic for their vibrators and sex toys).

As a person matures from pre-adult to sexual maturity, he can come to believe (especially if in a psychosocial depressed or other deficiency state) that the only way to feel good about himself is by orgasm, any kind of orgasm. At such an occurrence, one's personal development fuses sexuality-as-orgasm with the "only" psychosocial good feeling one has. This becomes one's identity and resulting is homosexuality or other paraphilia. Private personal "consent" is still fraudulent because such "consent" is obviously overdetermined and a secondary conditioning rather than a freely chosen stable desideratum.

Jaculasis, therefore, is a public health hazard, because it is a provocative addiction to orgasm by ever newer and ever more gross searching for what can never be found, because sex is neither love nor life-style and orgasm is mere physiologic reflex without substance in being. Period.

Jaculasis is to be recognized and then rejected. Only sporadic isolated developmentally curious masturbation is to be recognized and then as an amusing immature experience to be outgrown.

Samuel A. Nigro

The main criterion for commitment to anything is best determined by the willingness of those in charge of the anything to apply the principles which they propose to themselves. If those in charge of anything make exceptions for themselves, then they are frauds and do not deserve your commitment. In such circumstances, only pretend to go along with them and get out as discretely and quickly as you can.

Samuel A. Nigro

Or tell them to "practice what you preach."

Common speech is not the thing by which men express their emotions; it is only the thing by which they fail to express them.

G.K. Chesterton

. . .war is not the best way of settling differences; it is the only way of preventing their being settled for you.

G.K. Chesterton

Nothing can fail so completely, hopelessly, and finally as that which is solely based on success.

G.K. Chesterton

"Feelings" — and just about everything else, but especially feelings — are unworthy of having power unless sacramentally analyzed and synthesized:

1. By being baptized as a dignified event and giving faith.
2. By being confessed into a unified energy spectrum and giving hope.
3. By being transubstantiated into an integrated field and giving charity.
4. By being confirmed as an identifiable quanta and giving prudence.
5. By being spiritually singular and giving justice.
6. By being in ordered dimensions and giving courage.
7. By accepting the liberty of uncertainty and giving temperance.

By such sacramental living, Grace is obtained with the pursuing-happiness force of Holiness and one is free of all less. . . . This is the full use of one's soul. Neither "feelings" nor anything else should be given any power except by sacramental living!

Samuel A. Nigro

We all know that the worst of using strong language is that it produces weak language.

G.K. Chesterton

An open mind is really a work of foolishness, like an open mouth, mouths and minds were made to shut; they were made to open only to shut.

G.K. Chesterton

A blameless life,
St. Joseph,
May we lead,
by your patronage
from danger freed.

Josephites Everywhere

. . .the most sincere and sensible people were people who earned their own living.

G.K. Chesterton

We should do this everyday of our lives: Number one is laugh. You should laugh everyday. Number two is think. You should spend some time in thought. Number three is, you should have your emotions moved to tears, could be happiness or joy. . . If you laugh, think and cry, that's a full day.

Jim Valvano

Life is not just: How do I feel? It is moreso how do I present in matter, in form, in truth, in oneness, in good, and in beauty.

Samuel A. Nigro

As long as people want or believe what they see on T.V. or read as news, there will be violence.

Samuel A. Nigro

Overachievers, without drugs and orgies, have more fun.

Wallace Stegner

Teenage "love" is an exciting interval of fantasy, exhilarating fantasy, and addictive fantasy which respectively herald:

1. the awareness of sexual differences,
2. the hazards of complete selfishness,
3. the disappointment of dreams-come-true.

If teenagers could only understand all this and correctly place therein that which they are currently undergoing, they may acquire a protective caution such that adulthood is achieved with less physical and mental cost.

Samuel A. Nigro

There are many causes for the failure to comprehend Christ's teaching. . . but the chief cause which has engendered all these misconceptions is this, that Christ's teaching is considered to be such as can be accepted, or not, without changing one's life.

Leo Tolstoy

Our Savior came to save and not to destroy the lives of men; to give and plant peace among men; and if in any sense He may be said to send war, it is the Holy War indeed, for it is against the Devil, and not the persons of men. Of all His titles this seems the most glorious as well as comfortable for us that He is the Prince of Peace. It is His nature, His office, His work and the end and excellent blessing of His coming who is both the maker and preserver of our peace with God. And it is remarkable that in all the New Testament He is but once called Lion, but frequently the Lamb of God, and that those who desire to be the disciples of His cross and Kingdom, for they are inseparable, must be like him as St. Paul, and St. John tell us. Nor is it said that the Lamb shall lie down with the Lion, but the Lion shall lie down with the Lamb. That is: War shall yield to Peace, and the soldier turn hermit.

William Penn

Ask not what your age wants but what it needs. . .not what it will reward but what about which it cannot be saved. And then go and do it. Do it well. Do it thoroughly and find your reward in the consciousness of having done your duty and above all in the reflection that you have been accounted worthy to suffer something for Christ.

Orestes Brownson

Teen sex life is full of lies.

Pregnant teenager

A good-mood is self-fulfilling.

Samuel A. Nigro

The world is run by human action, not by human design.

Name Lost

It doesn't make any difference what we become when we grow up. We will still be treated like children.

An eastern German teenager in 1984 before the collapse of Communism and Socialism

Why study when my brilliant questions baffle the instructor?

Dick Larmer

Don't be discouraged because you're discouraged.

St. Francis de Sales

Real men use their brains. . . .

Name Lost

Act on your thinking, not on your feelings. You can only act on your feelings after you have *thought* them out.

Samuel A. Nigro

I've got my faults but living in the past isn't one of them. There's no future in it.

Sparky Anderson

I enjoy TV trash as much as the next slob. But the quality of truly trashy trash has declined.

Mike Royko

Take time to THINK
It is the source of power.
Take time to PLAY. . .
It is the secret of perpetual youth.
Take time to READ. . .
It is the fountain of wisdom,
Take time to PRAY. . .
It is the greatest power on earth.
Take time to LOVE AND
BE LOVED. . .
It is a God-given privilege
Take time to LAUGH. . .
It is the music of the soul.
Take time to GIVE. . .
It is too short a day to be selfish.
Take time to WORK. . .
It is the price of success.
Take time to DO CHARITY. . .
It is the key to heaven.

Name Lost

Never marry a feminist. She will ruin your boys and you won't find out about it until it is too late.

Name Lost

Don't like trees. . .they hem you in.

North Dakota farmer

Drinking alot of beer is really stupid. After spending all that money, all you end up with is a bucket of pee.

Name Lost

These are five intellectual virtues:
1) Wisdom — right reason of final causes.
2) Science — right reason of matter known.
3) Art — right reason of things made.
4) Understanding — right reason of habitual principles.
5) Prudence — right reason of things to be done.

St. Thomas Aquinas

What do you mean you're bored? The world will not entertain you. You have to find things to do for yourself. You have to entertain yourself. Go find something to do and stay out of trouble. We have no money. Entertain yourself.

Mom

. . .the matching of emotion with emotion. . .is not the essence of rational thought.

Sir Fred Hoyle

It is better to be a grave digger than an actor.

Edward Liu

(Actors and celebrities are fakes.)

I like a man who just doesn't get it.

Florence King

"Have a *courteous* time" and it will be a nice time.

Mom

God's best-answered prayers are sometimes our unanswered prayers.

Tanya Nero

Don't let anyone make a monkey out of you — think!

Dad

The day you no longer burn with love, many others will die of the cold.

St. Bonaventure

". . .erotic activity between males" is to be abolished "altogether."

Plato's Laws (841D to 842A, Thomas Pangle, translator)

The older you get, the dumber you get.

Dad (said every six months from age 12-20)

Hard work isn't easy.

Ara Parseghian

The difference between man and woman accounts for almost everything important that has happened. We must realize that when we try to make man and woman alike.

G.K. Chesterton

Easy come; easy go; so save your money! And never tell anybody how much you have and where you're keeping it.

Dad

Any group that must turn it's leadership over to women has ruined its men.

Name Lost

If you do not get up on time, clean yourself up, brush your teeth, make your bed and pick up your room, you cannot have a perfect day.

Samuel A. Nigro

Everyone has heard of racism, sexism, etc. Few have heard of *bookism* which is the anti-intellectual, anti-book approach to learning of many juveniles, especially boys, who seem to need to go around parading how tough they are by being ignorant.

Samuel A. Nigro

There are two things in which all men are manifestly unmistakably equal. All men are tragic. All men are comic.

G.K. Chesterton

It is not the name you call me that matters, only the name to which I respond.

Rabbi Hillel

The least masculine of vices is the admiration of brutality.

G.K. Chesterton

Are you unwilling to be anointed with the oil of God? It is on this account that we are called Christians: because we are anointed with the oil of God.

Theophilus of Antioch, C.A.D. 181

It is necessary for him that has been baptized also to be anointed, so that by his having received chrism, that is, the anointing, he can be the anointed of God and have in him the grace of Christ.

Cyprian, 254-255 A.D.

If men don't dominate as husbands and providers, then they form violent gangs and dominate as thugs and muggers and drug lords.

George Gilder

Nothing happens when nothing happens.

John F. Lewis

If you want to be the best at something, you've got to invent it.

Tom LaGarde

If you can't change your mind, then you are old before you are old.

Evelyn Nigro

Be good and you will have a jolly time; but you will not be happy. Fortunately, being happy is not so important as having a jolly time.

G.K. Chesterton

This argument business is the best fun in life.

G.K. Chesterton

A fan always sees the game *his* way.

Name Lost

Fatigue makes cowards of us all.

Paul Brown

One recognizes three types in three situations: the humble in anger, the hero in battle, and the friend in time of need. If you want to be friends with someone, first find out what company he keeps. If you speak at night, lower your voice; if you speak during the day look about and take care even though there is a wall behind you; if your foot stumbles, then one can mend the damage, but if your tongue stumbles, then death may be the consequence.

From the *Book of the Pius*

What good will it do you to have fellow citizens without conscience?

Moses Mendelssohn

To get their "act together," kids must first fall flat on their faces. The fall is either orchestrated by fine parenting teaching the child a lesson or self-inflicted by immature, learning-the-hard-way.

Samuel A. Nigro

The girls have the eggs and the boys have everything else.

Retarded adult woman on sex education

(Education is) the period during which I was being instructed by somebody I did not know, about something I did not want to know.

G.K. Chesterton

Reading maketh a full man, conference a ready man, and writing an exact man.

G.K. Chesterton

If there is anything that is serious, it is fun.

G.K. Chesterton

A feminist is weak, imitative, and dependant, for she repeats stale catchwords and lives on infectious emotion, but a woman almost always thinks for herself.

G.K. Chesterton

Music:
Melody is for the mind (enhances thinking).
Harmony is for the heart (soothes feelings).
Rhythm is for the rump (wiggles your butt).

Samuel A. Nigro

If you don't act like you believe, you soon believe like you act.

Bishop Fulton Sheen

What shall it profit a man if he has faith, but has not works? Shall faith be able to save him? . . .You believe that there is one God. You do well. But the devils also believe and tremble. But will you know, vain man, that faith without works is dead. . . . By works a man is justified and not by faith only. Even as the body without the spirit is dead, so also faith without works is dead.

James 2:14, 19, 20, 26

Being "nice" does not work. One must be transcendental!

Samuel A. Nigro

Work incarnates our prayer and expresses our love.

Cistercian Motto

If you do not keep a notebook and schedule as to what you're supposed to do and where you're supposed to be, you just may miss the train to heaven.

Name Lost

Self-esteem that depends on lies is itself a lie. Self-esteem depends on self-understanding which is *humility*.

Samuel A. Nigro

We should thank God for sex and everything else by not misusing or abusing it or anything else.

Samuel A. Nigro

In August 1943, the U.S. Army contained 31% Catholics; the Navy about 40%; and the Marines were over 50% — all this when the population of Catholics in the United States was barely 18%. For the Vietnam War, Catholics were 28% of all casualties — 35% if blacks were excluded, and

Catholics at the time were less than 25% of the population. Of course, Catholics should be good patriots for their country, but there is something wrong when they serve disproportionate to their numbers in whatever conflict.

Samuel A. Nigro

Reading is power. Real power. No one can take it away from you.

Name Lost

History is the greatest of all works of the imagination.

G.K. Chesterton

Misunderstanding always does harm.

G.K. Chesterton

Brother Fire, God made you beautiful and strong and useful; I pray you be courteous with me.

St. Francis of Assisi to burning coals as he was about to be tortured by Muslims

Ever notice how most really happy and well-off people are essentially traditionally-valued people?

Name Lost

Heresy always sets the mood against the mind. . .and the mood turns into a monomania.

G.K. Chesterton

Only mankind would abuse and pollute the planet by turning the marvelous, secretive, astounding, creative process of Nature into undignified recreation.

Samuel A. Nigro

It will be a typical Browns-Bengals game.

Otto Graham just before Browns-Bengals second-ever game

You can *feel* all you want. Feelings just are; they are neither right nor wrong. It is what you do with your feelings that counts. And feelings are notorious liars. . . . It is better to think.

Name Lost

It's just that I never shoot a deer until he pulls a knife on me first.

Grantland Rice on hunting

Open your eyes. Open your ears. Open your heart. Open your mind. But keep your big mouth shut. That is the best way to learn things.

Dad

If choice is not a transcendental phenomenon, then it is not a choice at all but more of a conditioned reflex.

Samuel A. Nigro

Induction only leads to a deduction. . . In this world, there is nothing but a syllogism — and a fallacy. . . . There is an IS.

G.K. Chesterton

To say that an atheist has a message is a contradiction in terms.

G.K. Chesterton

When society decrees that manhood or maturity is dependent upon ejaculation frequency, what other can be expected but obsessional, compulsive, addictive sexualness?

Samuel A. Nigro

Feelings are liars, so do not do what they tell you to do unless you have reasoned it out.

Name Lost

When one of your *characteristics* (rather than your *character* itself) becomes a way of getting something or manipulating another, then you are not only unfair but dishonest.

Samuel A. Nigro

You are only happy if you have found your soul.

Name Lost

To prove their believability, all talk show hosts and newscasters should perform their programs buck naked.

Ron Crocker

The more you study, the less free you become to know error.

Fulton Sheen

No machine can make your life better; it can only make you weaker and dependent; there is nothing of value that can be done for you, because it must all be done by you.

Thomas Fleming

If sexual, then every trembling hand could make us squeak, like dolls, the wished-for words.

Wallace Stevens

If you're not ready for babies, you're not ready for sex.

Janet Smith

. . .if you're dependent on people who do not know you, who control the value of your necessities, you are not free, and you are not safe.

Wendell Berry

Only a baby has the right to be understood without words. . .not a grown man or woman. . . . Adults must communicate.

Helen Trobisch

There are some desires that are not desirable.

G.K. Chesterton

. . .*the black hole*, an emotional quagmire characterized by an inner deadness — an inability to feel or express feelings — and overwhelming sense of powerlessness. . . . There is only one way out of the black hole, and that is through matching inner feelings with outer expression. When a man correctly matches feeling with behavior, he reconnects with his natural energy flow.

Joe Nicolosi

A warrior walks between terror and wonder.

Carlos Costenada

Purity is the only atmosphere for passion.

G.K. Chesterton

. . .we bless your simplicity but do not envy your folly.

Athenian response to Mellians' hope for help from others

The trouble with people is they run out of things to do.

Betty Howard

Today is a memory for tomorrow.

Karen Keily Debitetto

I'm not a hero because I did not choose to be in that position. A hero chooses to be put in a position in order to do right. If I had my choice, I would not have been there. I am not a hero.

Captain Al Hanes, airplane pilot after landing a commercial airliner under the direst of conditions

Avoid foolish and ignorant debates for you know that they breed quarrels. But a slave of the Lord must not quarrel, but should be gentle towards all, ready to teach, patient, gently correcting opponents with kindness. It may be that God will grant them repentance that leads to knowledge of the truth that they may return to their senses out of the devil's snare where they are entrapped by him for his will.

2 Timothy 2:23

When you give a bad dog a good name, he'll live up to it, and if you give a good dog a bad name, he'll live down to it.

William Most

Seriousness is idolatry.

G.K. Chesterton

Everything, however noble, that has shape has limitation.

G.K. Chesterton

Nothing is quite as annoying as someone continuing to talk when you are interrupting.

Name Lost

We should pray *what should be, will be.*

Tolkien

An Italian psychiatrist, R. Assagioli — one of the founders of a spiritual branch of psychotherapy — mentions numerous famous artists and scientists who lived chaste lives, and even gives direct examples of how the sexual passion was transformed into spiritual creativity with the result of beautiful opuses being born (the history of R. Wagner's opera *Tristan and Isolde*). As the areas of human relations can equally be considered as one of the most subtle spheres of spiritual and psychological creativity, the sexual energy, not wasted in the lustful and selfish sexual relations, can be a large power in the successful building of marital communion. This transformation is a fruit of conjugal chastity, which includes both: the periodic abstinence at certain times and the "channeling" of sexual desires into self-giving love in the conjugal intimacy. See *Psychosynthesis* by Roberto Assagioli, Hobs, Dorman & Co., Inc., New York, 1965, p. 274.

Gintautas Vaitoska

I have nothing to offer you but beers, boils, sweat and mud.

Winston Churchill at Woodstock supposedly

All females in the animal kingdom reserve sexual activity for reproduction purposes except human females! And the more females deviate from this planetary norm, the more they are out of synchrony with environment and nature. It is no wonder that psychosocial progression suddenly goes backward instead of forward when humans reject nature by contorting sexuality from its natural reproductive mode.

Samuel A. Nigro

Very few people make it without working very, very hard. And if they didn't work hard to get it, they still must work hard to keep it.

Samuel A. Nigro

Politeness is only the Greek for citizenship.

G.K. Chesterton

The inability to keep ideas separate from emotions or impulses is a major violation of the thinking of Western Civilization and is the major source of social tension.

Samuel A. Nigro

Courage is fear to say prayers and keep on moving. . .is the ability to focus on opportunity in the face of danger, to take disabilities and turn them into possibilities. . .to turn scars into stars.

Max Cleland

Well, kids when you reach your limits, there is only one place to go — beyond your limits.

Antoinette Bosco

Russia freed its slaves almost the same time that the United States did — so what happened to the Russian ex-slaves?

Name Lost

There are first of all *Wishbones* — those who wish somebody would do something about their problem. There are *Jawbones* — those who talk but do nothing else. There are *Knucklebones* — those who knock everything. And then there are *Backbones* — those who carry the load and do the work. Which are you?

sign in a senior center

The learners themselves do not know what is learned to advantage until the knowledge which is the result of learning has found a place in the soul of each.

Plato

I do not carve a statue out of marble; I release the form that is within.

Michelangelo

I can pay for almost anything you want except for wasted time. Once you waste time, you can never get it back.

Dad

When I grow up, I want to be a little boy.

Joseph Heller

Those who go about in masks are low persons.

Galileo

The fool changeth like the moon. . . . The wise man continueth as the sun. . . ."

Ecclesiastics 27:11 (as quoted by St. Bernard)

Woe unto us "whose soul is in our nostrils" (Isaiah 2:22)! Woe unto us who imitate the fool that "uttereth all his mind" (Proverbs 29:2)!
Woe unto us
Whose words flow out as unrestrained
As water through a sieve.

St. Bernard

The girl with a simple, unspoiled nature like Gwendolyn could hardly be expected to reside in the country.

Ernest

Life is short, the Art is long, occasion sudden, experience fallible, and judgment difficult. Not only must a physician show himself prepared to do what is needed, but he must make the patient, the attendants and the surrounding circumstances cooperate with him.

Hippocrates

Whatever occurring in the world, problems devolve to the failure to contemplate rationally and in the inability to accept criticism.

Samuel A. Nigro

There is no one more illiberal than a liberal whose feelings have been hurt.

Samuel A. Nigro

Chastity is the flowering of man and from it flows genius, heroism and holiness. . . . When that channel of purity is open, man flows it over to God.

Henry Thoreau

I do supportive psychotherapy for a few minutes on myself as I look in the mirror every morning.

Psychiatrist answering the question: "How do you keep sane working with all the disturbed people?"

Keep your bowels open. . .especially when you're traveling. . . .

Dad

There are some actions and emotions whose very names connote baseness, e.g. spite, shamelessness, envy; and among actions adultery, theft and murder. These and similar emotions and actions imply by their very names that they are bad. . . . It is, therefore, impossible ever to do right in performing them; to perform them is always wrong.

Aristotle

"Equality" is a will-o-the-wisp. It is almost an internal contradiction. People demanding it usually want some special treatment which in no way can be called "equality." Like "competence" and "freedom," *Equality* is not an absolute *but must be qualified*. For example: Competent to run a car and a house versus competent to fly a plane and manage General Motors? Freedom to speak, to beat one's child, or to defecate in public? Equality in sweetness or muscle? In math or cooking? In sexual response onset or duration? In ability or opportunity? Equality does not occur within any one group much less between the sexes.

Equality can be a destructive force when it becomes in one's mind what cannot be obtained in reality unless another holds back for the sake of the other. That is: "*Out of consideration* for the other, I(we) will do(not do) , so the other will be(feel) equal." Now, there is nothing wrong with this paradigm, in fact, it is done all the time. But it should not be called "equality" because it isn't! It is actually a double standard where, usually in sex equality efforts, men hold back and women plunge on (as long as men hold back).

Truly, for equality to be a fact, women must appeal to men to let it happen. Women, professing feelings or a right to be all they can be, must ask or require men to be less than what men can be. Again, there is nothing wrong with this, but it is closer to "intimidation" or "chivalry" than to "equality" regardless of raging or whimpering womankind. Subordination in nature occurs in all things. It is a self-entrapment to call it "inferiority" and carry on like a damn fool. In fact, Malcolm Muggeridge put it succinctly: ". . .all claims to equality (social, economic, racial, intellectual, sexual). . .intensify inequality."

Samuel A. Nigro

Equality applies to process not outcome. Or more precisely, equality applies to the opportunity to process. Equality applies to the opportunity to "be yourself." You can have equal opportunity to do your ultimate best in anything. . . that it may surpass others is too bad. Equality means you have equal opportunity to use your abilities. Equality does not mean you hold back so someone else can be or do the same as you.

Samuel A. Nigro

And there are the morbid states that are the result of habit, like pulling out hairs and nail biting, or eating coal and the earth, and male homosexuality, because, although these come naturally to some people, others acquire them from habit, e.g. those who have been victimized since childhood.

Aristotle

There are three sides to every argument: your side, the other side, and the truth.

Name Lost

If you don't take care of things, you should not have them. . .and after a while you will not have them.

Evelyn Nigro

Always carry something to write down ideas because that one idea may, if not forgotten, change mankind for the better.

Name Lost

There is no better test of a man's ultimate chivalry and integrity than how he behaves when he is wrong.

G.K. Chesterton

The first three rules for young drivers are: 1) Check the brakes, 2) Check the hazard lights, and 3) go in the right direction.

Dad

The only time one is "just existing" is when one is not acting transcendentally.

Samuel A. Nigro

I pray not to change God but to change me.

C.S. Lewis

We read to make sure we are not alone.

Name Lost

What becomes obvious to those of us treating children through adulthood is that those who do not control themselves sexually before marriage, cannot control themselves after marriage. Essentially, premarital and extra-marital sex can remove the capacity for sustainable, committed relationships. Premarital and extra-marital sex are incompatible with genuine love during the developmental years. Later, happy marriages are not forthcoming nor are happy single lives. The result is a failure of traditional family life, resulting in overwhelming numbers of intense psychological problems. This is not insignificant as any society discovers when it trivializes sexuality and demeans sexual differences by promoting "equality" because of detrimental effects on the family.

Samuel A. Nigro

What are we to do? Keep our tempers, primarily. And after that, look the situation in the face, and think.

G.K. Chesterton

There is no smaller package in the world than a man wrapped up in himself.

George Ruttler

Make haste slowly.

Boileau

In the battle that goes on for life,
I ask for a field that is fair
A chance that is equal with all in strife
The courage to do and to dare.

If I should win, let it be by the code
My faith and my honor held high
If I should lose, let me stand by the road,
And cheer as the winner rides by.

Knute Rockne

You grow up when you stop taking things for granted.

Name Lost

How do you tell an infield fly rule from a ground rule double?

Rachel Nigro Scalish

Much has been made of dreams in human history. However, the only times dreams have real relevance is when they are natural and at one with the transcendentals, which generally excludes any sort of dreaming which has occurred since the appearance of electronic video denatured phenomena.

Samuel A. Nigro

Learn to hustle; your life depends on it.

Name Lost

A real human being in concert with the earth will operate by virtues and transcendentals rather than by feelings.

Samuel A. Nigro

DRIVING

Brakes! Brakes! Look out for that guy. Keep your distance. Stay in your lane. Watch that curb. Don't tailgate. A disaster is always a half a second away. Stay alert. If you are confused or lost, put your hazard lights on. If you see an accident or a rushing emergency vehicle, put your hazard lights on. . . . Always use your hazards if confused. You won't get any tickets if you use your hazards either. Clutch! Clutch! Nobody gets mad at you with your hazard lights on. Look out for the jackasses. If someone is tailgating you put your hazards on and pull over; let the jackasses pass. Anyone who does one crazy thing will do another so stay away — they may even have a gun. You can run over little animals but watch out for deer. Gas! Gas! You need gas or you'll stall. Police will ticket you for that. . . . They'll let an old coot like me go but they'll ticket you. You see someone driving like that, remember people are allowed to be stupid. When a stupid jackass makes you mad, don't give him the finger; make the sign of the Cross and pray for him. If what they are doing is illegal, get their license number and make a note of it for the record — but if what they are doing is just stupid, they have a right to be stupid — stay away. You're going too fast. Give yourself plenty of time so you won't have to rush. Give yourself a head start so you can compensate for any delay. What's the problem? Why are you going so slow? Gas! Gas! You're a great driver — you haven't missed a pothole yet. Avoid having an accident even if you are absolutely right. . . . Always avoid accidents. . . . Let the other guy win because you win too. . . . Accidents are no fun even if you were in the right! Stop for three seconds and look both ways; left, right, left, right, left for stop signs. Your head is a radar beacon continually taking in all around you. One car length for every ten miles per hour. What is the rush to a red light? You're too close. You're too damn close. No margin for error. Don't be a jackass. If you are being courteous to some car you see in front of you, be certain you are not discourteous to ten cars behind you. Look ahead — way ahead — you can see the problems down the road. Keep your eyes on the road. Watch out for wet leaves — they are slippery. Look out for parked cars, the doors open fast. Pedestrians and bicycles have the right of way. Give old people a break. Every car should have three horns: a courtesy horn, a worry horn and an angry horn. . . . Since nobody has those, you have to know how to honk your message. Watch that curb! Truckers rarely give you a break. . . . Bastards. Keep your gas tank full. Hit the hazard lights! Trees will not move out of your way. If you run out of gas once you never will again. Always be courteous, especially to cops. What's the hurry? What's the hurry? Are you in a race? Clutch! Clutch!

Jonathan Nigro reciting all that his father told him when learning to drive

The things we need most for immediate practical purposes are abstractions.

G.K. Chesterton

The classes that watch most are those that work least.

G.K. Chesterton

Even if you are on the right track, you get run over if you just sit there.

Will Rogers

Boredom means you are not thinking of your soul.

Samuel A. Nigro

We should not fear the truth about ourselves.

John Paul II

The question is just what kind of life is examined and is worth living, regardless of all reasons and feelings. Considering all of one's being, just what kind of life is best? And what kind of life is best not only for you but for everyone, the world, the universe?

Name Lost

Words changed their ordinary meanings and were construed in new senses. Reckless daring passed for the courage of a loyal partisan, far-sighted hesitation was the excuse of a coward, moderation was the pretext of the unmanly, the power to see all sides of a question was complete inability to act. Impulsive rashness was held the mark of a man, caution and conspiracy was specious excuse for avoiding action.

Thucydides

Laughter has been from the beginning the one indestructible brotherhood.

G.K. Chesterton

Autonomy as self-sufficiency in true isolation from all others is a denial of a common humanity.

Peter Riga

Having fun just doesn't merely happen. Things have to be planned ordinarily. Sometimes luck is part of it — but usually you even have to *work* to have a good time.

Name Lost

What's purple and crawls? A wounded grape!
What's purple and goes slam, slam and slam? A four door grape!
Close your eyes tightly and count to ten.
Dark, isn't it?

Sylvian Smith

Four ducks were swimming in a row and one said "I'm not going any further." Which one said it? Don't be silly, ducks can't talk.

Sylvian Smith

A smart person, even if dumb, will pretend he is smart!

Samuel A. Nigro

A woman is only a woman, but a good cigar is a smoke.

early 1900 cigar advertisement

Trust in truth is the highest form of bravery.

Adam in *Paradise Lost*

I shall console myself with the reflection. . .that they who are ever taking aim make no hits; that they who never venture, never gain; that to be ever safe, is to be ever feeble; and that to do some substantial good, is to compensate for much incidental imperfection.

Cardinal Newman

While growing up, one must experience what he thinks is love about 100 times before he really knows what it is all about. . .which is why one cannot trust one's early infatuations because they only seem to be love.

Samuel A. Nigro

A true knight errant he and will wander in wild adventures trusting the prowess of his single arm while the weighty affairs of his kingdom slumber and his own safety is endangered.

description of King Richard in *Ivanhoe*

. . .Pious, proud, noble and generous.

description of Rowena in *Ivanhoe*

A dose like that within your guts, my boy, and every other wench is Helen of Troy.

Mephistopheles

Angels are quanta affirming spatial identities. In considering the giving and taking of energy, more prudence comes from considering the angels.

Samuel A. Nigro

My eloquence should capture every heart since prompting is the devil's special art.

Mephistopheles

Impartiality is a pompous name for indifference, which is an elegant name for ignorance.

G.K. Chesterton

Where there is no sense, there is no feeling.

Charles C. Nigro

When all the extraneous blather is stripped away, discovered is that contemporary liberals really do not care about objective data but that they can have the subjective feeling of doing good by pretending to care for others. The subjective feeling compels them to believe they are correct even though it will fly in the face of objective data derived from tradition, theory and outcome.

Samuel A. Nigro

The enemy knows the shape of your back and has never seen the color of your eyes.

A "coward" according to Huron Indians

A liberal is a person who has not the forthrightness to speak against what he knows is wrong finding more self-inflation by pretending to be accepting of everything. In other words, tolerance before courage.

Samuel A. Nigro

Okay, but first take off all your clothes, and run from my house all the way downtown and back stark naked, and I am yours.

What every woman should tell a guy who wants to have sex with her before marriage

If respectable people know what harm sensational stories did, they have no right to put poison in the sugarplums and let the small ones eat it.

Mrs. March

Dreams have value in direct proportion to the universal flow of nature within. Dream validity therefore has been destroyed because of the impact of television, movies and communications technology all of which are artificial and not at one with nature's flow. This contemporary deformation of dreams accounts for the loss of importance and helpfulness of dreams in modern times. Contemporary dreams are not at one with nature but contaminated with artificial schema creating worthlessness or irrelevancy.

Samuel A. Nigro

Early to bed, early to rise, makes a man healthy, wealthy and wise.

old proverb

We cannot escape our loneliness by throwing ourself into the bodies of those we desire. We cannot cling to the false sense of ecstasy that we feel during orgasm. Sexual desire ought not be the center of our dreams, the path to consolation. That is love's domain.

Love is the consequence of our deep commitment to the possibilities in others. Love is creation, trusting the future, the embracing of another human being in the belief that this embrace will produce something new and good. Desire ends in satisfaction. Love begins in commitment, leads to making love, and grows in the sounds of children laughing in the kitchen, blowing into a trumpet, giggling next to a father. That is what sex is all about.

Christopher de Vinck

Both. . .and sometimes a lot of other names that I don't say.

Coach Mike Fratello when asked if his Cleveland Cavaliers basketball team call him "Mike" or "Mr. Fratello"

Small reason was there to doubt them, but ever since that almost fatal encounter Ahab had cherished a wild vindictiveness against the whale. All the more fell for that in his frantic morbidness, he at last came to identify with him not only all his bodily woes, but all his intellectual and spiritual exasperations. The white whale swam before him as the monomaniac incarnation of all those malicious agencies which some deep men billeted in them so they are left living on with half a heart and half a lung. That intangible malignity which has been from the beginning at that most maddens and torments. All that stirs up the less of things. All truth with malice in it. All that cracks the sinews and cakes the brain. All the subtle demonisms of life and thought. All evil to crazy Ahab were visibly personified in Moby Dick. He piled upon the whale's white hump the sum of all the general rage and hate felt by his whole race from Adam down. And then, as if his chest had been a mortar, he burst his hot heart shell upon it. It is not probable that this monomania in him took its instant rise at the precise time of his bodily dismemberment. Then, in darting at the monster, knife in hand, he had but given loose to a sudden, passionate, corporeal animosity. When he received the stroke that tore him, he probably but felt the agonizing bodily laceration but nothing more. Yet, when by this collision forced to turn towards home. And for long months of days and weeks Ahab and anguish lay stretched together in one hammock, then it was that his torn body and gashed soul bled into one another and so interfusing made him mad.

Ishmal

The saddest spectacle imaginable to us is an anxious youth endeavoring to like only what the current intellectual mode approves.

Isabel Paterson

It is only through those actions which meet praise that a man may prosper.

Beowulf

Listen, my girl, your paycheck is your mother and your father; in other words, respect it.

Muriel Wells Hall

I, too, will have rules about sexuality when my children become teenagers:

Rule number one: Learn who you are.

Rule number two: Try as best you can to be patient.

Rule number three: Understand that you will never escape that small feeling of loneliness.

Rule number four: Understand that someone is out there waiting to fall in love with you.

Rule number five: Understand that you will find this person and be in love too.

Rule number six: Date as many people as you can.

Rule number seven: Understand that you are the only one who has to figure out how to handle your own sexuality.

Rule number eight: Understand that there are people who will try to turn everything that is beautiful into something ugly, including sex and the human body.

Rule number nine: Make love to the person you fall in love with.

Rule number ten: If you do not know who you are, you cannot possibly abide by rule number nine.

Rule number eleven: Remember that when your great-grandfather died, your great-grandmother clipped a lock of his hair and kept it in a small pouch around her neck, and she sang church songs all alone at night in her living room for ten years until she, too, died, a happy woman.

Christopher de Vinck

Natural law is that part of eternal law that resides in human nature. It is a subdivision of the eternal law which is God's rule for governing the universe. It contains three portions.

A. "Do good and avoid evil."

B. Precepts of:

(1) To persevere in one's own being, i.e. conserve one's own life.

(2) To accept and exercise biological functions.

(3) To seek good according to ascending reason — to seek truth, unity, mutuality, understanding and knowledge, and not to injure.

C. Human laws which aim at prescribing particular acts which natural law imposes for the common good. These basically are precepts bridging the gap between *deeds* and A and B.

Samuel A. Nigro

When one fantasy confronts another fantasy and when one set of facts confronts another set of facts, the only resolution can be by transcendental distinctions, remembering the saints, and embracing the angels as the ancients made sacrifices to their gods.

Name Lost

Ideas precede accomplishment.

Isabel Paterson

I'm a pansy for the jigs.

Jack Teagarden

It is only shallow people who do not judge from appearances.

Oscar Wilde

Hiya, man!

Louis Armstrong

Angels are the best ancient secret you were ever too embarrassed to use. They are better than the sheer, flickering nonsense on television or in movies. They are better than those mugging, intense actors that you see in the celluloid culture who are really nothing but pretend. If one can believe that any flickering light nonsense on television or in movies has anymore credibility than their good acting, one then can certainly believe in angels and their intervention. At least angels have a track record while television and movies are nothing but people pretending and evoking an emotional response which is disproportionate and certainly unjustified by the actors regardless of what they are pretending. Truly, the contemporary celluloid and flickering light culture is a fraud unworthy of impact and basically ineffective because it is fundamentally unreal. In contrast, angels will have an impact but only if one knows about them and invokes their energies.

Samuel A. Nigro

LOGICAL FALLACIES

Argumentum

Ad rem — arguing to the point. This is the way one is supposed to argue.

Ad hominem — arguing to the man. "How can you believe anybody like that?"

Ad ignorantiam — arguing to the ignorance. "Since no one knows, listen to me."

Ad populum — arguing to the people. Let's vote to determine what is true.

Ad captandum vulgus — arguing to the emotions of the crowd. "Who cares. . . crucify him!"

Ad individuum — arguing to the prejudice. "No white gal can teach black studies."

Ad misericordiam — arguing to sympathy. "Because they were victims, they are always right."

Ad hirsuitiam — arguing to the beard. "There are so many hairs to split, it must be the way I say it is."

Ad pulvinar — arguing to the couch. "I can read his mind — this is what he was thinking."

Ad auctoritate — arguing to the power. "Force makes it true."

Ad verecundiam — arguing to the hiding. "Well, so-and-so said this. . ."

Ad conquistador — arguing to the cruel. "Since you hurt my feelings, you brute, this is how it is."

Reductio ad absurdum — Extending analogies to absurdity.

Petitio principii — Begging the question — conclusion is already in the opening premise.

Shifting the burden of proof — "I assert this so prove me wrong."

Chronological snobbery — "It is old, therefore it is wrong."

Cliche thinking — Confuses distinctions.

False antithesis — All or none. . .no "in between" the extremes.

Hypothesis as fact

Post hoc ego propter hoc — "After this, therefore because of this."

Special pleading — Stack the deck with what is favorable only.

Straw man — Misrepresent the opponent's position.

Non-sequitur — That which does not follow — all fallacies are these.
Sweeping generalizations — "Everyone knows. . ."
Ipsedixit — "I have spoken!"

MINORITY OF ONE(!)

Being your own man even if it means preventing a unanimous decision:

— The answer is ____, sir.
— I can't help it, that is the way it is and the answer is ____.
— I always disagree darn it, I call them as I see them sir.
— That's the way I see them and that's the way they see them.
— I would follow my own view, though part of my reason would tell me that I might be wrong.
— You're probably right, but you may be wrong!
— I don't care if everybody says it, the answer is ____.
— You are pressing me to say something that I don't see or believe that way.
— Why do you want me to agree with something that just isn't so?

  the responses of individuals who maintained a minority-of-one as they resisted intense group pressure to modify and distort their judgment by going along with the group to agree with something they knew was wrong. One should know that they did this with frequent shrugging of shoulders, grinning embarrassedly, and by whispering their answers with great insecurity. These were sham experiences wherein everyone was in on the trick except the one being pressed to change his mind. Hundreds were manipulated into changing their minds. Only a few resisted the intense pressure. The above is how they did it.

People will allow anything to happen if the ideals to which they are motivated do not have transcendental aims. Every atrocity in human history has had as a pretext the benefit of some who will stand by. Moses killed thousands. Nero did it for sport. Cromwell ordered the massacre one time of over 30,000 people including infants in arms. Peter the Great was barbarous. Pol Pot, the Pharaohs, Hitler, Stalin, the Reign of Terror, commercialized slavery, the treatment of non-believers by Islam, and today: abortion. All atrocities and mass killings are always done to "benefit" a greater number.

Samuel A. Nigro

Most people are heartless about turtles because a turtle's heart will beat for hours after he's been cut up and butchered. . . I have such a heart too.

Santiago

Every stuffed shirt conceals a quaking heart.

Name Lost

Those genuinely free have chosen something greater than the mere following of their impulses. Indeed, the following of one's impulse is the ultimate conformity and is not freedom at all. True freedom is the choosing of Orthodoxy.

Samuel A. Nigro

The only moral superiority I claim is that of not defending the indefensible.

G.K. Chesterton

I myself cringe before (four-letter words) because of the contempt and hatred they express and their involving the perversion of the act of creation. To use such a word is to drag the sacred and the beautiful into the mire. . . . There can even be said to be an element of demonic in it.

Dorothy Day

In God's name, I beg of you to think.

Demosthenes

Feminism is a woman's contempt for herself.

Name Lost

Inequality is based on the inability to grasp virtue.

Name Lost

Feminism is women's self-deconstruction effort.

Name Lost

Never believe pro-abortion or pro-choice people about birth control unless you want to get pregnant. That is how they make their money.

Samuel A. Nigro

Happiness is a property of the soul, not the body.

Plotinus

What is your doctrine on the Destiny of Man?

Name Lost

The first question to ask anybody in an intellectual discussion.

I saw you shoot that light out. . . can you shoot it back on again?

Name Lost

I saw you kill that baby duck. . . if you were really strong, you could make it live again.

Name Lost

Youth is never a good judge of what is new.

Name Lost

If private feelings are private and no one else's business, why do some insist on telling us what our private feelings ought to be.

Name Lost

Sacraments keep one from politicizing. . . . Sacraments set one above it all.

Samuel A. Nigro

Some guys will treat girls like cigarettes — use them until they're almost nothing but ashes and then throw them away.

Samuel A. Nigro

Contemporary women's fashion is basically for a woman to dress as close as she can be to being naked without being naked.

Samuel A. Nigro

Since no one can dispense me from what I view as the danger to the health of my soul that this gang (the Nazi's) presents, I cannot change my decision. . . . If so many terrible things are permitted by this terrible gang, I believe it is better to sacrifice one's life right away than to place one's self in the grave danger of committing sin and then dying.

Franz Jagerstatter

The joy of a hypocrite lasts but an instant.

John Gerard

And having fulfilled the days, when they returned, the Child Jesus remained in Jerusalem; and His parents knew it not. And thinking that He was in the company, they came a day's journey; and sought Him among their kinfolks and acquaintances. And not finding Him, they returned to Jerusalem seeking Him.

Luke 2:43-45
(having a teenager)

I sought Him Whom my soul loveth; I sought Him and found Him not. I will rise and go about the city; in the streets and broadways will I seek Him Whom my soul loveth. I sought Him, and found Him not! The watchmen who keep the city discovered me: Have you seen Him Whom my soul loveth?

Song of Songs 3:1-3
(having a teenager?)

Those with a will to find good news for modern gays in ancient Greece or pagan Rome can certainly find isolated bits of evidence for their views. But the evidence will largely have to come from popular practices and secondary thinkers. Socrates, Plato, Aristotle, Xenophon, and Cicero (no mean philosophical crew), in spite of difficulties and complexities in interpreting them to a modern audience, cannot be enlisted as forerunners of modern gay liberation. Their arguments are far closer, as has been long thought, to what some now dismiss as merely bigoted sexual morality (conventional and traditional confinement of sexuality to marriage).

Robert Royal

Some education gives a stunted childhood limited to learning about crooks, killers, abortionists, sex addicts, fraudulent celebrities, and pretend history. This is no education at all. Such a child is psychologically constricted, tortured, controlled, exploited and discarded but not emancipated.

Name Lost

What I do today determines my past and my future. I must live one day at a time.

Alcoholics Anonymous saying

God will not help the helpless.

Alcoholics Anonymous saying

It took me a year out of college to realize how hard it was to be on my own and that, looking back, my parents were almost *always* correct.

Rachel Nigro Scalish

Women who do things nakedly are typically any combination of cold, nervous or excited. Thus they will swallow air and have a lot of flatus. The more they do in nakedness, the worse it gets. Therefore, whenever you see a picture of a naked woman (or man for that matter), you should be thinking "fart" and be glad you are not near them. People who go naked a lot have the worst smelling farts outside of stockyards.

Samuel A. Nigro

Loud is right?

Dad

ENVIRONMENTALLY AND PLANETARILY SOUND SEX EDUCATION (WHICH IS NOT SEX EDUCATION AT ALL BUT REPRODUCTION EDUCATION)

The Nice Way To Put It

Air purity, water cleanliness, and land management are not more important and not more necessary than compliance in nature with human behaviors of sex and violence. Animals (within nature) not only comply with the environment, but, behaviorally they have controlled sexuality with the goal of reproduction and have controlled violence to the goal of survival. The goals of humans should also be environmentally sound.

1. Every human being was started by sexual intercourse which is when the penis is inserted into the vagina so the male's sperm can reach the female's egg to start reproduction of a new human being. Sexual intercourse is a very special activity involving not only the physical action itself but it also involves, because we are human beings, much significant emotional responses from the male and female to each other. Because the natural function of sexual intercourse is reproduction, it is an activity which is best done between a married man and woman who are prepared to begin a family. This means both the man and woman understand that their sexual activity may result in a child.
2. The activity leading to sexual intercourse and sexual intercourse itself is an emotional experience. The high emotion felt by both man and woman is called an orgasm.
3. The best sexual intercourse is consensual — meaning both the man and woman have reciprocal feelings and each desire a closeness with the other. Forced sexual intercourse is wrong and also against the law. Forced sexual intercourse is called rape. Interestingly, rape rarely occurs in the animal kingdom, but does occur in humans primarily because human emotions are involved and not controlled well. As rape generally occurs when a human man forces sexual intercourse upon an unconsenting woman, the human emotions are ones of control and power. The same thing is when emotionally immature individuals are targeted by sexual

predators. The common denominator for all this is force as well as the lack of understanding that the result will be a child who ought to be conceived through a loving consensual relationship based on family unity.

4. Rape is violent and is the ugly side of sexual intercourse. Other activities which often are seen in today's media are also abhorrent to the idea that sexual activity is intended in marriage between a consenting man and woman which should result in a child.
5. Sex is not an occupation, preoccupation or prescription for anything. And if it ever becomes such, it is an addiction.
6. Impulses happen, but following them without reason is pollution.
7. Human sexual activity is mystifying to children and confusing to young adults. To understand the emotional component, which animals do not experience, children and young adults must first have a basic knowledge of human anatomy and physiology presented in more and more detail as the child grows into adulthood. No sexual education should begin without consideration of the appropriate age for the child and the child's own readiness to put together what has been learned in an emotionally calm and comfortable fashion.

The Same Thing But Told In the Explicit And Gruff Style Of Contemporary Media

If being in tune with the environment, the animal kingdom (of which we *are* a part), the planet and the universe as known, means a balanced compliance with nature on the planet, then mankind must maintain a balanced compliance with our animal nature too. Air purity, water cleanliness, and land management are not more important and not more necessary than compliance in nature with human behaviors of sex and violence. Animals within nature not only comply with the environment, but, behaviorally they have good control of sexuality to the goal of reproduction and of violence to the goal of survival. So should humans, to be environmentally sound.

We live in an age of anything goes, vulgarity and gruffness. Consistent with that is the following way to demystify sexual education for everyone:

1. Sexual intercourse is when the penis squirts in the vagina so the male's sperm can reach the female's eggs to start reproduction of a new human being. Almost all male animals in nature try to squirt only in the vagina or equivalent when the female indicates it is near time to reproduce. Every human being was started this way. It is kind of strange-sounding but it is very special and is best done only by married people so that a family life is offered to the new human being. In nature, each creature has a *best way* of raising young. For humans it has always optimally been a family of a mom, a dad and often other relatives.
2. When the penis squirts in the vagina, the man gets a head-rushing feeling with shortness of breath and a body shudder that feels good for several seconds. This is called orgasm. Sometimes it just happens and there is nothing wrong with that.

3. Females have an undeveloped penis called the clitoris. If it is played with a lot, it can be tricked to try to squirt like a real penis, and when that happens, the girl's body is fooled into thinking she is a male. If the female likes to do this it is called penis-envy or squirt-envy. This also is called orgasm. Sometimes it just happens and there is nothing wrong with that.
4. Some polluters teach sex education as orgasm education and as against reproduction. Actually when they do that, they teach "squirt ed" instead of sound behavior in confluence with the planet (which is *reproduction education*). Homosexuals and feminists like to teach orgasm education because it creates extreme selfish attitudes which convert people into being homosexuals and feminists. Whatever female orgasm occurs in nature, it most likely is a ripple effect associated with time of fertility.
5. In all nature, females control sexuality. Forced sex by males does not occur. Males concede sexual control to the female. Sometimes it seems otherwise but for the most part, females determine when, where and if. Sex initiations and pressures may be applied by the male, but violent or forced sex is unnatural. No male in the animal kingdom has sexual intercourse without willing compliance of the female except among humans, thus rendering forced intercourse to be pollution.
6. As already mentioned, in nature each creature has its own best way of raising young. For humans this has always been the optimal family. In this context and for the unity of the family, sexual intercourse can have a *unitive* purpose as determined by the female for her or her husband's special needs.
7. The press and media are often liars and schools do not tell the full story about sex. Never listen to anyone who is for abortion ("choice") about sex matters. If you listen to them now, you will need an abortion later. What they tell you does not work.
8. Television and movies turn you into Peeping Toms watching other people's fantasies while you waste your own life.
9. Sex is for making babies after marriage.
10. The penis goes into the vagina after marriage. That is the only place it goes.
11. For males, spontaneous loving orgasm almost always occurs with sexual intercourse and is the mental roar accompanying the simple neurophysiologic ejaculation reflex and is secondary to reproduction.
12. For females, spontaneous loving orgasm infrequently accompanies sexual intercourse and is the exhilaration of oneness secondary to unition (marriage for humans). However and for the most part, no females in the animal kingdom have orgasm comparable to males except among humans, thus rendering female orgasm as repeatedly sought for, to be pollution and an atypical imitation of maleness.
13. Males and females are metaphysically different. Be that way. Help each other be that way.
14. Real males primarily focus on matter, truth, and good.

15. Real females primarily focus on identity, oneness, and beauty.
16. Females in nature do not go around over-stimulating the males of the species unless they mean business — and sex is not just when the males want it but when a baby is wanted — that is Nature!
17. Feminists (who believe in the equality and equivalence of the sexes) ruin children (especially boys) and men; never be one; never marry one.
18. Males usually become uncivil, violent rogues unless they are hard working heads of their families (exceptions are priests and brothers).
19. Sex is not an occupation, preoccupation, or prescription for anything. And if it ever becomes such, it is an addiction.
20. Impulses happen, but following them without reason is pollution.
21. Masturbation in males is penis adoration and not found in nature.
22. Masturbation in females is penis envy and not found in nature.
23. The masturbation of pets and all animals (including humans) in the animal kingdom is animal cruelty.
24. The cultivation of orgasm for orgasm's sake in the animal kingdom is pollution (actually, humans are the only deviant ones who do this).
25. Infertile ejaculation is not the same as *responsibility*.
26. If you put your body into a sewer, you will get diseases you never heard of, and if you allow such to happen, you become a sewer yourself.
27. Multiple sex partners predispose to uterine cancer.
28. Contraception enhances the anti-environmental (anti-animal behavior) cultivation of orgasm as a way of life and it predisposes to breast cancer and infertility. So does abortion, but it messes up the body and mind even moreso.
29. The most important question in the world is *not* "how will I ejaculate today?"
30. The freedom of human animals allows one to choose to ignore all this, but when one does, he, she or they are violating nature, evolution and the planet and become "pollution" in the most personal sense. It is behavior pollution.
31. To be part of the fullness of the animal kingdom of which humans are a part, to respect the planet, and to be true to genuine maleness or femaleness as evolved, each human must elevate his or her sexual function to be consistent with right reason as informed by Nature and Nature's God. The best way to do that is by learning and using Natural Family Planning.

Regardless of what anyone else proposes, the preceding is the most basic factual description of "sex education."

Samuel A. Nigro

Men are men, but Man is a woman.

G.K. Chesterton echoing Verdi's "La donna e mobile"

If you do not practice laughing, it hurts. . .and later you then go mad.

Samuel A. Nigro

Don't waste your kisses!

Dad

Most people do not mean what they say but they mean more than what they say. Therefore people are almost always in a state of failed communication.

Samuel A. Nigro

Excuse me if I enjoy myself rather obviously.

Gabriel Syme

False pride is pride in anything other than what you are doing right now.

Samuel A. Nigro

Blessed are they who have seen and not believed.

Samuel A. Nigro on television and movies

If you catch one of your teachers in a lie, be very, very careful about believing anything he or she ever tells you again.

Name Lost

The composure of the army is the anger of a nation.

G.K. Chesterton

At that moment I lifted my feet to the strings of my father's old guitar, and I knew that somewhere in Heaven he was crying too — tears of joy for what God had done to answer my mother's prayers for all of us.

Tony Melendez, born without arms, playing
his guitar with his feet for Pope John Paul II

No man should leave in the universe anything of which he is afraid. . . Fight the thing you fear.

Gabriel Syme

But know for certain that it is worth fearing.

Samuel A. Nigro

Nobody likes a liar. . .be true to your self.

Carla Scalish

If there are no standards to rebel against, teenagers can only rebel against themselves with alcohol, drugs, recreational sex, dysocial self injurious acting out and suicide.

Jo Ann Gaspar

Be good, act right and do the best you can.

Edward and Radmila Vieder

Sometimes I've got it all together but then I don't know where to put it.

Betty Howard

Supervision is needed. If you don't supervise children they get hurt or victimized. If you don't supervise teenagers they get violent or sexual. If you don't supervise adults they will steal everything they can.

Name Lost

Sexuality not kept within the norms of nature is anti-social.

Name Lost

Only a woman who does not know how to be female would try to define herself by "equality." Not knowing how to be a real woman, she would want to be a man.

Samuel A. Nigro

Madness in great ones must not unwatched go.

from Hamlet

Oh shame, where is thy blush?

from Hamlet

Mad as the sea and wind when both contend which is the mightier.

from Hamlet

So full of artless jealousy is guilt. It spills itself in fearing to be spilt.

the mother of Hamlet

Venus smiles not in a house of tears.

from Romeo & Juliet

Keep your temper. Do not quarrel with an angry person, but give him a soft answer. It is commanded by Holy Writ and, furthermore, it makes him madder than anything else you could say.

Anonymous

If I were an archeologist, I would not mind getting older.

Samuel A. Nigro

"Success" is a lot of crap — just have a productive and virtue-filled day.

Samuel A. Nigro

Go where life takes you as if you are floating in a canoe — but paddling like hell with the virtues.

Name lost

The desperate temporary pathology of growing up always involves learning by experience and therefore the making of some just plain bad decisions. One can hope that whatever these are, they do not become permanent or injurious in a serious or sustained fashion.

Samuel A. Nigro

In all nature, femaleness is characterized by sexual behavior for reproduction. Is it not amazing how the human species can find ways to be at odds with the planet?

Samuel A. Nigro

Make haste slowly.

Caesar Augustus

By feminism, all women surrender to men by trying to join men equally.

Name lost

It does not take any longer to do it right than it takes to mess it up.

Evelyn Nigro

Never worry or fret about what you don't have. . .just keep working for it!

Name lost

Self-esteem usually depends on fantasy while humility depends on accurate self-perception.

Samuel A. Nigro

I am not upset, and will continue to deny how upset I am until I calm down.

Ashleigh Brilliant

What you too! I thought I was the only one with thoughts and feelings.

Ashleigh Brilliant

Please don't believe everything you hear about me regardless of how true it may be.

Ashleigh Brilliant

The only difference between yesterday and tomorrow is: today.

Ashleigh Brilliant

Freedom is not the goal, but you need freedom before you can decide what the goal is.

Ashleigh Brilliant

Thou canst not speak of that thou dost not feel.

Romeo

These times of woe afford no time to woo.

from Romeo & Juliet

Kids basically are worried about what is now being given to them as "sex" education. . . until they hear the absolutely necessary and necessarily comforting: "sex is to be done only to have a baby after you are married." That should be the opening and closing statements to any and every instruction given about sexual matters to youth at all ages.

Samuel A. Nigro

Eating slow is the essence of manners and civilization — so train yourself to eat a meal slowly at least once a day — savoring every bite and call it "relaxed dining."

Name lost

Stupidity has consequences. So does immorality.

Samuel A. Nigro

Never let anyone deprive of your right and opportunity to be civilized and cordial.

Evelyn Nigro

Self-esteem is preposterous.

Samuel A. Nigro

Humility is stark raving honesty.

Alcoholic Anonymous saying

The imposter demands toe noticed. His craving for compliments energizes his futile quest for carnal satisfaction. His bandages are his identity. Appearances are everything. He convolutes *esse quem videri* (to be rather than to seem to be) so that "seeming to be" becomes his *modus operandi*.

— Brennan Manning

CODE OF THE GOOD AMERICAN

- — I will control my tongue, and will not allow it to speak mean, vulgar, or profane words.
- — I will control my thoughts.
- — I will control my actions.
- — I will gladly listen to the advice of older and wiser people; I will reverence the wishes of those who love and care for me, and who know life and me better than I. I will develop independence and wisdom to think for myself.
- — I will try to find out what my duty is as a good American, and my duty I will do, whether it is easy or hard.
- — I will be honest, in word and in act. I will not lie, sneak, or pretend.
- — I will be loyal to my family. I will be loyal to my school. I will be loyal to my town, my state, my country.

National Education Association - 1941

Whenever you see an explicit sex scene always whistle out loud Loony Tunes because that is what is appropriate for anyone who is so undignified to act that way for public viewing.

Samuel A. Nigro

Never underestimate anyone. . . .

Frank Scalish

Self-esteem means that the dumb are believing their own lies.

Samuel A. Nigro

The age of psychological man is over. Modern man is just too sick now, too confused; he is beyond psychology! Modern man did it to himself, tearing apart the old order and inviting a revolution of nihilism. He has brought the biblical warning down upon himself, "sow the wind, reap the whirlwind."

Joseph Mauceri

Thanks are the highest form of thought.

G.K. Chesterton

Do not swear. Swearing scares the angels away. Say a gentle prayer instead.

Samuel A. Nigro

Get smart! Become immune or make yourself immune to television, movies and newsprint. Thereby you will be able to live *your own* life and a *real* life at that.

Samuel A. Nigro

There is no smaller package in the world than a man wrapped up in himself.

George Rutler

The more you are involved in NON-BEING (television, movies, celebrities, etc.), the LESS you are and the worse off you are going to be.

Samuel A. Nigro

Monkey see. Monkey do.

Aunt Rose

You're going to be crying in a minute.

Dad

Study like your life depends on it because it does.

Name Lost

Celebrities, even the ones you really like the most, are still basically actors and pretenders extraordinaire, should not take themselves seriously and neither should anyone else. After all, the most that could be said about any of them is that they are "faking it."

Samuel A. Nigro

Seconds are centuries, minutes ages. Men fire into each others' faces. There are bayonet thrusts, saber strokes, pistol shots. . . . Men going down on their hands and knees, spinning 'round like tops, throwing out their arms, gulping blood, falling; legless, armless, headless. There are ghastly heaps of dead men.

Civil War survivor's description

> All this again only now with women weakening the force so that more men will die. . . . All for some female soldier's career. So what will it cost us to give women complete military careers? Nothing but our sons.

Samuel A. Nigro

Sincerity, I believe, is the least of the virtues and perhaps the most insidious of all. For it is the one that substitutes for the good, an internal and subjective feeling as its main mark and justification.

James Schall

The existence of laughter is a most curious aspect of creation. Yet, there is laughter that mocks and is bitter. Both kinds of laughter unexpectedly transform both good and evil into something profounder than we might otherwise suspect. Laughter is mainly something heard. The ear may really be capable of hearing the sounds of eternity.

James Schall

In the temporal order, a *quantum* is the indivisible unit of receiving or giving energy. So is Confirmation. Fill all you can with goodness and laughter.

CHAPTER 7:

EXTREME UNCTION

In the physical order, a *singularity* is a point position at gravitational collapse wherein space-time curvature is infinite. Your human beingness is a singularity.

In the spiritual order, *Extreme Unction* is a *singularity* achieving *spirituality* by "detached warmth and gentleness" conveying *justice* with regard for and giving to all that which is due them because at infinity all is given which is due.

"It is finished."

Extreme Unction makes you a singularity — a spiritual affirmation of justice when you will get all due you.

Live Extreme Unction — a returning almost to whom we came from.

To be in the Father.
To Enter the Fullness of Life
and to participate in the Incarnation.

In physics, a *singularity* is a point position at gravitational collapse wherein the space-time curvature is infinite. So is Extreme Unction.

Extreme Unction is the Sacrament which, through the anointing and prayer of the priest, gives health and strength to the soul and sometimes to the body when we are in danger of death from sickness. Extreme Unction is a *singularity*.

Extreme Unction is a pattern of "detached warmth and gentleness." It coincides with the physical *singularity* at which point infinity is approached at gravitational collapse. The humanness principle here is *spirituality* enabling the activity of justice to be forthcoming because at infinity all is given which is due.

Detached warmth
and gentleness. . .

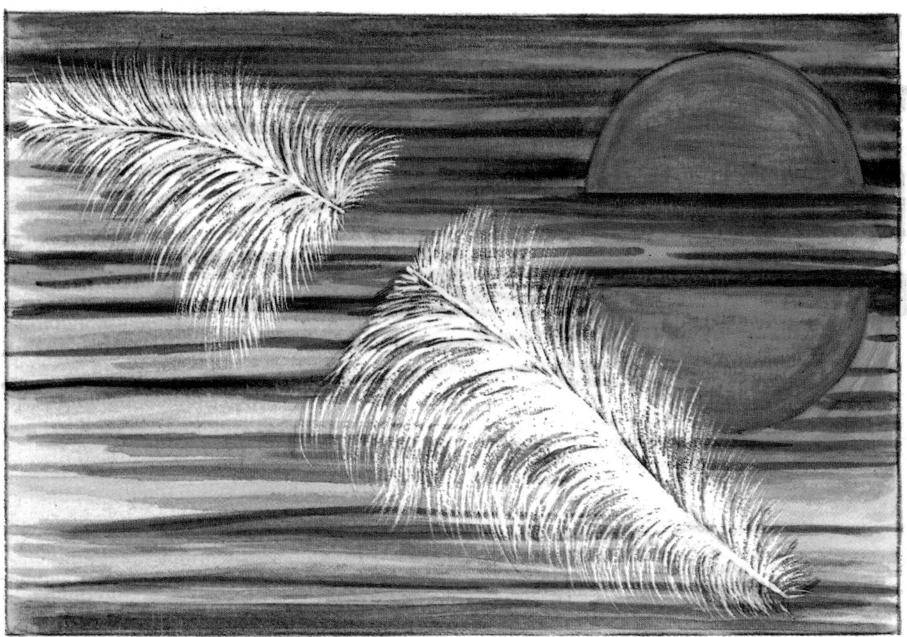

. . . One way to be a human being. Animals seldom keep their distance and often are rough, crude and overactive. But a human being has warmth (which is being "close"), detachment (which avoids being "too close"), and gentleness (which makes "love" more than a word). Altogether, detached warmth and gentleness make one's voice, touch, and manner to be more mild, more true, and more conducive to family, friends, and strangers having love for one another.

Detached Warmth and Gentleness

There is an old Zulu saying: "Softly, softly, catch monkey." I don't know what we'd do with a monkey — but a soft, low-key, gentle approach are tones which really need to be underscored and strived for. Warmth means that one is effectively friendly. It may be a hug, but detachment is absolutely essential, otherwise one can run into more serious problems with others hungry for affection. Keep your distance — people can be easily overwhelmed.

Gentleness reminds of the parable of the wind and the sun betting which could get the coat off the strolling gentleman. The wind blew and blew, and the man wrapped the coat around ever more tightly. The sun laughed during his turn shining brightly and warmly. After a brief interval, the man removed his coat. Warmth and gentleness work wisely together.

* * * * *

I expect to pass through life but once. If therefore, there be any kindness I can show, or any good thing I can do to any fellow being, let me do it now, and not defer or neglect it, as I shall not pass this way again.

William Penn

We are alone, absolutely alone on this chance planet: and amid all the forms of life that surround us, not one, excepting the dog has made an alliance with us.

Maurice Maeterlinck

You grow up the day you have your first real laugh at yourself.

Ethel Barrymore

That guy is the kind of person who gives his almost.

Norma Jenkins

People who are only interested in having fun cannot accomplish anything.

Mike Tyson (Heavy Weight Champion of the World)

God does not die on the day we cease to believe in a personal Deity, but we die on the day when our lives cease to be illumined by the steady radiance renewed daily of a wonder, the source of which is beyond all reason.

Dag Hammarskjold

Yesterday is but a dream, and tomorrow is only a vision, But today, well lived, makes every yesterday a dream of happiness, And every tomorrow a vision of hope. Look Well, therefore, to this day.

Sanskrit proverb

If happiness truly consisted in physical ease and freedom from care, then the happiest individual would be neither a man nor a woman; it would be, I think, an American cow.

William Lyon Phelps

Happiness is a butterfly, which, when pursued, is always just beyond your grasp, but which, if you will sit down quietly, may alight upon you.

Nathaniel Hawthorne

Everybody needs a hug. It changes your metabolism.

Leo Buscaglia

A man shows what he is by what he does with what he has.

Anonymous

Men want to improve only the world, but mothers want to improve their whole family. This is a much harder task.

Harriet Freezer

My best creation is my children.

Diane von Furestenberg

If we cannot now end our differences, at least we can help make the world safe for diversity.

John F. Kennedy

There is nothing stronger in the world than gentleness.

Han Suyin

Extreme Unction is the Sacrament which, through the anointing and prayer of the priest, gives health and strength to the soul and sometimes to the body, when we are in danger of death from sickness.

Baltimore Catechism

Beam me up, Jesus.

12-year-old girl dying of leukemia every time she received Communion/Extreme Unction

I think it's time to call on Jesus.

little boy to teacher trying to lead a classroom of children through a blizzard to safety

Good night. Pleasant dreams. God bless you. I love you. See you in the morning.

Samuel A. Nigro's night-time prayer to his children

A glimpse is not a vision. But to a man on a mountain road by night, a glimpse of the next three feet of road may matter more than a vision of the horizon.

C.S. Lewis

Treat a child as though he already is the person he's capable of becoming.

Haim Ginott

If your outgo exceeds your income, then your upkeep will be your downfall.

Ron Logan

Good sense is easier to have than use.

James Grady

Be safe. Study hard. Work vigorously for peace. Love (friendly) gently. Truth shall set you free. Persist in what is good. Fight fair and forget fast. Real laughter is divine. Happiness is doing nice things for others. Listen! Don't think you know when you really can know.

Samuel A. Nigro's reminder to children in college

The most difficult task in civilization is to civilize males. And only a good woman can do it.

Samuel A. Nigro

No woman can ever know what it takes to be a civilized man because a "civilized man" contradicts all maleness in the animal kingdom. And no man can ever know what it takes to be a good mother because no man has ever had to work so hard.

Samuel A. Nigro

In my suffering for you, (I) fill up those things that are wanting in the suffering of Christ.

Colossians 1:24

The Lord on his part has forgiven your sin: you shall not die. But since you have utterly spurned the Lord by this deed, the child born to you must surely die.

2 Samuel 12:14

Is any man sick among you, let him bring in the priests of the Church, and let them pray over him, anointing him with oil in the name of the Lord, and the prayer of faith shall save the sick man and the Lord shall raise him up and if he be in sins, they shall be forgiven him.

James 5:15

The reason people object to the Natural Law of St. Thomas Aquinas is that it will not let them do what they want to do. Natural Law tells people right from wrong, which is why they flounder around looking for something else.

Samuel A. Nigro

The soul grows wings as it beholds values.

Plato

Time is the one fact of life that is inescapable. We may lose love, happiness, friends, work and health, but not time. To a certain extent, "growing old" means being more and more conscious of time and less and less conscious of life. Part of the euthanasia debate springs from the perception that certain people are just not dying "on time." The truth is, we neither are born or die "on time."

Donald DeMarco

The greater the man, the deeper his love.

Leonardo de Vinci

Our hearts are restless until they find their rest in Thee.

St. Augustine

My true weight is my love. . .and I will float up to Thee.

St. Augustine

We do not have to agonize over death if we are committed to life as Mary was.

Samuel A. Nigro

I can't get too excited about anything that won't fit in my coffin.

Fred Allen

The Bible says: "Peter died leaning on his staff," and someday the same will be said of me.

Lou Holtz, Notre Dame Football Coach

You are never so important that you cannot be replaced. . .except in God's vision.

Mom (Evelyn Nigro)

Life to me, of course, is Christ, but then death would bring me something more.

Philippians 1:21

Unless a wheat grain falls on the ground and dies, it remains only a single grain; but if it dies, it yields a rich harvest.

John 12:24

I think science has a real surprise for the skeptics. . . . Nothing in nature, not even the tiniest particle, can disappear without a trace. Nature does not know extinction. All it knows is transformation. . . . Everything science has taught me — and continues to teach me — strengthens my belief in the continuity of our spiritual existence after death.

Wernher von Braun

Death doesn't bother me. I just don't want to be there when it happens.

Woody Allen

It is suffering, more than anything else, which clears the way for the Grace which transforms human souls.

Pope John Paul II

For dust thou art, and unto dust shalt thou return.

Genesis 3:19

He is not the God of the dead, but the God of the living. . . .

Mark 12:27

It is impossible that anything so natural, so necessary, and so universal as death, should ever have been designed by Providence as an evil to mankind.

Jonathan Swift

Judge none blessed before his death.

Ecclesiasticus 11:28

The last enemy that shall be destroyed is death.

1 Corinthians 15:26

O death, where is thy sting? O grave, where is thy victory?

1 Corinthians 15:55

Blessed are the dead which die in the Lord from henceforth: Yea saith the Spirit, that they may rest from their labors; and their works do Follow them.

Revelation 14:13

Christians NEVER say goodbye!

C.S. Lewis

There is joy in the amusing astonishment at our beliefs — never contradicting nature but regularly going beyond our finiteness and splendorously surpassing our natural substance.

Samuel A. Nigro

My God, my God, why did you abandon me?

Matthew 27:46

We wouldn't want to just run out on the people.

Sister Dorothy Kazel

Grant, oh Lord, that I might commune in the peace of your presence, so that when my hour is to come, I shall pass through a transition all but insensible, from You to You; from You, the Living Bread, the Bread of Man, to You, the Living Love, already possessed by those of my beloved ones who, in that love, have gone before me to sleep.

Francois Mauriac

If the physician presumes to take into consideration in his work whether a life has value or not, the consequences are boundless and the physician becomes the most dangerous man in the state.

Christopher Huffeland

The doctor,. . .if not living in a moral situation. . .where limits are very clear,. . .is very dangerous.

Auschwitz survivor

The mind must be enlarged to see the simple things.

G.K. Chesterton

We can't hunt God; He hunts us and his story is sad.

Robert Lowell

. . .that is one of the purposes of cemeteries: to unite in love the living with the dead, to remind us that time does not exist in eternity, to create a necessary compact, to prepare us for death while simultaneously causing us to hug life.

Barbara Grizzuti Harrison

St. Peter was crucified upside down. . . . He saw the landscape as it really is, with stars like flowers, and the clouds like hills, and all men hanging on the mercy of God.

G.K. Chesterton

The real world has a capital "W" and no "L."

Samuel A. Nigro

A little sincerity is a dangerous thing, and a great deal of it is absolutely fatal.

Oscar Wilde

Angels are much more believable, logical, and rational than fortune-tellers, futurists, astrologers, and other feeling-filled enthusiasts who delude themselves into believing their fantasies. The reality of angels cannot be logically denied while astrology et cetera are based on gnosticism, which is nothing more than individual enthusiasm about one's own emotional steam.

Samuel A. Nigro

. . .very few of the things that happen to us are purposeless or accidental (and this includes suffering and grief — even that of others),. . .sometimes one catches a glimpse of the link between these happenings.

Iris Origo

We need to relate to each other like we are rescuers for each other. When you shake hands, grasp firmly and gently, like it is the first hand you've touched since being buried in rubble for a week.

Samuel A. Nigro

Without God as their proper object, faith becomes credulity or incredulity; hope becomes optimism or pessimism; love becomes eroticism or cruelty or both.

George Rutler

The lion roared to the mouse: "You don't scare me — you don't scare anybody!" and the mouse replied: "I've been sick."

Anonymous

Fear flees evil and misses the chance to fill it with love.

Anonymous

There is so much more to life than merely growing up.

Samuel A. Nigro

Steam is water gone crazy with the heat.

Charles C. Nigro

Never talk about illness to a hypochondriac.

Anonymous

What is the cash value of this idea?

William James

What is the transcendental value? Cash has nothing to do with it.

Samuel A. Nigro

I readily believe those witnesses who get their throats cut.

Paschal

Madness is a preference for the symbol over which it represents.

G.K. Chesterton

If I believe in immortality, I need not think about it. But if I disbelieve in immortality, I must not think about it.

G.K. Chesterton

Everything is bearable because we die. There is nothing serious under the sun except love of fellow mortals and of God.

Malcolm Muggridge

You matter because you are you, and you matter to the last moment of your life.

Dame Cicely Saunders,
Founder of St. Christopher's Hospice

Was it not necessary that the Christ should suffer and enter into his glory?

Luke 24:26

Live your own life, for you will die your own death.

Latin Proverb

I never stopped saying the Hail Mary.

American Pilot Jeffrey Fox in television interview
answering the question as to what he did as a
prisoner of war in a terrifying Iraqi prison

For those who believe in Jesus, life has not ended but merely changed.

1 Thessalonians 3:14

At morn, at noon, at twilight dim,
Maria, thou last heard my hymn.
In joy and woe, in good and ill,
Mother of God, be with me still.

Edgar Allan Poe

The incorporeal and the invisible may be unimaginable by us, but they are not unthinkable or unintelligible. Angels are no more incomprehensible than minds or intellects are, whether embodied or not.

Mortimer J. Adler

They are kind of like words.

The only justification for affirming the existence of something unperceived and, perhaps, imperceptible, is that whatever it is that needs to be explained cannot be explained in any other way.

William of Ockham

Everything is easy if you know how. . . .

Charles Nigro

Stop moaning about it. . . . Don't let it get you down. . . . Life is too short to dwell one more minute on that. . . .

Evelyn Nigro

Genuine freedom is in choosing what is right, because choosing wrong is so easy the latter is not really choosing but more of a conditioned response which is not a choice at all.

Anonymous

I'm not going to play by their set of rules, but by ours. I'm going to do my best to replace whatever hatred they have in their hearts.

Medical officer in charge of an American
warship filled with wounded prisoners in World War II

True freedom is being your transcendentals.

Anonymous

Is this (anything at all) necessary for salvation?

Anonymous

Jes fine.

Fremont the Bug's response to everything.

It is a far, far better thing that I do, than I have ever done; it is a far, far better rest that I go to than I have ever known.

Sidney Carton in *Tale of Two Cities* before the guillotine falls
as he sacrifices himself for his friend and his wife

Forget not Death, Oh man! For thou may'st be of one thing certain — he forgets not thee.

Persian saying

Roaming in thought over the Universe, I saw the little
that is Good
steadily hastening towards immortality,
And the vast all that is call'd Evil I saw hastening to
merge itself,
and become lost and dead.

Walt Whitman

He that would die well must always look for death, everyday knocking at the gates of the grave; and then the gates of the grave shall never prevail upon him to do him mischief.

Jeremy Taylor

There is a post-death, post-physical, meta-death, meta-physical reality. But the barrier called Life must be overcome in order to get there. The barrier is increased by sin and decreased by grace. On closer examination, this barrier is a wilderness with a very clear trail through it known as Roman Catholicism. It is a trail of Natural Law, transcendentals, virtue, and living the Sacraments. It is only by these means that one can reach the Beyond.

Samuel A. Nigro

Through this anointing
may the Lord in his love and mercy help you
with the grace of the Holy Spirit. Amen.
May the Lord who frees you from sin
save you and raise you up. Amen.

Rite of Extreme Unction

I am an optimist. It does not seem too much use being anything else.

Winston Churchill

The Incarnation is the humanization of a divine path to an existence we can only faintly feel by the most ecstatic moments of our lives. The Incarnation is the blazing divinization of a human trail which we must follow to get to our potential ultimate destination which is back to God from Whom we came.

Anonymous

The past has a future.
Christians know that. . . .

G.R. Elton

It is precisely the soul that is the traveller; it is of the soul and of the soul alone that we can say with supreme truth that "being" necessarily means "being on the way" (en route).

Gabriel Marcel

Fear of death is essential for human living.

Anthony F. Zimmerman

It may be that after this life we shall perish utterly, but if that is our fate, let us live so that annihilation will be unjust.

Etine de Senancour

Always go to other people's funerals, otherwise they won't come to yours.

Yogi Berra

Hope for the best, but prepare for the worst.

English Proverb

If you die in an elevator, be sure to push the UP button.

Sam Levenson

All men should strive to learn before they die
What they are running from, and to, and why.

James Thurber

Do not get excited over the noise you have made.

Desiderius Erasmus

Life is too short to belittle.

Benjamin Disraeli

Your gentleness has made me great. You have made wide steps for my feet, to keep them from slipping.

2 Samuel 22:36-37

If you wouldst live long, live well; for folly and wickedness shorten life.

Benjamin Franklin

Go to bed the same day you get up.

Miles B. Carpenter, age 93

The essence of life: fight as if there were no death.

Geuy de Rothschild

In the long run, we'll all be dead.

John Kenneth Galbriath

(Or alive in Christ Jesus.)

I don't think we are in Kansas anymore, Toto.

Dorothy

A light touch is the mark of strength.

G.K. Chesterton

Death is not the end, there remains litigation over the estate.

Ambrose Bierce

When people can stand up, they're thinking of killing you.
Whereas when they're ill, there is no doubt about it, they're less dangerous.

Celine

Hold up your limp arms, steady your trembling knees, injured limbs will not be wrenched, but will grow strong again.

Hebrews 12:13

We are not going to worry about making a living, we're going to worry about why you are here.

Sister Ignatia Gavan, Co-founder of Alcoholics Anonymous

Go with God.

Arthur O'H

I only know scientifically determined truth, but I am going to believe what I wish to believe, what I cannot help but believe — I expect to meet this dear child in another world.

Louis Pasteur, 1895 — of his dying daughter

I throw myself on your mercy and your pleasure, *save the honor of God.*

St. Thomas Becket

Extremes meet.

Proverbs

Marcus the Physician called yesterday on the marble Zeus. Though marble and though Zeus, the funeral is today.

Nicharchus, Circa 100 A.D.

It is in vain, old man, that you seek within yourself the cure of all your miseries. All your insights only lead you to the knowledge that is not in yourselves that you will discover the true and the good. The philosophers promised them to you and have not been able to keep their promise. Your principal maladies are pride which cuts you off from God, sensuality which blinds you to the earth, and you seem to do nothing but foster one of these maladies.

Paschal

Don't you know God can cure cancer just like a toothache.

Father Solanus Casey

We do well to remember how short, after all, it is till our suffering and our time of merit will be over.

Father Solanus Casey

Please provide the date of your death.

A letter from the U.S. Internal Revenue Service

Seek the best of what has been thought and said.

Mathew Arnold

If you're laughing, you cannot die.

Name Lost

The goal of humanity is to consume goods? The goal of an individual is to adjust happily? The destiny of a human being is sexual satisfaction? What is an individual all about?

Name Lost

"Why are you crying?" the young Francis of Assisi, seeking his future, had asked the weeping monk. "Because," the old man said, "Love is not loved." . . .nor belief believed. . .still that is my destination.

Patricia Hampl

Spiritual life is not a quest. . .it is a disappearing act.

Patricia Hampl

Savage indignation no longer tears his heart.

Epitaph for Jonathan Swift

Are you sure your husband is dead? I can't jump out of windows like I used to. . . .

Groucho Marx

Pray for my soul.

Henry VIII on his death bed

But your Highness, you abolished purgatory!

A minister to the king

Pride looks down, and no one sees God but by looking up.

Peter Kreeft

Prayer is a kind of death, a rehearsal for death. In praying we die ourselves, our wills, our ordinary consciousness and desires and concerns, even our ordinary world, and enter God's world, aligning our minds and wills with God's.

Peter Kreeft

Naked I came into this world and naked I shall return.

Job

There are two kinds of people in the end: those who say to God, "Thy will be done," and those to whom God says in the end, "*Thy* will be done."

C.S. Lewis

The essence of Christianity is not Christianity; the essence of Christianity is Christ — He rose from the dead!

Peter Kreeft

We can no more choose our final end than we can prove our first principles such as the law of non-contradiction; for we must always pre-suppose them. The consequences of this technical, logical point are enormous from the practical and religious points of view: It means that God, our final end, is not avoidable, not an "option" like a movie or a meal, not something for "Religious people" (whoever they are), but "the only game in town" (or, as C.S. Lewis puts it, "the only fruit (good) this universe can grow — the only fruit any possible universe can grow").

Peter Kreeft

Choice results from the decision or judgment which is, as it were, the conclusion of a practical syllogism. Hence, that which is the conclusion of a practical syllogism, is the matter of choice. Now, in practical things the end just stands in a position of principle, not of conclusion. . . . Whereforce, the end, as such, is not a matter of choice.

St. Thomas Aquinas

. . .volition is of the end, but choice of the means.

Aristotle

In other words, we will an end but choose a means. The end is always there.

Easy come, easy go in money and what you think is love.

Charles C. Nigro

Man is an end, things (wealth) are means. For man to serve things is to reverse the order of reality. . . . In summary, God is to adored, man loved, and things used.

Peter Kreeft

And any other way does not work very well.

Thank you for giving us a place in paradise.

Dante DiFiore

The point of life is not death but to end up in a beatifying union with God.

Ralph McInerny

To love someone means saying to him, "You shall not die."

Gabriel Marcel

There we shall rest and see, see and love, love and praise. This is what shall be in the end without end.

St. Augustine of Beatific Vision

Everything declines, everything shatters, everything passes, and only memories remain.

French Adage

May God grant us this grace — to be led by death to the Bridegroom!

Dietrich von Hildebrand

Love is not changed by death and nothing lost, and all in the end is harvest.

Edith Sitwell

Remember, man, you are dust and into dust you shall return!

Ash Wednesday warning

Grant eternal rest, oh Lord, onto thy servant and let perpetual light shine upon him.

Requiem Prayer

Behold, the Bridegroom cometh.

Matthew 25:6

Yet, not my will be done, oh Lord, but Thine!

Luke 22:42

We live our lives in the very midst of death.

Notkar of St. Gall

Behold, I make all things new!

Revelations 21:5

Death is then no cause for mourning, something to be avoided, for the Son of God did not think it beneath his dignity, nor did He seek to escape it.

St. Ambrose of Milan

If I knew I was going to live this long, I would have taken better care of myself.

Mickey Mantle

God did not decree death from the beginning; He prescribed it as a remedy. Human life was condemned because of sin to unremitting labor and unbearable sorrow and so began to experience the burden of wretchedness.

There had to be a limit to its evils; death had to restore what life had forfeited. Without the assistance of Grace, immortality is more of a burden than a blessing.

St. Ambrose of Milan

One day, you look about and decide for yourself that you are going to be free of that which enslaves you. You are to choose forever the good in the face of suffering. At that moment, you begin to be beautiful by always embracing the planet's Natural Law reflectively; you become one with yourself, family, neighbors, community, humanity, the planet, and the universe by always extending beyond your epidermal confinement; you become truth by always giving witness to the reality of beings; you become an identity with human beingness itself by always giving only that power to feelings which are justified by reason; and you become matter itself by living virtuously. On that day, and forever after, nothing can bother you, not tragedy or foulness, not excitement or boredom, not beast or human, not enemy or family. You will be free.

Samuel A. Nigro

Funeral ceremonies are not a tribute to the dead, but to the living.

G.K. Chesterton

Most of the world's work is done by people who don't feel very well.

Winston Churchill

Tell them in Lakedaimo passer-by carrying out this order, here we lie.

Epitaph at Thermopylae

Cave, *adsum* — Beware, I am here.

Name Lost

Whomever death takes would have to trust in God's judgment.

Beowulf

Death would be better than shameful life.

Wiglaf

Presuming their state to be equal, it is more useful to have a practitioner who is a friend than a stranger.

Celsus on medical care

They ought of kilt us, but they ain't whupped us.

Faulkner's redneck

It's so crowded nobody goes there anymore.

Yogi Berra

How are ye blind, ye treaders down of cities, ye that cast temples to desolation, and lay waste tombs, the untrodden sanctuaries where lie the ancient dead; yourselves so soon to die!

Poseidon's warning to all conquerors

Lord, I *know* that what you want is best for my life. If what you recently want is ____, you don't have to take ____ I give to You ____. You are second to nothing. Even though this doesn't make sense to me, I give You this friend that I love so dearly.

Susan Stanford Rue's prayer of Goodbye

And the prayer of faith will save the sick man, and the lord will raise him up. . . .

James 5:15

Lord/Jesus/Christ/Son/of/God/have/mercy/on/me/a/sinner.

Russian Jesus prayer; each word is said to your heart beat (anytime, all the time, for any reason)

One who keeps death before his eyes conquers despair.

Desert Monk

When my third snail died, I said, "I'm through with snails." But I didn't mean it.

A little girl

My consolation is to have no consolation on this earth.

St. Theresa of Lisieux

Behold what will be at the end without end.

St. Augustine

. . .the flesh is a sacred thing.

G.K. Chesterton

Glorified and sanctified be His great name in the world which He has created according to His will. May He establish His kingdom during your life and during your days, and during the life of all the house of Israel, speedily and soon, and say ye, Amen.
Blessed, praised and glorified, exalted, adored and honored, extolled and lauded be the name of the Holy One, blessed be He; though He be high above all the blessings and hymns, praises and words of solace which are uttered in the world, and say ye, Amen.

Kaddish of Jewish Liturgy

Death? How can it be a problem? Everybody does it.

Name Lost

The older I get, the better I used to be.

Connie Hawkins

If immortality be untrue, it matters little if anything else is true or not.

Henry Thomas Buckle

I trust that we shall, once in Heaven, see each other full merrily.

St. Thomas More to his executioner

Time had a beginning as a singularity 15 billion years ago per Albert Einstein's general theory of relativity. At another singularity, space-time will end, and ostensibly one cannot predict what will happen. In actuality, the result will be a black hole, according to contemporary physics. However, at that singularity, the black hole can be escaped if one travels faster than the speed of light — simply done spiritually by being a Catholic.

Samuel A. Nigro

Is today the day, Lord?

Name Lost

If you make every game a life-and-death proposition, you're going to have problems. For one thing, you'll be dead a lot.

Dean Smith, North Carolina basketball coach

I acknowledge before you, my God and God of my ancestors, that my cure and my death are in your hands. May it be your will to grant me complete recovery. And if I die, may my death be an atonement for the sins, transgressions and violations which I have committed before you. And set my portion in Paradise and let me merit the world to come reserved for the righteous. Hear, oh Israel, the Lord is our God. The Lord is one.

Jewish Prayer anticipating death

Time is yours, but eternity is mine.

A.L. Thomas on what God tells us.

God or nothing.

Erik von Kuehnelt-Leddihn

Thou, Lord, callest me, and I am coming to Thee. I come, not by my merits, but through Thy mercy alone, for which I beseech Thee by virtue of Thy blood!

St. Catherine of Sienna near her death on April 29, 1380
and whose blessed body has never known corruption

For the name of Jesus and the defense of the Church, I embrace death.

Last words of Archbishop Thomas Becket as he was slain
by the sword in Canterbury Cathedral, December 29, 1170

The whole world would not suffice this "nature" of man. If the whole world were given to him, he would have to say, and would say: It is too little.

Josef Pieper

(Yes! There is more.)

Love doubles one's strength, makes one inventive, renders one interiorly free and happy.

Father Ingelmar Unzeitig, Martyr priest of Dachau

At the sunset of our lives, we shall be judged by our love.

St. John of the Cross

It was the will of God, and God wants only the good.

Johannes Maria Lenz, Jesuit survivor of Dachau

Love of God is the source of the right love of neighbor.

Maximilian Kolbe

That's where all the good people are. . . .

Charles Nigro on cemeteries

Only God can satisfy us because God *infinitely exceeds all other pleasures*.

St. Thomas Aquinas

Christian doctrine is primarily concerned with the doctrine of salvation, not with interpreting reality or human existence. But it implies as well certain fundamental teachings on specific philosophic matters — the world and existence is such.

Josef Pieper

He who perseveres to the end shall be saved.

St. Augustine

On death, things become common, only to be reacquired again for a time by someone else.

James V. Schall

Clouds gather at evening.

Name Lost

That is the only thing I do believe in. my whole life has been a prayer.

Horace Williams on his death bed when asked by his nurse, "Professor, aren't you going to pray? Do you believe in God?"

If odd of God
to choose the Jews
More odd of God
to be in me.

David C. Leege

We live after all in a shadowland, for earth is not our permanent home.

C.S. Lewis

Somewhere in the world there is defeat for everyone. Some are destroyed by defeat, and some made small and mean by victory. Greatness lives in one who triumphs equally over defeat and victory.

John Steinbeck

Life is under no obligation to give us what we expect.

Margaret Mitchell

Time is a dressmaker specializing in alterations.

Faith Baldwin

Honey, faith means that when you pray for rain, you bring an umbrella.

an AIDS patient

"Make it difficult." What to ask the Lord if one could live one's life over.

Name Lost

We are broken to be more beautiful.

Name Lost

My father always said that if we ask "why me?" of the bad things, we have to ask it of the good, too.

Diane Berger

What is man's purpose? What is his place in the cosmos? What happens after death? Why do the big ones always get away?

Paul Quinnett

Final Antiphon For Catholic Burial Prayer

May the angels lead you into paradise;
may the martyrs come to welcome you
and take you to the holy city,
the new and eternal Jerusalem.

May choirs of angels welcome you
and lead you to the bosom of Abraham;
and where Lazarus is poor no longer
may you find eternal rest.

Oh, my dear children, don't you understand that nothing matters but your Transcendentals?

Dad

In nature, reasons exist for animal parents to regurgitate food for their young because the young cannot chew and will choke. This is important for every parent to know about their child and eating habits. To keep your child from choking, children must be taught to chew food well and eat slow. If under 6 years old, they should not eat peanuts, hard candy or anything with seeds. Everything should be cut into small pieces and mashed up, even if thought soft such as raisins and grapes. Everything should be chewed well, mashed with teeth and never gulped. If a child cannot eat properly or develops gulping and gorging habits, he should go without solid food for a day emphasizing that he needs to learn to chew food well. While humans do not regurgitate food for the young, in a very real sense it has to be done in one way or another. Choking children (and adults!) has been a tragic reality for centuries. One should study Saint Blaise.

Samuel A. Nigro

We are losing our lives, our real lives, sitting here watching these actors pretend on television. There is nothing there that's real!

Name Lost

Impressionism means believing one's immediate impressions at the expense of one's more permanent and positive generalizations. It puts what one notices above what one knows. It means the monstrous heresy that seeing is believing.

G.K. Chesterton

You are able to strengthen others only insofar as you are aware of your own weakness.

John Paul II

It was our infirmities that He bore,. . .we had all gone astray like sheep, each following his own way; but the Lord laid upon him the guilt of us all.

Isaiah 53:4-6

The spiritual, mystical dimensions of the Church are much greater than any sociological statistics could ever possibly show.

John Paul II

But man, proud man,
drest in a little brief authority,
most ignorant of what he's most assur'd,
his glassy essence like an angry ape
plays such fantastic tricks before high heavens
as make the angels weep.

Shakespeare (*Measure for Measure*)

Ye gods, alas, why call on things so weak for aid? Yet there is something that doth still cry out when one of us hath woe!

Euripides

Lift one thought in prayer for S.T.C. that he with many a year with toilsome breath found death in life may here find life in death.

Samuel T. Cooleridge

Abandon all hope ye who enter here.

Dante - sign on the entrance to hell

A secret land awaits me. . . .

Faust

Angels are singularities in and at spiritual infinity. If good and beauty are to be maintained, more justice comes from considering the angels!

Samuel A. Nigro

All things corruptible are but a parable. Eternal womanhood leads us above.

Mystical Chorus from Faust

. . .destiny will take him where he is to go and will lead him to the end that is to end him. . . . That is all I know. . . .

Madam DeFarge

Murder will out and nothing can prevent God's honor spreading.

Chaucer

I am looking for any loopholes I can find.

W.C. Fields near the end of his life when asked about his reading the Bible all of the time.

Yeah. . .to another world.

Dimmesdale

However long you live, I never can wish you a greater happiness than this.

Mrs. March

Truth. . .I love much.

The last words of Leo Tolstoy

(A picked rose may). . .serve to symbolize some sweet moral blossom that may be found along the track or relieve the darkening close of a tale of human frailty and sorrow.

Nathaniel Hawthorne

Thou art too late. With God's help I shall escape thee now.

Dimmesdale

He died as he lived. . . without noticing.

Alexander Dumas the Younger about his father's death

I will no longer need your remedies. . . .

Dimmesdale

They speak of eternal reconciliation and eternal life. . . .

Turgenev's description of the flowers that grow on the grave of the Nihilist (Bazarov)

This is what I think of you. . . . You will go forth from these walls but will live like a monk in the world. You will have many enemies, but even your foes will love you. Life will bring you many misfortunes but you will find happiness in them and will bless life and will make others bless it which is what matters most.

Father Zossina to Alyosha

Tonight I'd just like to be wrapped in life and quilts, squeezed into a small place beside my family under the seven stars of the Big Dipper, and that's how I'd like to be buried someday.

Christopher de Vinck

When we have come to the end of a thing we have come to the beginning of it.

G.K. Chesterton

Its mind was sad, wandering and death-dwelling. . .his doom near at hand which the old man must salute and seek his soul award parting asunder life from body. . . .

Beowulf

You are the last remnant of our race. Destiny has taken all my kinsmen to the Godhead. . . earls and their valor. I shall follow them.

Beowulf's final words to Wiglaf

As he was very close to death, a young boy entered the room. The man was in turmoil, throwing himself deeper and deeper into an agony he could not understand. The young boy was the dying man's son. The child reached over and took his father's hand. The boy then pressed his father's hand into his own face, and the boy wept. Seeing this, the father suddenly understood. At that moment he understood. He saw a light, a bright light. He watched his son weep, and the father knew that there, weeping before him, was the world and all the world had to offer us human beings: love. The boy simply loved his father. That is all. That is everything, and everything to come.

Christopher de Vinck

I cannot tell you the sadness I felt when I learned from your August issue that I had died. On 23 February 1994, the date of my reported demise, I was in Egypt as part of my sabbatical. I do not remember feeling poorly; in fact, I do not remember how good it felt to be alive. Since my return from the sabbatical, my appearances can be deceiving. I will miss me, as there is no one that I know and love better.

Thomas Everitt Wilson, 68, correcting a University of North Carolina Alumni Report

Time bereaves everyone.

Name Lost

. . .I knew that a positive, passionate, living, and everlasting joy is the only reality.

Paul Claudel

Out of donations received, the officials pay themselves first.

Isabel Paterson

That is about what occurs with organized charities having endowments. They support a lot of kind friends in cushy jobs.

Isabel Paterson

At last I emerged again to see the stars. . . .

Dante leaving Hell

I came back from the holiest waters new, remade, reborn. . . . Healed of winter's scars. . .perfect, pure and ready for the stars.

Dante leaving Purgatory

The underlying force that creates and unites humanity is the love that moved the sun and the other stars.

Dante leaving Heaven

What you become is the transcendental itself — that angelic part of you which then will carry your name resounding forever in eternity.

Name Lost

The whole of anything is never told. . . .

Henry James

It's the wallpaper or me. One of us has to go.

Oscar Wilde as he lay dying in the grungy room of his death

. . .the men signed of the Cross of Christ go gaily in the dark.

G.K. Chesterton

Free will as positive doctrine was the original affirmation of Christianity. . . when death was regarded rather as an event in time emancipating the soul from temporality to a wider sphere, free will entered into faith.

Isabel Paterson

Any man's death diminishes me because I am involved in mankind and therefore never send to know for whom the bell tolls. . .it tolls for thee.

John Donne

A writer is driven far out passed where he can go. . .out to where no one can help him.

Ernest Hemingway

And Extreme Unction does the same for everyone else.

A fellow ain't got a soul of his own but only a piece o the big one. . .and then. . .then it don't matter. Then I'll be around in the dark. I'll be ever where. Wherever ye look. . .wherever there's a fight. So hungry people can eat, I'll be there. . .wherever there's a cop beatin up a guy, I'll be there. . . .

Casey

If you're in trouble or hurt or in need, go to poor people. . .they're the only one's who'll help. . .the only ones.

Ma Joad

A man gits a knife into ya and ya jis gonna do somethin and I done it with a shovel and I would do it agin and I ain't proud o it neither. . . . Now let's git goin. . . .

Tom Joad

We all see the moon. We all, at one time or another, recognize in the moon a pull toward a distant space that offers us a moment's grace and a certainty that we are going to be OK.

Christopher de Vinck

Put back thy sword into its place, for all those who take the sword will perish by the sword.

Matthew 26:52

The lie is the father of violence.

Reverend Vincent O. Miceli

Violent delights have violent ends.

Shakespeare

You cannot serve both God and money.

Matthew 6:24/Luke 16:13

He touched her hand; the fever left her, and she got up and began to wait on him.

Matthew 8:15

I am not worthy that you should come into my house. Just say the word and my servant shall be healed.

Luke 7:6-7

We are all here only in passage.

Venetian gondolier

We enter here. . .into an unknown realm, into a foreign realm, the realm of joy. A hundred times less known, a hundred times more foreign, a hundred times less ourselves, than the kingdoms of sorrow. A hundred times more profound, I believe, and a hundred times more fecund. Happy the man who may one day have some idea of it.

Charles Pegui a few days before his death

The faculty of being shy is the first and most delicate of the powers of enjoyment.

G.K. Chesterton

The yardstick of immortality guides and succors real Catholic life. What else matters?

William Marra

Sam: I would like to fly but I would not want to be a bird.

Sue: That's good. I don't think the birds would be happy with you either.
I'm glad I'm not a bird too; it would probably kill my back.

Sit tibi terra levis — may the earth lie light upon you... et lux perpetua luceat ei — and let the perpetual light shine upon him.

Burial Prayer

A minor operation is one that is on someone else.

Name Lost

Tragedy is the incense offering to God since the Fall.

Samuel A. Nigro

Do you believe in Heaven? Heaven is, my sons! Do you not believe in Hell? Hell is my sons!... You can kill me: my body I leave behind, but my soul will rise to Heaven... I pardon you and in Heaven I will pray for you.

Cruz Laplana Laguna, Bishop of Cuenca, Spain to the Communist sympathizing Republicans who were to murder him during the Spanish Civil War in 1936

What a beautiful night this is for me! I go to the house of the Lord!

Florencio Asensio, Bishop of Barbastro, Spain just before his murder, Communist Republicans during the Spanish Civil War in 1936

Keep your death before your eyes each day.

St. Benedict

I live and you will live.

John 14:19

I try to take life as it comes, and just hope it keeps coming.

Ashleigh Brilliant

Now cracks a noble heart... Good night, sweet prince, and flights of angels sing thee to thy rest.

from Hamlet

For there is still a vision for the appointed time; it speaks of the end, and does not lie. If it seems to tarry, wait for it; it will surely come. . . .

Hab 2:3

Listen, I will tell you a mystery! We will not all die, but we will be changed!

1 Corinthians 15:51

Congratulations, you're home!

Brennan Manning on Extreme Unction

Our courteous Lord does not want His servants to despair because they fall often and grievously; for our falling does not hinder Him in loving us.

Julian of Norwich

Often breakdowns lead to breakthroughs.

Mary Michael O'Shoughnessy

Quit keeping score all together and surrender yourself with all your sinfulness to God who sees neither the score nor the scorekeeper but only His child redeemed by Christ.

Thomas Merton

I know I should do something. We just came from e hospital. Their mother died an hour ago. I just don't know what to do.

Man on a subway when asked by others to restore order by telling his three wrestling, screaming, shouting children to come back and sit down.

God did not make death, and he does not delight in the death of the living. For he has created all things that they might exist. . . . God created man for incorruption, and made him in the image of his own eternity, but through the devil's envy death entered the world, and those who belong to his party experience it.

Wisdom 1:13-14; 2:23-24

Death, after all, is totally democratic, every man contemplates his death and no man can escape it. . . . Powerful thoughts occur of one's own annihilation, the end of one's mind, one's power, "the end of me."

Joseph Mauceri

Euthanasia is *making* people die, rather than letting them die. . . . Put bluntly, euthanasia means killing in the name of compassion.

Rita Marker

I know of nothing that is safe except, possibly death.

Basil Grant

Since the Fall, there can be no synthesis without entropy.

Samuel A. Nigro

We will never pass away.

William Marra

The bell invites me, therefore hear it not, for 'tis a knell that summons thee to heaven or to hell.

Macbeth

Here no one lies buried.

Peer Gynt's epitaph for himself

Ah Christians, heavenly shoot, ye strangers on earth, who seek a city in heaven, who long to be associated with the holy angels, understand that ye have come here on this condition only, that ye should soon depart. Ye are passing on through the world, endeavoring to reach Him who created it.

St. Augustine

How little we need is one of the great wonders of our species. How much there is given is another.

James V. Schall

In the temporal order, a singularity is a point position at gravitational collapse wherein the space-time curvature position is infinite. So is Extreme Unction. You can be saved.

CHAPTER 8:

HOLY ORDERS

In the physical order, *dimensions* are space coordinates and time. Your human beingness is dimensions.

In the spiritual order, *Holy Orders* is "non-reactive listening" *dimensions* (of poverty, chastity, and obedience without time) in confluence with human *life* (personified by the Father). It conveys *fortitude* — the courageous practice of virtue in pursuit of good and avoidance of evil, especially when facing adversity.

"Woman behold your son. Behold your mother."

Holy Orders makes your dimensions — a facing adversity with fortitude in Life with the Father.

Live Holy Orders — a reliving of the experience of Jesus.

To be on the Cross.
To Enter The world of Liberty and to participate in the Incarnation.

In physics, *dimensions* are space coordinates (length, width, height, or equivalents) and time. So is Holy Orders (poverty, chastity, and obedience without time).

Holy Orders is the Sacrament by which bishops, priests, and other ministers of the Church are ordained and receive the power and grace to perform their sacred duties. Holy Orders are *dimensions*.

Holy Orders is wherein the universe is "non-reactively listened" to in the *dimensions* of poverty, chastity, and obedience without time, evoking and emoting the human principle of *life* (personified by the Father) activated by *fortitude*, i.e. the courageous practice of virtues in pursuit of good while confronting adversity.

Non-Reactive Listening

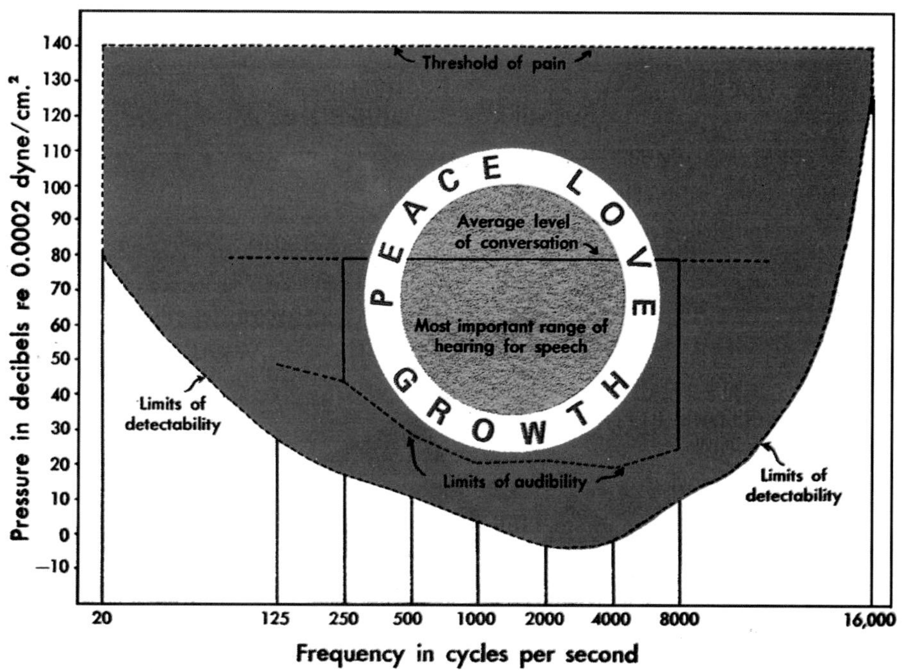

. . . One way to be a human being. Animals hardly listen; they mainly react, and reaction spoils the listening; But a human being accepts voluntary communications from another by allowing full expression without cues of acceptance or rejection. Such non-reaction allows the other to bring forth ideas, feelings, wishes, and fantasies which, if listened to, give understanding — the basis of growth, love, and peace.

Non-Reactive Listening

Listen with good eye contact, but not reacting. Allow him or her to elaborate fully what is important. Probing questions include: "Where have you been? How was it? What do you mean by that?" Or say nothing — but "I'm listening — tell me about it."

We must listen at the pace and peace of the other. We cannot hurry them in talking. We cannot rush to rescue either. Sometimes silence says a lot especially: "I have time for you. . ." or "I have poverty, chastity, obedience, and timelessness for all."

* * * * *

> We are obliged to yield many things to the Catholics — (for example) they possess the Word of God which we received from them; otherwise we should have known nothing at all about it.
>
> Martin Luther on the Bible

> Life is not so short but that there is always time for courtesy.
>
> Ralph Waldo Emerson

> It gives me great pleasure to converse with the aged. They have been over the road that all of us must travel, and know where it is rough and difficult and where it is level and easy.
>
> Plato

> Interminable arguments between heretics and Catholics generally have no other effect than to upset either one's stomach or one's brain.
>
> St. Irenaeus, circa 150 A.D.

> No matter how witty or how superficially rewarding, habitual sarcasm is too expensive a luxury. It costs too much in terms of human relationships.
>
> Anonymous

> His thoughts were slow, his words were few, and never formed to glisten.
> But he was a joy to all his friends — you should have heard him listen.
>
> Anonymous

> Life is not a 100-yard dash, but more a cross-country run. If we sprint all the time, we not only fail to win the race, but never even last long enough to reach the finish line.
>
> Joseph A. Kennedy

> The less you talk, the more you're listened to.
>
> Abigail Van Buren

> Stare. It is the way to educate your eye.
>
> Walker Evans

> The severest test of character is not so much the ability to keep a secret as it is, but when the secret is finally out, to refrain from disclosing that you knew it all along.
>
> Sydney J. Harris

The Church keeps us from being one of the masses — we are the counterpoise to crazy governments and to those who would rule and ruin us.

Samuel A. Nigro

About 250 A.D., Cyprian (Bishop of Carthage) wrote a book entitled: *On The Unity of The Catholic Church*, explaining how the unity of the Church is founded on the unity of the body of Bishops in union with the Roman See.

Pier Franco Beatrice

I would not believe in the Gospel were it not for the authority of the Catholic Church.

St. Augustine in the 4th Century

What a lovely surprise to finally discover how unlonely being alone can be.

Ellen Bursty

You can always tell something when it is non-Catholic — it makes you feel "good" without having to think or without having to be good.

Samuel A. Nigro

Friends are those rare people who ask how we are and then wait to hear the answer.

Ed Cunningham

There is not a social, political, or religious privilege we enjoy today that was not bought by the blood, tears and patient suffering of the minority. It is the minority who have stood in the vanguard of every moral conflict and achieved all that is noble in the history of the world.

John Bartholemew Gough

Even a family tree has to have some sap.

Los Angeles Times Syndicate

Holy Orders is the Sacrament by which bishops, priests, and other ministers of the Church are ordained and receive the power and grace to perform their sacred duties.

Baltimore Catechism

Confessors are doctors of the soul.

Dominic Savio

POPE PETER'S PRIMACY

When Christ was seized, they fled, after all the miracles they had seen. The one who stayed behind, who was the leader of the others, denied Him.

St. John Chrysostom circa 400 A.D.

Peter, the first pope, was the central character among the twelve apostles. His preeminence becomes obvious as we study the Bible.

Peter is the first apostle called by Jesus (Matt. 4:18).

It was Peter that Jesus called to come over the water from his boat (Matt. 14:28-29).

Peter was identified by Jesus as the rock on which the Church would be built (Matt. 16:18).

It was to Peter that Jesus gave the keys of the kingdom of heaven (Matt. 16:19).

It was to Peter that Jesus said, "Whatever you bind on earth shall be bound in heaven; and whatever you loose on earth shall be loosed in heaven" (Matt. 16:19).

It was to Peter that God sent the angel with the special revelation of Jesus' Resurrection (Mark 16:7).

It was to Peter first that the risen Jesus appeared (Luke 24:34), and from Peter's boat Jesus taught the multitudes (Luke 5:3).

It was Peter to whom Jesus said, "confirm your brethren" (Luke 22:23).

It was to Peter that Jesus entrusted the care and feeding of the Church — flock, lambs, and sheep (John 21:15-17).

Peter presided at the election of Matthias to replace Judas as an apostle (Acts 1:25), was the first to preach the Gospel to the Jews in Jerusalem (Acts 2:14), and performed the first post-Pentecost miracle when, in Jesus' name, he cured the lame beggar at the Temple (Acts 3:1-11).

It was Peter who replied to the Sanhedrin in the name of the whole Church (Acts 4:8-12), and he made the decision to admit Gentiles into the Church (Acts 11).

It was Peter who, after much argument at the Council of Jerusalem, stood up and said the words that made all present hold their peace (Acts 15:6-12).

It was Peter's decision that James ratified at the Council of Jerusalem (Acts 15:13-21).

Peter judged the case of Ananias and Sapphira (Acts 5:1-11).

It was to Peter as the chief apostle that Paul went after his conversion on the Damascus Road, staying with him for fifteen days (Gal. 1:18).

Every time the Bible gives us a listing of the apostles (Matt. 1);2-5; Mark 3:16-19; Luke 6:14-17; Acts 1:13, Peter is named first.

Peter is referred to 195 times in the pages of the Bible — the name of the next most frequently mentioned apostle, John, appears 29 times.

(Catholic Answers Newsletter, August 1989)

> Concerning these things, let us likewise look at that tradition in teaching and faith which was the Catholic Church's from the beginning, which the Lord gave, the Apostles preached, and the fathers guarded. For in this the Church has been founded and anyone who falls away from it neither is nor any longer is called a Christian.
>
> Athanasius, circa 330 A.D.

> Genuine Good coincides, in the long run, either overtly or covertly, with Rome. Beware of those ideas, however fashionable or pleasing, which are not compatible with the faithful Apostles.
>
> Samuel A. Nigro

> Success has nothing to do with what you gain in life or accomplish for yourself. It's what you do for others.
>
> Danny Thomas

> There are no rights without responsibilities.
>
> Pope John XXIII

The world belongs to those who get up early.

The Early Bird

By inflection you can say much more than your words do.

Malcolm S. Forbes

Those who know the least know it the loudest.

Joan Tosti

He who fishes for compliments can expect to be handed a line.

Ivern Ball

Many can rise to the occasion, but few know when to sit down.

Evan Esar

It requires wisdom to understand wisdom; the music is nothing if the audience is deaf.

Walter Lippman

We do not really want a religion that is right where we are right. What we want is a religion that is right where we are wrong.

G.K. Chesterton

Our Apostles knew, through our Lord, Jesus Christ, that there would be dissensions over the title of bishop. In their full knowledge of this, therefore, they proceeded to appoint the ministers I spoke of, and they went on to add an instruction that if these should fall asleep, other accredited persons should succeed them in their office.

Clement of Rome in 97 A.D.

Christ did not write a book. He founded a Church.

Michael Pakaluk

(That is all He founded. He did not found a country, government, or economic system either.)

The Catholic Church is the only thing which saves a man from the degrading slavery of being a child of his age.

G.K. Chesterton

Truth rests with God alone, and a little bit with me.

Yiddish Proverb

We learn about Christ in the Scriptures; we learn about the Church in the Scriptures. If you accept Christ, why do you not accept the Church?

St. Augustine

I am incurably convinced that the object of opening the mind, as of opening the mouth, is to shut it again on something solid.

G.K. Chesterton

The Roman pontiffs as the Vicars of Christ on earth have not willy-nilly imposed their ideas on the Church, but have responded to the Holy Spirit's distillate as it drifts through the baffles of life.

Samuel A. Nigro

Religious liberty might be supposed to mean that everybody is free to discuss religion. In practice it means that hardly anybody is allowed to mention it.

G.K. Chesterton

No prophecy in Scripture is the subject of private interpretation.

2 Peter 1:20

You have one teacher, Christ.

Matthew 23:10

Nothing of an *individual* is inspired. The Church is inspired.

William Smith

Some may well ask why, if we have Scripture we need the Tradition of the Church. The reason is that Scripture is so profound that not all understand it in the same way: different people understanding it differently. This man and that man understand it this way and that, explaining and interpreting its meaning according to their viewpoint. There are as many opinions as there are men holding them. It is necessary because of the variety of errors that have arisen that a line be drawn, to explain the meaning of the prophets and Apostles, along with the rule of Catholic and ecclesiastical tradition.

St. Vincent Lerins, circa 445 A.D.

It is for thee to hold fast the doctrine handed onto thee, the charge committed to thee.

2 Timothy 3:14

If "the gate is narrow and the way is hard," (Matthew 7:13-14) then yelling "I have been saved" a couple of times is just not going to do it.

Samuel A. Nigro

See how faith comes from hearing, and hearing through Christ's word.

Romans 10:17

This is my covenant with them, say the Lord: My spirit that is upon you, and my words that I have put in your mouth, shall not depart out of your mouth, nor out of the mouth of your children, nor out of the mouth of your children's children, says the Lord, from now until forever.

Isaiah 59:21

But the word of the Lord lasts forever. And this word is nothing other than the Gospel which has been preached to you.

1 Peter 1:25

The Apostles indeed have prescribed nothing about this (re-baptizing heretics) but the custom (of not requiring re-baptism) must be considered as derived from their Tradition since there are many things observed by the Catholic Church which are justly held to have been laid down by the Apostles, although they did not write them down.

St. Augustine

As the Father sent me, so I am sending you.

John 20:21

It is plain that the Apostles did not pass on everything to us in their writings, but many things were passed on orally. These are equally worthy of being believed. Hence let us regard the Tradition of the Church as the subject of our belief. Such and such a thing is a tradition: seek no further.

St. John Chrysostom, circa 400 A.D.

And he said to them, go into the whole world and preach the gospel to every creature. He who believes and is baptized shall be saved, but he who does not believe shall be condemned.

Mark 16:15-16

All scriptures inspired by God can profitably be used for teaching, for refuting error, for guiding people's lives and teaching them to be holy.

2 Timothy 3:16

This is not the same as saying that *only scripture* is inspired and profitable.

Michael Pakaluk

Make sure that you let God's Grace work in your soul by accepting whatever He gives and give whatever He takes from you.

Mother Teresa

It is not the things themselves which trouble us, but the opinions which we have about these things.

Epictetus (First Century A.D.)

There is only one mediator between God and man, Jesus Christ.

1 Timothy 2:5

We are Christ's ambassadors.

2 Corinthians 5:20

We must make use of Tradition; for all things are not to be found in Scripture.

St. Epiphanius, circa 350 A.D.

He who listens to you, listens to me; he who despises you, despises me.

Luke 10:16

The church here in Babylon, united with you by God's election, sends you her greeting, and so does my son, Mark.

1 Peter 5:13

It is not good to have several masters: let there be one chief, one king.

Homer

Thou art Peter and upon this rock I will build my Church.

Matthew 16:18

Simon, Simon, behold, Satan has claimed power over you all, so that he can sift you like wheat; but I have prayed for thee (singular) that thy faith may not fail; while, after awhile, thou hast come back to me (after the denial), it is for thee to be the support of thy brethren.

Luke 22:31-32

I am Christ's soldier; I am not allowed to fight.

Martin of Tours, circa 339 A.D.

Lord, to whom shall we go? Thou hast the words of eternal life.

John 6:69

Wheresoever the bishop shall appear, there let the people be, even as where Jesus is, there is the Catholic Church.

Saint Ignatius of Antioch, circa 80 A.D.

You never have to explain what you never said.

Patrick Buchanan

If any man preacheth unto you any gospel other than that which ye received, let him be anathema... For I make known to you, brethren, as touching the gospel which was preached by me, that it was not after man. For neither did I receive it from man, nor was I taught it, but it came to me through revelation of Jesus Christ.

Galatians 1:6-13

Your obedience to your bishop, as though he were Jesus Christ, shows me plainly enough that yours is no worldly manner of life, but that of Jesus Christ himself.

St. Ignatius Antioch in 100 A.D.

Test everything, retain what is good.

Thessalonians 1:5-21

Neither for these only (the Apostles) do I pray, but for them also that believe in me through their words; that they may all be one.

John 17:20-21

Our hearts are restless until they rest in you.

St. Augustine

I, therefore, a prisoner in the Lord, beseech you to walk worthily of the calling wherewith you were called... There is one body and one Spirit, even as also ye were called in one hope of your calling; one Lord, one faith, one baptism, one God, and Father of all.

Ephesians 4:1-6

Upon this rock I will build my Church and the gates of hell shall not prevail against it.

Matthew 16:18

The Church is the ultimate custodian and arbiter of Sacred Scripture and Sacred Tradition.

William Smith

Whoever preaches with love, preaches effectively.

Saint Francis de Sales

I have lived, Sir, a long time, and the longer I live, the more convincing proofs I see of this truth — *that God Governs in the affairs of men.*

Benjamin Franklin

If they have persecuted me, they will also persecute you.

John 15:20

I am a Christian and we do nothing vile.

Saint Blandina, circa 177 A.D.

But have confidence, I have overcome the world.

John 16:38

God hath reconciled us to Himself through Christ, and hath given to us the ministry of reconciliation. . . For Christ, therefore, we are ambassadors; God as it were, exhorting through us.

2 Corinthians 5:18-20

Real Good has only one "o."

Samuel A. Nigro

Religious devotion does not destroy: it perfects.

Saint Francis de Sales

Go ye, therefore, teach ye all nations. . . Teaching them to observe all things, whatsoever I have commanded you. And, behold, I am with you all days, even to the consummation of the world.

Matthew 28:19-20

If you deal well with objectivity, you will not have much problem with subjectivity.

Samuel A. Nigro

He that heareth you heareth me; and he that despises you despises me; and he that despises me despises him that sent me.

Luke 10:16

And when they had ordained to them priests in every church, they commended them to the Lord, in whom they believed.

Acts 14:22

Behold, how good it is, and how pleasant, where brethren dwell as one!

Psalm 132

Impose not hands lightly upon any man.

1 Timothy 5:22

Whosoever will come after me, let him deny himself, and take up his cross, and follow me. For whosoever will save his life, shall lose it; But whosoever shall lose his life for my sake and the gospel's, the same shall save it. For what shall it profit a man, if he shall gain the whole world, and lose his own soul?

Mark 8:34-37

You are built upon the foundation laid by the Apostles and prophets, and Christ Jesus himself is the foundation stone.

Ephesians 2:20

When we were sensible of danger, we had daily prayer in this room for divine protection. Our prayers, Sir, were heard and they were graciously answered.

Benjamin Franklin

Genuine trustworthiness translates into those committed to poverty, chastity, and obedience (to God). Anyone not so firmly committed cannot, at some level some time, be fully trusted.

Samuel A. Nigro

I envy those of you who are Catholics. You seem to have learned one of the great secrets in life, which is how to make a wheel for the long haul, and not feel compelled to re-invent some 28,000 of them, which, according to the *Oxford Encyclopedia of World Christianity*, is how many identifiable Protestant denominations and sects have been established since Martin Luther wasted a good nail posting his 95 theses on the door of Wittenberg Chapel.

Minister David Hartman

See into how many morsels those are divided, who have divided themselves from the unity of the Church.

St. Augustine

Christ did not say to his first company: "Go forth and preach garbage unto the world" but gave them, rather, truth to build upon.

Beatrice of Dante

Everyone who hears these my words, and acts upon them, shall be likened to a wise man who built his house on rock.

Matthew 7:23-24

. . .a fallible being will fail some-where.

Samuel Johnson

There are no false prophets, only slow learners.

James K. Fitzpatrick

Where Peter is, there is the Church.

St. Ambrose, circa 370

How can I unless some man shows me.

Acts 8:30

Do for others what you want them to do for you: This is the meaning of the law of Moses and the teaching of the Prophets.

Matthew 7:12

We should not forget that in the long run, the pope in Rome is a greater enemy of National Socialism (the Nazi Party) than Churchill or Roosevelt.

Heinrich Himmler (head of the Nazi Secret Service)

. . .The Son of Man has no place to lie down and rest.

Matthew 8:20

If one of you wants to be great, he must be the servant of the rest. . .

Matthew 20:26

To be in communion with the Bishop of Rome is to be in communion with the Catholic Church.

Cyprian of Carthage, circa 250

THE ROMAN CATHOLIC CHURCH
Want to be a member?
Want to be a leader?
. . . the greatest organization ever in human history.
Can you think of any other organization as old yet magnanimous, charitable, committed, non-political, rational, humanity-promoting, agelessly revolutionary, genuinely free and cultured, filled with ancient secrets, sacrificing, identity confering, truth seeking, oneness creating, good demanding, beauty promoting, life dedicated, male/female complementing (rather than competing), environmentally sound by Natural Law, and helping anyone and everyone in all ways i.e. catholic Catholic?
The Roman Catholic Church — synonymous with PEACE:
productive tranquility based on order emanating from truth established according to norms of empathic justice, sustained by charity under the auspices of gentle liberty.
Want to be a member?
Want to be a leader?

Samuel A. Nigro

In extreme necessity, all goods are common.

Old Roman Catholic Dogma

Do not make my Father's house a market place!

John 2:16

He for the world but little cared;
And at his feats the world was scared;
A crazy man his life he passed,
But in his senses died at last.

Epitaph for Don Quixote

Every other (local) church must concur with this Church (Rome) on account of its special pre-eminence.

St. Irenaeus, circa 170

Neither prison nor chains nor sentence of death can rob a man of the Faith and his own free will.

Franz Jagerstatter

Let us love our enemies, bless those who curse us, pray for those who persecute us. For love will conquer and will endure for all eternity. And happy are they who live and die in God's love.

Franz Jagerstatter

I follow no one as leader except Christ alone, and therefore I want to remain in union in the Church with you, that is, with the chair (office) of Peter. I know that on this rock the Church is founded.

St. Jerome (the first to set the New Testament to writing), circa 400

Journalists are totally dependent on others — therefore they are the biggest bunch of parasites in the world. They only report news instead of make it. . . In order to feel good about themselves, they need bad news which provides an arrogant, self-aggrandizement. Somehow, they can only "report" good news, but if it is bad news, they tend to make it and be part of the story themselves. Thus reporters ask questions to enhance themselves rather than only provide the truth and the facts of the matter.

Samuel A. Nigro

Bureaucracy defends the status quo long past the time the quo has lost its status.

Laurence J. Peter

Culture becomes deformed when its major institutions are so preoccupied with novelty, fashion and progress that they fail to communicate the wisdom of the past.

Donald DeMarco

Credo quia absurdum — I believe because it is absurd.

St. Augustine

The Fountain of Youth is the Roman Catholic Church by its virtues, transcendentals, and Sacramental life.

Samuel A. Nigro

The foundation myth in The Republic of Plato suggests we should believe that we live in a just order and do what is best for us when all is ordered to the good. At the beginning of Acts, it says, "Why stand you there looking up?" The myths we swear by tell us what we are.

James Schall

Opponents of Christianity will believe anything except Christianity.

G.K. Chesterton

God did not become man so that man could become a theologian.

Saint Ambrose

If you do not believe in religion, then you have no business saying anything about it.

Samuel A. Nigro

Life is probably round.

Vincent van Gogh, after being in the Roman Pantheon

Atheism is the supreme example of a simple faith.

G.K. Chesterton

Humanity has been blessed with a ponderously slow, intractable, self-correcting process — known informally as Natural Law and formally as the Roman Catholic Church.

Anonymous

The Church is the source and deposit of transcendentals. If you live transcendentally by Sacramental life in all you do, nothing can bother you for very long and you are always part of positive engagement in life.

Samuel A. Nigro

A religion that can exist in spite of its clergy MUST be divine.

Samuel A. Nigro

To maintain their own identity, God-is-dead theologians must come up with something different — otherwise it is they who are dead.

Samuel A. Nigro

What does your religion do for you? Give personal solace? Coping skills? A better world? Virtue? Values that last or expediency? Do you build cathedrals every day? Does your religion create problems or solve them?

Anonymous

How Catholic can the Church be without a language that crosses and defuses national and linguistic barriers which rend the world?

Anonymous

When it comes to good priests and good religious, I doubt we will ever do better than eleven out of twelve.

Anonymous

There is no person so narrow as the person who is sure that he is broad; indeed, being quite sure that one is broad is itself a form of narrowness. It shows that one has a very narrow ideal of breadth.

G.K. Chesterton

The believers in miracles accept them (rightly or wrongly) because they have evidence for them. The disbelievers in miracles deny them (rightly or wrongly) because they have a doctrine against them.

G.K. Chesterton

The Church's role is always to tell what is wrong and what is right!

Anonymous

For whatever else the fundamentalist is, he is not fundamental. He is content with the bare letter of scripture — the translation of a translation, coming down to him by the tradition of a tradition — without venturing to ask for its original authority.

G.K. Chesterton

That virtue cannot be taught is an ancient truism documented repeatedly by experience. But "what virtue is" can be taught, nay must be taught, if virtue is ever to be known or recognized for what happens.

Anonymous

You cannot deny that you are aware that in the city of Rome the episcopal chair was given first to Peter; the chair in which Peter sat, the same who was head — that is why he is also called Cephas — of all the apostles; the one chair in which unity is maintained by all.

Optatius, 367 A.D.

If I have spoken wrongly, bear witness to the wrong, but if I have spoken rightly, why do you strike me?

John 18:23

The person who possesses one virtue, possesses them all.
And the one who lacks a single virtue, lacks them all.
For prudence cannot be cowardly, nor unjust, nor
intemperate, since where any of these qualities actually
exist, prudence cannot (exist).

St. Augustine

Roman Catholicism is a METHOD of living as well as a theology and philosophy.

Samuel A. Nigro

My grace is sufficient for you, for my power is made perfect in weakness.

2 Corinthians 12:9

Simply put, the Bible commands our attention as a convincing witness to the truth of our spiritual inadequacy and God's supreme adequacy. The Bible performs its vital function admirably, and to require more of it will only in the end detract from the truth it was designed to promote.

Richard Becker

Ubi Petrus, Ibi Ecclesia — Where Peter is, there is the Church.

Anonymous

If you can't sleep, all you got to do is start to read a book. If it is really bad, I grab a Bible. The devil doesn't like me reading that book, so he puts me to sleep right away.

Betty Howard

. . .the central paradox of religious faith: the secret of happiness lies in removing the right to be happy. . .

Christopher Lasch

. . .one cannot prove the Scriptures by quoting Scriptures. They are not self-validating.

Father Richard Murphy

There is a difference between the words of Scripture and the Word of God, and nowhere in the classic creeds is there any mention of "believing" in a book; we are called to believe in a person.

Richard Becker

Reason is itself a matter of faith. It is an act of faith to assert that our thoughts have any relation to reality at all.

G.K. Chesterton

Money, sex, and power are the basic destroyers of trust, which is why the only genuinely trustworthy people are those who can faithfully keep their promises of poverty, chastity, and obedience.

Samuel A. Nigro

No scientist is going to explain this world! Go to church.

Anonymous

. . .preach the words in season and out of season.

2 Timothy 4:2-3

Our students are supposedly smarter, more free and more independent than ever but they cannot read the same works in the same time students did five and more years ago. Television is one of the main causes limiting their ability to remain focused on a book for a mere two hours of reading at one sitting. It is very sad.

Cornelius O'Boyle, University of Notre Dame
professor of Great Books Program, 1995

If you judge, investigate.

Seneca

If mankind can create plows and airplanes, bins full of food, computers and nuclear energy, then a Higher Being (stifle your arrogance) can readily create the world.

Anonymous

Liberty is traditional and conservative; it remembers its legends and its heroes. but tyranny is always young and seemingly innocent, and asks us to forget the past.

G.K. Chesterton

And as to you Death, you bitter hug of mortality, it is idle to try to alarm me.

Walt Whitman

Everyone keeps saying "if I knew then what I know now. . ." It's time to face the fact that we're going to be stupid for the rest of our lives, so why fight it? Learn from it, and laugh at it.

Michael D. Nigro

The Church must not allow itself to be swept away by the movements of the age.

Karl Barth

Will power comes in two directions: positive and negative. The negative comes with an addicting excitement. The positive comes with a seemingly silly enjoyment which sets one genuinely free.

Anonymous

The world will only be more just to the extent that it is more chaste.

Georges Sorel

Authority is the only alternative to slavery. Thinking without reference to authority has left us without any claim to liberty.

G.K. Chesterton

For whoever hath sinned without the Law, will perish without the Law; and whoever hath sinned under the Law, will be judged by the Law. For it is not they who hear the Law that are just in the sight of God, but it is they who follow the Law that will be justified. When Gentiles who do not possess the Law carry out its precepts by the light of nature, then, although they have no Law, they are their own Law, for they display the effects of the Law inscribed on their hearts. Their conscience bears witness to them, and their own thoughts argue the case on either side, against them or even for them, on the day when God judges the secrets of human hearts through Christ Jesus.

Romans 2:13-16

You must be different. You must not be just a doctor, or just a lawyer, or teacher or parent or spouse. You must bring to your life, and the lives of those around you, the love of God that Christ came to share with all of us. Ultimately, you will not be judged by your brains, your beauty, your wealth, or your degree from Notre Dame; but rather by the rare spiritual values such as charity, self-sacrifice, honor, honesty, a sense of fairness, and love.

E. William Beauchamp, to graduating class of University of Notre Dame

Our society is obsessed with first impressions. We may not have a second chance to make a first impression, but a teacher may have additional chances to make what is far more important — a lasting impression.

Donald DeMarco

Of all the forms of charity. . . in the hospitals, those of some Catholic Sisters were the most efficient. More lovely than anything I've ever seen in art. . . are the pictures. . . of those modest Sisters going. . . among the suffering and the dying. . . . They were veritable angels of mercy.

Abraham Lincoln in his Civil War diary

Pride impels everyone to develop, add on, correct, amend, emend, elaborate, and to aggrandize one's self by an imagined "improvement" of all that has gone before. For many, their's is an identity process which depends on making truths different than what has been given. And thus we have theologians.

Samuel A. Nigro

Don't pay attention to what people say. Pay attention to why they say it.

Archbishop Fulton Sheen

The priest performs the essential work of the apostles:
1. by effectively proclaiming the Gospel;
2. by gathering together and leading the community;
3. by remitting sin;
4. by celebrating the Eucharist;
5. by exercising Christ's work of redeeming mankind and glorifying God perfectly.

Bishop Donald Wuerl

For God is not unjust, that he should forget your work and the love that you have shown in his name, you who have ministered and do minister to the saints. But we want everyone of you to show to the very end the same earnestness for the fulfillment of your hopes; so that you may become not sluggish but imitators of those who by fate and patience will inherit the promises.

Hebrews 6:10-12

Open a Protestant Bible, and you will find there are seven complete Books awanting — that is, seven books fewer than there are in the Catholic Bible, and seven fewer than were in every collection and catalogue of Holy Scripture from the fourth to the sixteenth century. Their names are Tobias, Baruch, Judith, Wisdom, Ecclesiasticus, 1 Maccabbes, 2 Maccabbes, together with seven chapters of the Book of Ester and six verses from the third chapter of Daniel, commonly called "the Song of the Three Children." These were deliberately cut out, and the Bible bound up without them. The criticisms and remarks of Luther, Calvin, and the Swiss and German reformers about the seven Books of the Old Testament show to what depth of impiety those unhappy men have allowed themselves to fall when they broke away from the true Church.

Henry G. Graham

Make every effort to supplement your faith with virtue, virtue with knowledge.

2 Peter 1:5

If one embraces fully the Roman Catholic life, i.e. the amusing, bewildering, quaint, simple, playful, prayerful Church-following style, ignoring the self-conscious silliness of it all, thereby occurs an amazing rebellion against the seductive, contagious evils of the age resulting in:

(a) a child-like joy which is as free as one can ever get;
(b) a oneness with humanity and the planet which is as close to Nature as one can ever get; and
(c) a transcending beyond constricting material components thereby enabling a Supernaturalness which is as unearthly as one can ever get.

You will laugh more and love faithfully. You will produce more. You will be less bothered by anything. (These are the psychological benefits)... And you get Heaven.

You will not find it to be simple silliness at all but the strange effectiveness of genuine ancient secrets.

Samuel A. Nigro

The religious man was born to be saved; psychological man was born to be pleased.

Philip Rieff

You should never try to teach a pig to sing: it can't be done, and it annoys the pig.

Robertson v. White, 633 F.Supp. 954, 959 (W.D.Ark. 1986)

The Law of Nature dictated by God himself is superior to any other. It is the binding over all the Globe, in all Countries, and at all Times. No human laws are of any validity if contrary to this, and such of them are as valid derive all of their force and all their authority mediately and immediately from this Original. Upon these two foundations, the Law of Nature and the Law of Revelation, depend all human laws. Human laws are declaratory of the act in subordination to Divine Law.

William Blackstone

The earth is like any musical instrument and must be played by the instruction manuals, in the case of the earth: Natural Law.

Anonymous

Nothing works very well for very long without virtue.

Anonymous

. . .organization is always disorganization.

G.K. Chesterton

Catholic doctrine and discipline may be walls; but they are the walls of a playground.

G.K. Chesterton

Give a man a fish and you feed him for a day. Teach a man to fish and you feed him for a lifetime.

Chinese Proverb

God, deliver me from sour-faced saints, please!

St. Theresa Avila

Another manifestation of Original Sin is the need for people to change things always believing they are making an improvement.

Anonymous

No one serving as God's soldier entangles himself in worldly affairs, that he may please him whose approval he has secured. And again, one who enters a contest is not crowned unless he has competed according to the rules.

2 Timothy 2:4-5

After observing all the trouble the world's peoples are in, you know the Church is right.

Anonymous

If one embraces the mundane, everyday minor truths, the great truths take care of themselves.

Anonymous

Christianity is not a philosophical speculation, a sociological synthesis, or a public relations scheme. It is a revelation from God.

John Cardinal O'Connor

Once virtue and transcendentals are ignored, all that is left are violence, orgasm and lies (the opposites of poverty, chastity, and obedience).

Anonymous

When you want to test the depth of a stream, don't use both feet.

Chinese Proverb

When the fox begins to preach, look to your geese.

German Proverb

Make a crutch of your cross.

English Proverb

Remember, a closed mouth gathers no foot.

Steve Post

Never let people see the bottom of your purse or of your mind.

Italian Proverb

So keep your eye on God by knowing, loving, and serving Him.

Anonymous

Male/Female Differences

Male

Transcendetals - masculine-tm

Res -matter organizing
-procreative dimension
-fathering
-corporeal principle

Verum -truth enhancing
-social orienting
-reality principle

Bonum -good promoting
-work
-choice principle

activating style
centrifugal
sacrifice

Female

Immanentals-feminine-tf

Aliquid -form/identity/essence
-forming
-mothering
-activating principle

Unum -oneness
-unifying desirables
-family orienting
-relational principle

Bella -beauty
-elevating beyond
-total humanity
-ascendant principle

unifying style - unitive dimension
centripetal
give life

The transcendental actuality of all created being has seven components:

1. *Ens* (Latin) — what has existence.

2. *Res* (Latin — which is the *corporeal body*, i.e. the confluence of the being with the matter completing it. It is the most visible dimension for those in the material world. In nature, nature rules, neurochemistry and all, on how the being manifests itself in nature. Bodies are needed to relate. They are our physical being by which men interact with all.

3. *Aliquid* — which is the *identity* or *form* of the being, i.e. the confluence of the being with its *essence* — for humans, not ethnicity, not color, nor anything but human beingness — the total embracing of humanity for us — in a word "catholic" —(all for and with all).

4. *Verum* (Latin) — which is the *truth* of the being, i.e. the confluence with real life and not television shows, movies, magazines, newspapers or figments of imagination from oneself or others.

5. *Unum* (Latin) — which is the *oneness* of the being, i.e. the confluence of the being with itself and all desirability related to it: its integrated, whole entirety.

6. *Bonum* (Latin) — which is the *good* of the being, i.e. the confluence of the being with proper function in nature, or for mental beings, with proper choice in Natural Law (or Rational Environmentalism).

7. *Bella* (Italian. . . preferred by the author to the Latin "Pulchritude" for multicultural reasons and the economy of two syllables) — which is the *beauty* of the being, i.e. its confluence with ascendancy or the "bringing out the best of itself and all around it."

BE A REAL MAN OR REAL WOMAN IN TUNE WITH THE UNIVERSE! — Bubbles of sanity in an ocean of chaos.

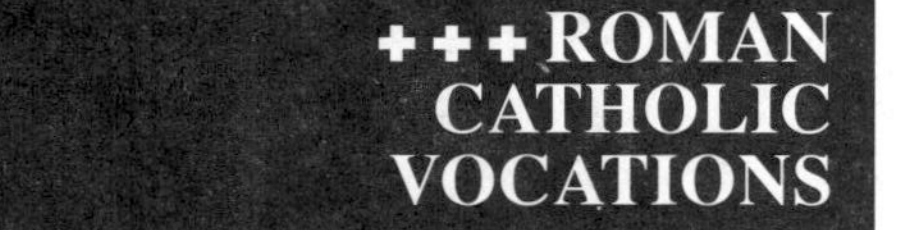

THE TRANSCENDENTAL PERMANENCE OF MEN:

-MATTER – (Res) — Organizing matter in all being

-TRUTH - (Verum) — Seeking, finding, enhancing truth and reality for self and society.

GOOD - (Bonum) — Promoting good by properly choosing in accordance with the animal kingdom, the planet and the universe.

THE IMMANENTAL PERMANANCE OF WOMEN:

-IDENTITY - (Aliquid) — forming the identity and essence of human beingness in all others.

-ONENESS - (Unum) — establishing unity with the desirables of all, enabling all to embrace all.

-BEAUTY - (Bella) — bringing out the best in one's self and all others all the time.

Know that the key to human relationships and all life is not sex, no matter what anyone claims. Priests, sisters and all believers know the keys to life and relationships are the TRANSCENDENTALS of all created being:

•Ens (Latin) — what has existence

•Res (Latin) — which is the corporeal body, i.e. the confluence of the being with matter completing it. It is the most visible dimension for those in the material world. In nature, nature rules, neurochemistry and all, on how the being manifests itself in nature. Bodies are needed to relate. They are our physical being by which men interact with all.

•Aliquid (Latin) — which is the identity or form of the being, i.e. the confluence of the being with its essence — for humans, not ethnicity, not color, nor anything but humanbeingness — the total embracing of humanity for us — in a word "catholic" — (all for and with all).

•Verum (Latin) — which is the truth of the being, i.e. the confluence of the being with reality and not fantasy — or for us humans, the confluence with real life and not television shows, movies, magazines, newspapers or figments of imagination from oneself or others.

•Unum (Latin) — which is the oneness of the being, i.e. the confluence of the being with itself and all desirability related to its integrated, whole entirety.

• Bonum (Latin) — which is the good of the being, i.e. the confluence of the being with the proper function in nature, or for mental beings, with proper choice in Natural Law (or Rational Environmentalism).

•Bella (Italian. . . preferred by the author to the Latin "pulchritudo" for multicultural reasons and the economy of two syllables) — which is the beauty of the being, i.e. its confluence with ascendancy or the "bringing out the best of itself and all around it."

Holy Orders

POVERTY

-For life. . . the Father.
-Doing sacrifice for the good of others.

CHASTITY

-For genuine liberty. . . Jesus the Son.
-Uplifting strength maintaining natural oneness.

OBEDIENCE

-For the faithful pursuit of happiness. . . the Holy Spirit
-Promoting 2000 year-old truths & always being ahead of one's time.

THE ONLY TRUTSTWORTHY MEN AND WOMEN +++

Committed to the Transcendental God & His Founded Church

No problem. But remember, where there is no solution, there is no problem.

Simon Peres

My watchmen are blind, all of them unaware; they are dumb dogs, they cannot bark; dreaming as they lie there, loving their sleep.

Isaiah 56:10

Power tends to corrupt and absolute power corrupts absolutely.

Lord Acton

Never bolt your door with a boiled carrot.

Irish Proverb

Listen like hell all the time.

Spencer Tracy

Any fool can see the case for liberty; it is precisely the very intelligent who are left watching with some suspicion the general indifference to authority.

G.K. Chesterton

It is much easier to organize than to think.

G.K. Chesterton

Avoid, as you would the plague, a clergyman who is also a man of business.

Saint Jerome

Let not the authority of the writer offend thee whether he be of great or of small learnings; but let the love of pure truth draw thee to read.

Thomas a Kempis

Be still and know that I am God.

Psalms 46:10

(So stop shouting.)

Render unto Caesar the things which are Caesar's and unto God the things which are God's.

Matthew 22:21

Believe those who are seeking the truth; doubt those who find it.

Andre Gide

Sell not virtue to purchase wealth.

English Proverb

Trust, but verify.

Old Russian Proverb

Never is he more active than when he does nothing; never is he less alone than when he is by himself.

Publius Cornelius Scipio (Africanus) also known as Hannibal

All prayers are answered. We need to distinguish between a prayer unanswered and one not answered how or when we would like it to be.

Lloyd Ogilvie

Never trust a reporter with a nice smile.

William Rauch

Our prayers should be for blessings in general, for God knows best what is good for us.

Socrates

Those skilled in war subdue the enemy's army without a battle.

Sun Tzu

There is good in everybody. Boost — don't knock.

Warren G. Harding

Be aware that a halo has to fall only a few inches to be a noose.

Dan McKinnon

Pray to God only for those things which you cannot obtain from man.

Pope Xystus I

Take care that no one hate you justly.

Publius Cyrus

The secret of patience: Do something else in the meantime.

Anonymous

I like to speak of prayer as listening. We live in a culture that is terribly afraid to listen. We'd prefer to remain deaf. The Latin root of the word "deaf" is "absurd." Prayer means moving from absurdity to obedience. Let the words descend from your head to your heart so you can begin to know God. In prayer, you become who you are meant to be.

Henri J.M. Nouwen

Be a good listener. Your ears will never get you in trouble.

Frank Tyger

The way to become boring is to say everything.

Voltaire

You must not expect old heads upon young shoulders.

English Proverb

Latin tells you something is going on and it keeps one focused and refocused on the message of the church: that there are deep secrets in the Being of All.

Samuel A. Nigro

Now I recall to your minds, the Gospel that I preach to you, which also you receive, wherein also you stand, through which also you are being saved if you hold it fast, as I preached it to you. . .

1 Corinthians 15:1-4

Assuredly, no philosophy outside the influence of Christianity could make intelligible the benevolence by which the superior being desires, without compromising his own status, the good of the inferior being. No such (non-Christian) philosophy could comprehend that. . .the good Shepherd loves his sheep to the point of giving his life for them.

Pierre Duhem

Latin makes one aware that there are unknowns and other ways of doing things — that there are mysteries beyond us. Latin gives an aura of: "There is more than meets the eye and it is difficult to understand and that is all right."

Name Lost

There is an embitterment that comes almost automatically with non-Christian beliefs. . . an embitterment readily discernible in the emotional distortions and convictions which seem to always accompany those who profess nothing but this world one time or many times. This bitterness is engendered from the unfair pointlessness of such a world. The universe does not fulfill unless sanctified by Christ.

Samuel A. Nigro

No matter whatever else is done, keep telling the Bishops to "DO YOUR DUTY."

Anonymous

Act as men of thought. Think as men of action.

Henri Bergson

If they were to keep silence, I tell you the very stones would cry out.

Luke 19:39-40

Before the rooster crows today, he will deny me three times.

Matthew, Mark and Luke

It is for thee to hold fast to the doctrine handed on to thee, the charge committed to thee.

2 Timothy 3:14

Self, self has half filled Hell.

Scottish Proverb

Moral codes are always obstructive, relative, and man-made. Yet they have been of enormous profit to civilization. They *are* civilization. Without them, we are invaded by the chaotic barbarism of sex, nature's tyranny, turning day into night and love into obsession and lust.

Camille Paglia

WESTERN CIVILIZATION

The concepts of Western Civilization have been getting bad press recently. This can only be if people do not know what the concepts of Western Civilization are. . . which means that our educators are doing a worse job than the press and media. After 40 years of distortion and suppression of Western civilizing concepts, what else can be expected besides the collapse of civilization?

Indeed, what has been touted as the failures and crimes of Western Civilization in reality have been its lack of implementation or its betrayal.

Those who decry Western Civilization will find themselves using it and invoking it whether they want to or not when they attempt to present alternatives. Indeed, the biggest challenge for anyone who is allegedly against Western Civilization is: What is your alternative? And intellectually defend it. Unwittingly, when they try to do this, they will be practicing Western Civilization. This is because Western Civilization provides the fundamental structures of existence, and vice versa.

Perhaps it devolves down to Socrates' admonition that "the unexamined life is not worth living" (or a more contemporarily relevant tautology: "the emotional-only life is not worth living") to which can be added "the unexamined proposition is not worth believing." A corollary of this (and a truism) is: When you examine your life (really examine it!), you end up with the concepts of Western Civilization.

So what is Western Civilization — Absurd to summarize in a paragraph or two, but, let us try.

Western Civilization is scholarship, rules, standards, deliberated criticism and a fundamental focus on virtue and transcendentals. Ideas and actions will be challenged unrelentingly and nothing will be without criticism. Western Civilization is "Socratic dialogue" open to all, about all, without demand for agreement and with the prohibition of violence. It is to care about everything by everybody by thinking.

A few undeniable Western Civilization concepts (and Western Civilization is being espoused whenever any of these are invoked): Faith, hope, and charity; transcending; prudence, justice, fortitude, temperance and all derived virtues; international law, private property, objective rules, liberty, just war, civil rights and duties, rational environmentalism (Natural Law), family, monogomy, monotheism, personhood, science, democratic capitalism, ethics; and the processes of analyzing by which all ideas are then discarded, corrected, amended, and then absorbed in transcendentals for all; and then all is put in writing and placed in a library for further study.

A clear example of Western Civilization: Music — written, uplifting, analyzed, and not only performed but transcribed and stored in a library.

Indeed, a case can be made that a library is the sine qua non of Western Civilization — and vice versa.

Another example: Universities, i.e. centers of learning focusing on "universals" (the transcendentals, of course, even if unnamed) by which reason and scholarship embrace the universe as it is in reality. There is no dualism of "this is real" and "this is religion" as if the two do not have to be the conformable. No, Western Civilization demands a unity, and there can be no incompatibility between reality and truths held. Indeed, this very fact distinguishes Western Civilization from its alternatives (which are always its opposites) and it also has given Western Civilization its power over matter.

Western Civilization is a sponge absorbing all offered or discovered after filtering it through a virtue-transcendental analysis. It is a demand for the analysis of transcendental differences conforming to reality and reasoning as objectively as possible.

Western Civilization is bridge-and-gate-building seeking to embrace and define existence by common Humanity and common Beingness. It cares for Being not constricted nor confined but open to whatever new idea challenges the tried and true still faithfully adhered to. Western Civilization is the cerebral approach accommodating all ideas, analyzing them, and putting them in a library, resulting in a Noosphere — a layer of thinking or a thinking envelope about the earth.

Western Civilization helps one to transcend beyond what one is, to the fullness of Humanity — and if not, then its opposite: tribalism — or constricted self-conceit — is the result.

The opposite of Western Civilization is constricted tribalism — where only the group matters and not total Humanity. The opposite of Western Civilization is bigotry — where a person gets so caught up in his own characteristics that he dehumanizes and disgraces himslf by withdrawing from the fullness of Humanity. For such tribal-oriented people, the concept of virtue is usually limited to a selfish inwardness ignoring the rest of humanity and total Existence. In addition, the transcendentals of matter, form, truth, oneness, goodness, and beauty, are rendered secondary to the tribe. An opposite of Western Civilization is the lack of a thoughtful middle class. Another opposite is that which separatists (self-exalting groups) are and promote. Un-Western, un-Civilization is epitomized by the not-examined life wherein one professes emotionalism and subjectivism, confining one's self to decrees that are incompatible with reality by belligerently and imperialistically saying, "It is this way because I say so. . . don't examine me."

Thusly, untruths, prevarications, and the unnatural are characteristics of un-Western un-Civilization (and whatever results from this will prove that "untruth is the root of all evil").

The specific piece of behavior characteristic of un-Western un-Civilization: Someone unable to admit to being wrong.

Some examples of un-Western un-Civilization: the rages of racists: the marauding aggrandizement of Black Study groups; the puerile punning, illogic, tolerated plagiarism, and pseudoscholarship of feminist "academics"; the duplicity of tyrants; the historical appropriations and distortions by Mohammed; the actions of the homosexual group ACT UP; The Book of Mormon; the rabbi invading the Catholic convent in Poland; feminism's anti-male sexism which is unique in history by its group-based, consciously-organized willed hatefulness of the other sex; animalism; verbicide; pornography; "New Age" PaganoChristianity; and non-being in any form.

Regardless of decriers, Western Civilization is not white, European, or even Western. It is nothing less than the processes of the fullness of Humanity or fullness of Being — and perhaps "Full Humanity" or "Full Being" would have been better names.

Western Civilization is only rejected by those who do not really know what it is. In essence, it is derived from Nature and therefore it is Natural Law applied.

The concepts of Western Civilization need to be studied, promulgated, promoted and embraced in the struggle and examination of life. Those who do so will find joy regardless and also progress will be the end-result. Those who do not do so will rail like savages motivated to argue blindly rather than transcend, encompass, and embrace the world.

ADDENDUM:

Western Civilization embraces all Mankind and is therefore Catholic.

In fact, another accurate name for Western Civilization is Secular Catholicism. The real meaning of the word "catholic" is "everyone." Everyone means everyone. Real Catholics think of themselves as Everyone — regardless of race, color, creed, and any difference between individuals. This is done by virtue, transcendentals, and by living the sacraments — everything else is secondary. When this is done, difficult as it is, differences that separate individuals and groups are transcended, and humanity is embraced supernaturally as Catholic and catholic — which is why liberals and scientists prejudicially struggle to resist "Western Civilization," i.e. It is Catholic.

For those interested, Western Civilization becomes Roman Catholicism (rather than Secular Catholicism) by merely asserting that it is most rational that God would communicate to humanity primarily by reason through a Church and a Book rather than by subjective emoting and "anything goes."

Samuel A. Nigro

> The Church admits its own evil — something no other group does. Hmmm. . . — and then it defies all who would do wrong.

Samuel A. Nigro

> Continuity with the past is a necessity, not a duty.

Oliver Wendell Holmes, Jr.

> If the world is not rational, science is not possible; if the world is not contingent, science is not necessary.

L. Newbigin

> The quality of specificity lies at the level of the relationship between matter and form, while the quality of contingency concerns the levels of the connection between essence and existence. The road of contingency is therefore one which cannot be traversed by science alone; the use of philosophy is required.

Paul Haffner

> Unlike an angel who needs no conquests and unlike an ape uninterested in them, man thrives on conquests which are the fruit of a mysterious union in him of matter and mind.

S.L. Jaki

I am a Catholic man and a priest; in that faith I have lived and in that faith I intend to die. If you esteem my religion treason, then I am guilty; as for other treason, I have never committed any, God as my judge.

Edmund Campion, S.J. at his being condemned to die by Queen Elizabeth I

Anytime you see a turtle atop a fence post, you know it had some help.

Alex Haley

No reasoning can engage those unconcerned whether they are right or wrong.

Pierre Duhem

Eternal as it is, logic can afford to be patient.

Pierre Duhem

What God has separated no man should join together.

S.L. Jaki

How about a little verve?!

Name Lost

You are never so important that you cannot be replaced.

Evelyn Nigro

With the progress of the times, the knowledge of the spiritual fathers increased; for, in the science of God, Moses was more instructive than Abraham, the Prophets more than Moses, and the Apostles more than the Prophets.

Pope Gregory the Great

Thou hast learned from many who can witness to it, the doctrine which I hand down; give it into the keeping of men thou canst trust, men who will know how to teach it to others besides themselves.

2 Timothy 2:2

WHAT EVERY TRUTH-LOVING PERSON SHOULD KNOW ABOUT GALILEO

1. Galileo did not discover heliocentricity. Some ancient Greeks and Romans did with Aristotle and Ptolemy trying to refute it.

2. Galileo added nothing new to Copernicus' elaboration of heliocentricity. Copernicus was a Polish priest who really promoted and studied the sun as center of the star system as then known; he was never in conflict with Rome because he knew he was dealing with an unproven hypothesis and never made grandiose statements because of it. However, Galileo attempted to prove heliocentricity by using mathematical calculations about the tides of the earth. Galileo's calculations were inadequate and indeed heliocentricity was really not thought to be proved to scientific level of acceptance until mid-19th century. In fact, the Church had every reason to reject Galileo on the basis of the evidence he was providing. Galileo happened to be right but not because of his "proofs." He had no right on the basis of his calculations to demand the Church change its interpretation of Scripture.

3. Galileo was rather pompous and unapproachable when thinking he was right. For example, he was obsessed by perfect circular orbits and much of his work was actually opposed by Francis Bacon.

4. Galileo was know-it-all blind to Kepler's elliptical orbits and Kepler's three laws verified time and again to the present day. Johannes Kepler (died 1630) accepted the heliocentric hypothesis and was vehemently condemned by the Protestant faculty at Tunbingen University some ten years before Galileo was condemned by the Church.

5. Galileo was condemned not for heliocentricity but because he claimed his mathematical calculations proved heliocentricity when they did not, and that because of his calculations the Church must reinterpret Scripture. Essentially, the Church said: You have not proven it. Stop claiming so until you do. Stop demanding Scripture be reinterpreted on the basis of your inadequate evidence.

6. Objectively, Galileo was neither a martyr nor an unselfish pursuer of truth. He was not condemned by a pope but by a cardinals' court because he made religious claims linked to his physical evidence which was inadequate to prove what he was claiming at the time.

7. Galileo was never tortured but was honorably detained and mildly reproved. . . and he died peacefully in his own bed.

8. Most anti-Church comments about the Galileo incident are either entertainment or stupid anti-Catholicism, neither historical nor instructive, except how bigoted and ignorant people can construct and reconstruct history to suit themselves and promote their own agenda.

The greatest wrong in the Galileo case was not Galileo's confused capitulation; or his arrogant, erroneous reasoning; or his reliance on other's methods without attribution; or his pretending to discover what Copernicus (a Polish priest always in good standing with Rome) had already proclaimed; or his "founding" science but then not using it well enough to make his claim (Amazing, if Galileo was the first real scientist, he was also the first to ignore real science).

The greatest wrong was not in the Church's demand for better analysis and proof of Galileo's assertions; or its refusal to evaluate and revise scriptural interpretations because of Galileo's grandiose insolence; or the Church's affirmation of tradition in the face of what could have been merely a loud fad until really proven.

No, the greatest wrong lay not in what Galileo or the Church did.

The greatest wrong lay in those who reported (and still report) on the Galileo case tendentiously to promote their own agenda be it anti-Catholicism, anti-religion or just plain misanthropic know-it-all, better-than-thou show biz by which they obviously were (and are) hoist by their own petards.

Samuel A. Nigro

When I was fully confident the Church of Rome was the only, true Church, I joined her.

John Henry Newman

Man is too noble to serve anyone but God.

Cardinal Stefan Wyszynski

Who hears you, hears me.

Luke 10:16

Whoever does not take up his cross and follow me, is not worthy of me.

Matthew 18:38

Whoever separates himself from the Church. . .is separated from the promise of the Church. . . He cannot have God as his Father who does not have the Church as his Mother.

Saint Cyprian

If I had to choose one word to define being a Catholic, it would be "more" — more faith, but more aggravation; more hope, but more pain; more joy, but more sorrow — more of everything. I attribute this heightened sense to being immersed in the "real thing," to being embraced by the Mother instead of the Aunt, to being out of the frying pan and into the fire of God's love.

Sally Box — convert

You have the New Testament and the Old Testament, and the Shepherd of the Church to guide you; let this be enough for your salvation.

Dante Alighieri, 1201 A.D.

As in each diocese, there is one bishop who is the head of the Church among that people, so in the whole Church and over all Christian people, there is one supreme bishop, namely the Pope of Rome, successor to St. Peter, that the Church militant may bear the likeness of the Church triumphant where One presides over the whole universe. . . The priesthood is the spiritual power conferred on the ministers of the Church by Christ for the purpose of dispensing the Sacraments to the faithful.

John of Paris, O.P., 1306 A.D.

It is surely harmful to souls to make it heresy to believe what is proved.

Galileo, 1642 A.D.

One of the great artifices the devil uses, to engage men in vice and debauchery, is to fasten names of contempt on certain virtues, and thus fill weak souls with a foolish fear of passing for scrupulous, should they desire to put them into practice.

Paschal, 1662 A.D.

The Church of the Lord is built upon the rock of the Apostle among so many dangers in the world; it therefore remains unmoved.

St. Ambrose, 380 A.D.

If anything could sustain and support a wise man in this life or help him preserve his equanimity amid the conflict of the world, it is, I think, meditation on the knowledge of the Bible.

St. Jerome, 380 A.D.

He prays too little who only prays when he is on his knees. But he never prays who, while on his knees, is in his heart roaming the fields.

St. John Cassian, 400 A.D.

Let us now come to the sacraments of the new covenant. They are baptism, confirmation, the blessing of the bread which is the Eucharist, penance, extreme unction, ordination and marriage. Of these, some offer a remedy for sin and confer helping grace. Others strengthen us with grace and virtue.

Peter Lombard, circa 1100 A.D.

The Roman Church remains the head of all the churches and the source of Catholic teaching. Of this there can be no doubt. Everyone knows that the keys of the kingdom of heaven were given to Peter.

St. Thomas Becket, circa 1170 A.D.

Upon his faith and teaching, the whole fabric of the church will continue to be built until we all reach the full maturity in Christ and attain to unity and faith and knowledge of the Son of God.

St. Thomas Becket, circa 1170 A.D.

All important questions that arise among God's people are referred to the Judgment of Peter in the person of the Roman Pontiff.

St. Thomas Becket, circa 1170 A.D.

A priest has the primacy of Abel, the patriarchate of Abraham, the government of Noah, the order of Melchizedek, the dignity of Aaron, the authority of Moses, the perfection of Samuel, the power of Peter, the unction of Christ.

Peter Bloisus, 1212 A.D.

My life is poverty, chastity, and obedience — no money, no honey, and a boss. I just live the corporal and spiritual works of mercy. It's great!

Brother Richard Roemer

For as I see it, it is not so much from books as from the living and permanent voice that I must call prophet.

St. Papias, circa 125 A.D.

A priest blesses, he is not blessed except by bishops; he imposes hands, he does not ordain. . . A deacon does not bless. . .a deaconess does not bless, nor do any of the things which priests and deacons do: she alone minds the doors and ministers to priests when they baptize women, for decency's sake.

Constitutions of the Apostles, circa 350 A.D.

God's cause is often hurt by people who are trying to save God.

Edward Dowling, S.J.

It seems to me necessary to wait until someone comes to instruct us how we ought to conduct ourselves toward God and Men.

Socrates

If the author had been less industrious, this book would be twice as long.

Evelyn Waugh about one of his novels

If Christianity is historical, Catholicism is Christianity.

Cardinal Manning

Men should be changed by Religion, not Religion by men.

Bishop of Viterbo

For it is not the faithful who hear the Law that are just in the sight of God, but it is they who follow the Law that will be justified.

Romans 2:13

The real Christ is dangerous and untame. He defies our laws: born of a Virgin, transubstantiating bread and wine into His Body and Blood, passing on the power to do so to a select group of men, resurrecting from the dead, ascending into Heaven, and remaining with His Church until today. He demands our submission and our incorporation into Him, if we are to escape the ruin brought us by our first ancestor. In a word, He is terribly uncomfortable.

Charles A. Coulombe

It is only in romances that people undergo a sudden metamorphosis. In real life, the main character remains exactly the same.

Isadora Duncan

No wise man ever wished to be younger.

Jonathan Swift

QUIET PLEASE, THE BOSS IS ASLEEP.

Sign on office door of Stephen Hawking

Being free from the fetters of Dogma means holding opinions without knowing why.

G.K. Chesterton

In short, a man does not know what he is saying until he knows what he is not saying.

G.K. Chesterton

Thou shalt call me Father and shalt not cease to walk after me.

Jeremiah 3:19

Have we not all one Father? Hath not one God created us? Why then doeth everyone of us despise his brother?

Malachi 2:10

Yahweh, the teacher of mankind
knows exactly how we think,
how our thoughts are a puff of wind.

Psalm 94:10

You shall serve strange gods day and night who will give you no rest.

Psalm 40:4

What can be made clean by the unclean? And what truth can come from that which is false?

Sirach 34:4

Without a dream, people perish.

Name Lost

All I know is how to use my hands, but I still must not starve my mind. I try to feed my brain books, the proper books. If people starve their minds, they will die.

Migrant farm worker

Q: Why are you Catholic?
A: What else is there?

Walker Percy, convert

The Old Testament describes God as "Father" only eleven times. Jesus, by contrast, uses the term at least 170 times. This unfailing use of this form by Jesus leads us to believe that calling God "Father" was a central part of Christ's revelations.

Chris Kaczor

Reason is a whore.

Martin Luther

And without it, you are a fool.

Samuel A. Nigro

"The Bible and only the Bible" is an absolutist and anti-historical slogan of anthropological subjectivism, presumption, and terror.

Name Lost

The Roman Catholic Church is appropriately defined as Basic Being Realism.

Samuel A. Nigro

Saints are the only celebrities worth imitating.

Name Lost

Out of step, out of date, and out of this world!

A Roman Catholic priest's description of his vocation

Those who bad mouth Western Civilization are actually bad mouthing themselves.

Name Lost

HAVE YOU EVER MET A BISHOP BEFORE?

St. Basil: These tortures. . .what would they do to me? Not having a body except so to speak the first blow. Of these things only, are you Lord. But death would be an act of kindness for it would bring me nearer to God, for whom I live and for whom I have been created and to whom in the greater part I have died and towards whom I hasten. . .

Imperial Emissary (threatening St. Basil to accept a heresy): I am astonished. No one until now has spoken to me in such words. . .

St. Basil: Perhaps you have never met a Bishop before. Where God is endangered and exposed, there all other things are considered as nothing.

NO, I GUESS NOT.

A celebrity feasts on public attention, a role model thrives on personal commitment. The former thirsts for the adulation of the crowd, the latter is content with the obscurity of the home.

Donald DeMarco

A thing is true in so far as it conforms to its proper idea in God's knowing mind and in so far as it actualizes the ideal toward which it is ordered by God's knowing mind.

St. Thomas Aquinas

A good priest is higher than a King.

Name Lost

The Bible's purpose is not to teach how heaven goes but to teach how to go to heaven — under direction of the Church.

Name Lost

Blessedness, beatitude, is what all of us are seeking all the time *in* and *by* everything we seek. Blessedness is always our end, whether our means is pleasure or power or riches or virtue or wisdom or honor or anything else. Blessedness is the *summum bonum*, "the greatest good." Everyone seeks it, but not everyone finds it, because not everyone knows where it is. St. Augustine says, "Seek what you seek, but it is not where you seek it." Not everyone has a road map. Jesus gives us the road map for our lives.

Peter Kreeft

I must follow them, I am their leader.

A man marching to the barricades in Paris, 1848

When men turn their backs on the lie, the lie ceases to exist purely and simply. Such a contagious disease (lies) can only exist when men cooperate with it. Our way must be a refusal knowingly to give support to the lie in any way whatsoever.

Alexander Solzenietzen

We should take our estimation of human good not from the foolish but from the wise.

St. Thomas' answer to the popular skeptical question, "who's to say?"

Happiness is joy in truth.

St. Augustine

. . .those who believe that they believe in a living God, and who live as though He had never existed: these are the real atheists.

Octavio Paz

Money, unlike happiness, is good only when spent, not kept.

Peter Kreeft

You can't beat a horse with no horse.

Name Lost

No one can answer the truth except concerning what he knows.

St. Thomas Aquinas

So, before you believe anybody, find out what they really know.

The bad guys ignored the Church back then, just like you guys do today. . .

Universal Catholic retort

Absolute authority is no more than the service to the people of God. . . .It is sweet and gentle. . . .It never speaks a language of force, but it is expressed in the love of brethren and in the truth.

Pope John Paul II

True law is right reason in accord with Nature. Changeless and everlasting, it imbues all men. By its commands, it summons to duty. By its prohibitions, it averts from wrongdoing. To alter this law or to repeal any part of it is forbidden by all that is holy while to abolish it is impossible. We can be free from it neither by the Senate nor by the people nor need we look outside ourselves for its exposition and interpretation nor will there be one law in Rome and another in Athens, one now and another in ages to come. Rather, a simple sempiternal and immutable law will hold among all nations and for all time. And there will be one master and commander over us all: God, the author, promulgator and enforcing judge of this law.

Cicero

. . .the same yesterday, today and forever. . .

Hebrews 13:8

All differences of opinion are theological at bottom.

Cardinal Manning

I have found my vocation at last. My vocation is love. . . Charity gave me the key. . .

St. Therese of Lisieux

No one has the right to make up stories and call it history; anyone who does ought to be shot.

Name Lost

Thinking is the conversation of the soul.

St. Thomas Aquinas

Resigned virtue in the face of suffering is what the Roman Catholic Church is all about anyway.

Name Lost

You are my friend if you do the things I command you.

John 15:14

God instituted prayer to communicate to creatures the dignity of causality.

Paschal

God's love is hierarchically ordered, as ours should be. Does anyone really think we should love people no more than animals?

Peter Kreeft

There is no point to praising, blaming, counseling, encouraging, or commanding a machine.

Peter Kreeft

God wrote two books: nature and scripture.

Medeval Maxim

You are separated from Christ, you who are trying to be justified by law; you have fallen from Grace.

Galatians 5:4

Take care not to be misled. Many will come in my name saying "I am He" and "the time is at hand." Do not follow them.

Luke 21:8

Women becoming priests is like the Church trying to become Jesus.

Name Lost

Superiority is being able to accept one's own unique qualities with composure.

Name Lost

Faith without works of justice is not sufficient for salvation; neither is righteous living secure in itself of salvation, if it is disjoined from Faith.

St. Gregory of Nyssa, 360 A.D.

Live with it.

Vince Lombardi

Where obedience is lacking there grace is lacking too.

Thomas Merton

Once God makes sense and becomes rational in one's own mind, everything changes!

Samuel A. Nigro

Where am I from? Well, I stay in Cleveland, but I live in Rome.

Name Lost

You are alone. But how you handle that fact determines your loneliness.

Name Lost

If you say one thousand times that you are a Christian and continually sign yourself with the cross of Christ, but do not give alms according to your means, and you do not want to have love and justice and chastity, the name of Christian will profit you nothing. . .

Caesar of Arleys, 542 A.D.

The Faith is old and the devil is bold
Exceeding bold indeed
And the methods of doubt that are floating about
Would smother a mortal creed.
But we who sit in a sturdy Faith still can drink strong ale
Can put all away to infallible truths that always shall prevail.

Hilaire Belloc

Many want the benefits which only Western Civilization can give but are incapable of understanding that these benefits are intrinsically linked to knowing, understanding and implementing the principles of Western Civilization. Having not embraced the principles, they end up condemning that which they have not tried. And not having tried the principles of Western Civilization, they can never obtain that which they say they want. You cannot have the benefits without living the principles.

Samuel A. Nigro

The commitment of the Roman Catholic Church to truth, oneness, goodness, and beauty is without peer on the planet and in all history. This is an amazing persistence in spite of temptations. Accompanying this is an amazing historical observation: that those in opposition to the Church invariably end up making covert exceptions to their own professed opposing principles which are usually framed in terms of emotional correctness rather than truth, oneness, goodness, or beauty. Indeed, unless exception is made for themselves to their own anti-Church principles, they will be forced to recognize their own errors.

Samuel A. Nigro

It is oldest, immeasurably the oldest, throne in Europe (in the world); and it is the only one that a peasant could climb. . . I speak of the pure peasant advanced for pure merit. This is the only real elective monarchy left in the world; and any peasant can still be elected to it.

G.K. Chesterton on the Papacy

We can all love mankind if we remember not to judge them by their leaders.

G.K. Chesterton

It is no disgrace to Christianity, it is no disgrace to any great religion, that its counsels of perfection have not made every single person perfect. If after centuries, a disparity is still found between its ideals and its followers, it only means that the religion still maintains the ideal, and the followers still need it.

G.K. Chesterton

. . .an honest man must always respect other religions, because they contain parts of his religion — that is, of his largest vision of truth.

G.K. Chesterton

The difference between two philosophies is like the difference between two solutions of a geometric problem. The difference between two religions is like the difference between the smell of onions and the smell of the sea.

G.K. Chesterton

The world has not repeated proverbs because they are proverbial, but because they are practical.

G.K. Chesterton

. . .if every human being lived a thousand years, every human being would end up either in utter pessimistic skepticism or in the Catholic creed.

G.K. Chesterton

The wise man's understanding turns him to his right; the fool's understanding turns him to his left.

Ecclesiastes 10:2

Fame is like a river, that beareth up things light and swoln, and drowns things weighty and solid.

Sir Francis Bacon

The Catholic Church is the only *the* church.

Lenny Bruce

I have fought the good fight, I have finished the race, I have kept the Faith. Henceforth there is laid up for me the crown of righteousness, which the Lord, the righteous judge, will award to me on that day, and not only to me but also to all who have loved his appearing.

2 Timothy 3:7-8

There is only one religion in the world. Beyond it, there are only storytellers and philosophers — and never, 'til Bethlehem, could the twain meet.

G.K. Chesterton

I have not come to bring peace, but a sword. . .

Matthew 10:34

Eighty-six years have I served Him and He has done me no wrong. How can I blaspheme my King who has saved me?

St. Polycarp at his martyrdom

It is good to live, but that life for which we yearn is better. And good it is to see the light of day, but to see the true light is better. And all these things are good; but the reason we flee from them is not that we long for death, or hate God's words, but because of the surpassing greatness of other things.

Pionius at his Martyrdom

I must have in mind the Catholic Church, which is dispersed from the East even unto the West.

Bishop Fructuosus of Tarragona, the first martyr of Spain
in 259 testifying to the presence and universality of the Church

Consider your birthright. Think who you are. You were not made to live like brutes, but to pursue virtue and knowledge.

Wallace Stegner

Kissing someone is like sucking on a 30 foot tube with shit at the other end.

Medical school biology professor

Are you ignorant that the custom has been for word to be written first to us, and then for a just decision to be passed from this place?. . . For what have we received from the blessed Apostle Peter, that I signify to you.

Pope Julius to Eusebius of Constantinople, 340 A.D.

Tear then with any torture you wish this weak body of mine. Over that you have power but over my soul you have none.

Bishop Philip of Heraclea at his martyrdom

To change place is not to change your nature. The greedy who demand more lose all. Danger often comes from where we least expect. There is always someone worse off than you.

Aesop

Some bishops only talk the language of, the craziness of, the fashion of the age, thereby rejecting the cornerstone as they fail in their duty.

Name Lost

My standing alone does not make the truth a whit weaker.

Pope Liberius to Emperor Constantine, 355 A.D.

He was a man sure, foursquare, complete, unassuming, humble before his God, at home upon the earth, neighbor to the sky. Hence he was unconquerable.

Warren H. Carroll about Alfred the Great

Match foes, stroke for stroke.

Name Lost

Let no one seek for a third hand. . .

Athanasius

I am telling you that he who lives in comfort and yet accepts alms is not a religious man.

St. John Chrysostom

Monks are the athletes of Christ.

Warren H. Carroll

No one can love his neighbor on an empty stomach.

Woodrow WIlson

Peter has spoken through Leo!

Cry of the Bishops at Council of Chalcedon, 451, upon hearing the full reading of Pope Leo's tome statement on the incarnation and the divine and human Natures of Christ

Father, if thou art willing, remove this cup from me; nevertheless not my will, but thine, be done.

Luke 22:40-42

"Greater love no man has than to lay down his life for his friends" (Jn. 15:13). What a privilege as well as a lifetime challenge: to be Christ the priest-savior for contemporary mankind!

John H. Miller, CSC

After the final fall of Rome when marauding bands swept unchecked through previously "secured" and "pacified" regions, the counter-values of the Christians emerged and began to take flesh in society. The most obvious carriers of these values were bands of monks who set themselves down by rivers and streams and made a promise of stability, a vow to spend their lifetime in their communities. The motto of these men, followers of Benedict of Nursia, was of course Pax, and their ideal was that work was prayer.

Eileen Egan

Thank God! I knew something was on your mind. I thought you wanted a divorce.

Frank Bruder to his Kosher-home-keeping Orthodox Jewish wife, Judith, when she told him she was to become a Catholic

If you're going to do something wild like become a Christian, at least be an Episcopalian. They have more class.

Frank Bruder

An old Jewish story concerns a woman who stopped going to the Synagogue. One day the Rabbi went to her house and asked to sit with her by the fireplace. For a long time, neither spoke. Then the Rabbi picked up the tongs, took a glowing coal from the fireplace, and set it on the hearth. As the two watched the coal slowly lost its glow and died. A few minutes later the old woman said, "I understand. I'll come back to the Synagogue."

Mark Link

Will no one rid me of this troublesome priest?

Henry II

It is better to curse the darkness than to light the wrong candle.

Motto in fireworks factories

Eastern wisdom has a natural attraction for astonishingly stupid people.

G.K. Chesterton

The more you think of yourself, the more you aggrandize your own particular characteristics. The more you constrict yourself into your own kind, the worse it is for everybody else and for yourself too, because to the degree you delimit yourself to your own kind, the less fully human (make that "Catholic") you are.

Samuel A. Nigro

The *carpe diem* religion is not the religion of happy people, but of very unhappy people. Great joy does not gather the rose buds of May; its eyes are fixed on the immortal rose whom Dante saw.

G.K. Chesterton

You can do me no greater kindness than to suffer me to be sacrificed to God while the place of sacrifice is still prepared. Thus forming yourself into a chorus of love, you may sing to the Father in Jesus Christ that God gave the bishop of Syria the grace of being transferred from the rising to the setting sun. It is good to set, leaving the world for God, and so to rise in Him. . . Beg only that I may have inward and outward strength, not only in mind but in will, that I may be a Christian not merely in name but in fact. For, if I am one in fact, then I may be called one and be faithful long after I have vanished from the world. . . Christianity is not the work of persuasion, but, whenever it is hated by the world, it is a work of power.

I am writing to all the churches to tell them that I am, with all my heart, to die for God. . . Let me be thrown to the wild beasts; through them I can reach God. I am God's wheat; I am ground by the teeth of the wild beasts that I may end as the pure bread of Christ. . . Fire and cross and battling with wild beasts, the breaking of bones and mangling of members, the grinding of my whole body, the wicked torments of the devil — let them all assail me, so long as I get to Jesus Christ.

Neither the kingdoms of this world, nor the bounds of the universe can have any use for me. I would rather die for Jesus Christ than rule the last reaches of the earth. My search is for Him who died for us, my love is for Him who rose for our salvation.

St. Ignatius of Antioch

Natural Law is a universal pattern and action, applicable to all men everywhere, required by human nature itself for its completion.

John Wild

You don't know what you're asking.

Jesus to Mary

Take away the supernatural and what remains is the unnatural.

G.K. Chesterton

There is no question about it: Information and whatever-one-talks-about affects the brain chemistry. So, be careful of what you expose yourself to and of what you expose to others, especially youths. You can affect their chemistry.

Samuel A. Nigro

Nothing fails like success.

G.K. Chesterton

Man proposes, God disposes.

Russian Proverb

O Jesus/our great High Priest/hear my humble prayers
on behalf of your priests.
Give them a deep faith/a bright and firm hope/
and a burning love/which will ever increase/
in the course of their priestly life.
In their loneliness/comfort them/
In their sorrows/strengthen them/
In their frustrations/point out to them that it is through
suffering/that the soul is purified/and show them
that they are needed by the Church/they are needed
by souls/they are needed for the work of redemption.
O Loving Mother Mary/Mother of Priests/take to
your heart your sons who are close to you/because
of their priestly ordination/and because of the power
which they have received/to carry on the work of
Christ/in a world which needs them so much.

Be their comfort/be their joy/be their strength/and
especially help them to live and to defend the ideals
of consecrated celibacy. Amen.

John Joseph Cardinal Carberry
Archbishop of St. Louis

Common things are never commonplace.

G.K. Chesterton

Oh, Jesus Christ, is it you again? (watch your emphasis)

Name Lost

Receive all guests as Christ.

St. Benedict

Why not become all flame?

Abbot Joseph to a troubled colleague

The end of all our exploring
And know the place for the first time.

T.S. Eliott

When you come to a place where have to go left or right, go straight.

Sister Ruth

Ghosts don't exist in some cultures. They think time exists.

Martin Broken Leg

For a Father of the Church, such as St. Augustine, there was no particular difficulty about the idea of miracle. In a way everything is a miracle. At the marriage of Cana, Jesus made water into wine and everybody was astounded; but rain becomes wine in our vines everyday, and we take it all as a matter of course. Nevertheless, it is God who creates the rain and the vine and the wine; but He does it regularly, and we get so accustomed to it that we cease to wonder.

Etienne Gilson

Tradition is truer than fashion.

G.K. Chesterton

Too much involvement in *res* (sex, structures, and sociopolitical stuff) interferes with living in a real life embracing and projecting the other transcendentals.

Samuel A. Nigro

Not he who fears but he who loves is the true believer.

Zacharias Frankel

Hope for the best but be prepared for the worst.

Boy Scout advice

Socrates insisted many times that the true philosopher to attain truth and to be like God, should have as little as possible to do with things of the body.

William G. Most

The act of the believer terminates in the reality, not in the proposition.

St. Thomas Aquinas

The fatal thing about facts is that they do not last. It is the only idea that lasts.

G.K. Chesterton

If you can't pray it open, don't pry it open.

Lydell Rader

The biggest problem in human relationships is confusing the person with their ideas.

Samuel A. Nigro

If only I could find this Book
whose origin is eternal,
whose essence is incorruptible,
whose knowledge is life,
whose script is indelible,
whose study is desirable,
whose teaching is sweet,
whose depth is inscrutable,
whose words are ineffable,
yet all are a single Word!
Truly, whosoever finds this Book
will find Life,
and will draw Salvation from
the Lord.

St. Bonaventure c. 1250

The Church has nothing to do with nations — the Church existed before nations. The Church is pre-national, not "international."

Samuel A. Nigro

The Catholic is scarcely ever frightened of the Protestant picture of Catholicism; but he is sometimes frightened of the Catholic picture of Catholicism.

G.K. Chesterton

Whenever the Church imitates the state and the culture of the state, that is when the Church errs.

Samuel A. Nigro

Go out and seek.

Song of Solomon 3:2

. . .swift as the eagle, fleet as the stag. . .to do the will of thy Father.

Sayings of the Fathers

If religion is illuminated by tolerance, if it should and can go hand in hand with morality, then we not only do one another no harm, but come closer to one another, until our religions run practically side by side.

Simon Deit to his son Phillip at the
latter's conversion to Catholicism

The absolute truth depends on truth.

Name Lost

And after the fire, there was a still, small voice.

1 Kings 19:12

The first law of history is not to dare to utter falsehoods; the second, not fear to speak the truth.

Pope Leo XIII

The good or the evil does not lie in the wisdom but in the one who sees it and in whether or not she profits by it with humility; for if humility is present, no harm can be done not even by the devil. And if humility is not present, even if the visions be from God, they will be of no benefit.

St. Theresa of Avila

Rebuke them sharply that they may be sound in faith.

Titus 1:13

A woman could never be Pope because the Pope is infallible only part of the time.

Father Stanley Rudcki

Words are the only things that live forever.

G.K. Chesterton

A book not worth reading twice is not worth reading once.

C.S. Lewis

Amen, I say to you, there is no one who has given up house or wife or brothers or parents or children for the sake of the Kingdom of God who will not receive back an overabundant return in this present age and eternal life in the age to come.

Luke 18:29-30

Wherefore, labor the more, that by good works you make sure you are called and elected.

2 Peter 1:10

Be doers of the word and not hearers only, deceiving your ownselves.

James 1:22

Truth is sacred; and if you tell the truth too often nobody will believe it.

G.K. Chesterton

The aim of argument is differing in order to agree; the failure of argument is when you agree to differ.

G.K. Chesterton

If you wish to enter into life, keep the Commandments. . .

Matthew 19:17-18

It would be "perilous" to confuse religious freedom as a principle of civil order and Christian freedom inside the Church.

Monsignor George A. Kelly phrasing a
principle of John Courtney Murray

Many of my friends say, "Forget about Israel and the Jews — they will never allow themselves to be Jewish *and* Catholic. We will never convert the Jews." I suspect they are correct, but I would add that in our own way, we Catholics are Jewish, which means we cannot turn our back on ourselves. In the same manner, Islam is linked to Rome in ways overlooked to the sad fate of millions because they have misunderstood the origin of the Koran which Mohammed got, in part, from the Church. We Catholics cannot turn our backs on our Muslim brothers and sisters anymore than the Jews.

Samuel A. Nigro

Your thoughts should be wholly directed to all that is true. All that is honest, pure, admirable, decent virtues worthy of praise. Live according to what you have learned and accepted. What you have heard me say and do. Then will the peace of God be with you.

Philippians 4:7-9

In the eyes of rabbinic law, non-Jews do not have the same status as Jews unless they renounce idolatry and observe the "Seven Commandments of the sons of Noah. The Seven Universal Commandments were developed by the rabbis of the talmudic era. They are: (1) recognition of the rule of law in society; (2) the prohibitions against idolatry; (3) against blaspheming God; (4) against murder; (5) against sexual impropriety; (6) against theft; and (7) against cannibalizing animals, that is, ripping a limb from a living animal for food.

David S. Ariel

See. All Roman Catholics *are* Jewish.

When humanity is simply human, it is simply heathen.

G.K. Chesterton

A man telling the truth has careless eyes.

G.K. Chesterton

"Catholic" means that one is linked to *all* being because God is in all being. Only the Natural Law deals with being as such unfettered by anything less than Catholicity.

Samuel A. Nigro

It is not a matter of "I think/you think," but a matter of what nature and nature's God teaches through the Church.

Francis Arinze

If the errors of the Church are enough to condemn it by some then so much more condemned must be the government, the press and media, and big business.

Samuel A. Nigro

What is your view of the universe? The answer to that question determines what is real, serious, and expected from the person.

Samuel A. Nigro

A priest. . .when he intends to perform an exorcism over persons tormented by the devil, must be properly distinguished by his piety, prudence, and integrity on life.

Roman Ritual

Nothing doing!

Fr. William S. Bowdern, S.J. (when told he was to exorcise the possessed child in St. Louis in 1949)

You've got it.

Archbishop Joseph E. Ritter

Disney — that avalanche of poison — and we Catholics thought that only the British frightfully torched and roasted priests.

Samuel A. Nigro

Life is like a night at a bad inn.

St. Theresa

The major question is: How do you live in God's geography and the world's at the same time? The answer is Transcendentally.

Samuel A. Nigro

The most pathetic people are those who have abandoned their ancestors for something less and are caught up in the craziness and sinfulness of the age. . . And the most pathetic aspect of that is their superficialness such that they do not even know it.

Samuel A. Nigro

First of all, you must understand then that no prophesy of Scripture is a matter of one's own interpretation.

2 Peter 1:20

The error, however, of those who say that the Vicar of Christ and the Pontiff of the Roman Church does not have primacy over the Universal Church is similar to the error of those who say that the Holy Spirit does not proceed from the Son. For Christ Himself, the Son of God, consecrates and marks her as His own with the Holy Spirit, as it were with His own character and seal. . . And in like manner the Vicar of Christ by his primacy and foresight as a faithful servant keeps the Church Universal subject to Christ.

St. Thomas Aquinas

When someone's leaving the Roman Catholic Church is analyzed, it is usually found to be a tribute to the Roman Catholic Church.

Samuel A. Nigro

No man can be a hero to his valet.

Carlyle

When men forget the transcendentals, nothing works, nothing is right, and nothing is real.

Samuel A. Nigro

Followers of Roman Catholicism have the basis to "do things right," and thereby achieve the Good Life and, in the same process, be ready to complete the "Trip of one's life." This is to enter the STATIMUUM, or what this believing psychiatrist calls "Heaven." If there are "black holes" in the universe in which matter compresses to an incredible nothing, there must also exist a spiritual expansion encompassing all — a "white totality." Not a space-time continuum, but a spiritual STATIMUUM (from "statim," Latin for "immediate"). The STATIMUUM: The never-ending ecstacy of Love and Truth surfeited eternally and infinitely — only feebly adumbrated by the best personal feelings ever experienced — Truth and Love that stand the test of time — Roman Catholicism — those who speak for Loving Truth — those who witness Loving Truth.

Samuel A. Nigro

Nothing compares to the spirit of a good religious person, i.e. a good priest (Pope John Paul II) or a good nun (Mother Theresa). It is the best of pioneering, the best of altruism, the best of creativity, the best of helping others, the best of what heroes and heroines have to offer. The imitation of Jesus and Mary concentrates, exhilarates, and elevates like nothing else. Poverty, chastity, and obedience together is to reject corrupting-power, to accept rejecting-opponents, and to acquire legitimate-leadership. Also, only those genuinely committed to poverty, chastity, and obedience can regularly be accepted as trustworthy!

Name Lost

Would the genuine Messiah merely duplicate other religions? Would not the new Loving-Truth be contradictory to the old violence, slavery, brutality, intolerance, dishonesty, anti-freedom, anti-truth, anti-intellectual, anti-dialogue, suppression of individuality, undemocratic styles, bartering of peoples, animalized sexuality, harems, eunuchs, concubines, clitorectomies, infanticides, euthanasia, intoxicating drugs, Moloch burning of babies, dictators, tyrants, terrorism, hostage-taking, mobs, torture, suttee, mutilations, satanism, kali, bizarre unnatural birth control, and hate-filled grotesque, idolatry of the non-Western pre-Christian world? Do not social trends witness the return to such old derangements whenever Catholicism is rejected in practice if not in belief? Desert functional Roman Catholicism and achieve disaster? Does not history show barbarism when people are without the Church? Is that not what happens when the teachings of the Church are rejected? Gradually you wake up and find you are amidst a pack of dogs, so you look elsewhere finding the world perpetually wrong and the Church perpetually right — and you leap, nay run, much wiser, to the One, Holy, Catholic, and Apostolic Church — the Phylum of Life, Liberty, and the Pursuit of Happiness — Loving Truth.

Samuel A. Nigro

The Evangelical Counsels are poverty, chastity, and obedience. Poverty means one has not been coopted by money; chastity means one hasn't been coopted by sex; and obedience means one is committed to a transcendental life and will follow the only group which promotes such: The Roman Catholic Church.

Name Lost

New Age religion, like all Paganism, is a simple Materialist's effort to be spiritual.

Samuel A. Nigro

Where the Church is, there is civilization.

Name Lost

Christianity is a battle — not a dream.

Wendel Phillips

The trouble with power is that it violates and disrupts Oneness. Oneness actually is inversely proportional to power. While the reality of power cannot be denied, power nevertheless is an anti-transcendental and anti-natural approach to life.

Samuel A. Nigro

All ISMS turn into paganism except Catholicism.

Samuel A. Nigro

Spart is pretty much like gumption or fight. Like the Spart of St. Louis, that plane Lindbergh flowed to Europe.

Dizzy Dean

I know now the Catholic Church is the church of the poor, no matter what you say about the wealth of Her priests and bishops. Daily, I saw people coming from Mass. Never did I set foot in a Catholic Church but that I saw people there at home with Him. First Fridays, Novenas, and Missions brought the masses thronging in and out the Catholic Churches. They were of all nationalities, all classes, but most of all they were the poor. The very attacks made against the Church proved Her divinity to me. Nothing but a divine institution could have survived the betrayal of Judas, the denial of Peter, the sins of many of those who pressed Her faith, who were supposed to minister to Her poor.

Dorothy Day

You do not know what a home the Catholic Church is. No one can tell, no man can tell what she is to women. . . their teaching. . . their discipline. . . their hopes. . . their home. For what training is there compared to that of the Catholic nun? I have seen something of different kinds of nuns. I'm no longer young and do not speak from enthusiasm but from experience. There is nothing like the training these days which the Sacred Heart or the Order of St. Vincent's gives to women.

Florence Nightingale

Roman Catholic churches are the hinges of civilization.

Name Lost

Don't worry about the horse being blind, just load the wagon.

John Madden

The beginning and end of Protestant Christianity is in arguing with the Roman Catholic Church.

Samuel A. Nigro

Who is against her but all men, and who is beside her but thou.

Swinburne about Rome and liberty

There are two kinds of people in the world: Roman Catholics and those spending an inordinate amount of time trying to find reasons not to become Roman Catholic.

Name Lost

Amicus Plato, amicus Aristatolis, magnus amica veritas.
Friend of Plato, friend of Aristotle, most of all friend of truth..

The Motto of Sir Isaac Newton

The Church is always in advance of the world. That is why it is said to be behind the times. It discussed everything so long ago that people have forgotten the discussion.

G.K. Chesterton

The Church is the natural home of the Human Spirit.

Hilaire Belloc

One cannot take a vacation from history.

Charles De Gaulle

All boats leak. You've got to find the one that leaks least.

Wally Kuhn

We have to take the fact of our own birth on faith.

G.K. Chesterton

The only tradition in Protestantism is an allegiance to the anti-Catholicism of the Reformation.

Name Lost

I say as do all Christian men, that it is a divine purpose that rules, and not fate.

King Alfred of England

The Cross stands while the Earth revolves.

Name Lost

Only the Church preserves a civilized and cultured life.

Samuel A. Nigro

Where is your *pallium*?

Universal comment to know-it-all priests and religious not in concert with Rome

Ethereal Catholicism is a grandiose miasmatic tolerance for everyone's ideas and beliefs except what used to be their own from Rome. With Ethereal Catholicism comes a grandiose subjective sense of better-than-thou which is really nothing more than a suicidal manifestation of pride.

Samuel A. Nigro

(Nations) are courted by Him less than nothing. . .

Isaiah 40:17

The whole fabric of the enchanted realm of Raphael's Vatican pictures rests upon one simple but far-reaching thought. It is that of the greatness in triumph of the Church; her greatness in her wisdom, and her center, the Papacy; her triumph in the wonderful ways in which God continues to guard and protect the successor of Him to whom the promise was given; "thou art Peter and on this rock I will build my Church, and the gates of Hell shall not prevail against it."

Ludwig von Pastor

Three distinguished Inquisitors were sent to interview Catherine (of Sienna). They began by calling her a "wretched little female" (which is no more than what Catherine habitually called herself) and ended by singing her praises and telling the doctor of theology who was present: "Let her answer for herself; she does it much better than you."

Warren H. Carroll

Remember me in your prayers, and may God, by your intercession, reveal to me which belief is more pleasing to Him.

Sultan al-Kamil as he escorted St. Francis back to the Crusader lines, not permitting Francis to enter a furnace to prove the truth of his faith by ordeal

The most important thing a priest can do is pass on the Apostolic message in season and out of season — not the message of themselves or anyone else but the message of Jesus and the apostles. The people have a right to this message. The people will suffer without it.

Daniel McAffrey

And still the gates of hell will not overcome it.

Luxenburg Pastor Johann Brachmond in 1940 at the priests' barracks in Dachau in front of hundreds of other clergymen after an S.S. Stormtrooper Platoon Leader cursed and swore obscenely against God, Christ and his Church

Divine filiation protects against mental illness.

George Maloof

Power	*Authority*
From a "self" — a feminist, a Woman's Selfish Movement	From an "author" — the Father of all — a transcendental God
Revels in control	Revels in rational appeal
Represents itself	Represents an author
Remakes history to a positive fantasy ruining others	Keeps faith with positive historical reality
Coerces	Convinces
Constricts	Transcends
Corrupts	Saves or at least cleanses
Liberal	Conservative
Commits to the future by abandoning the past	Commits to the future without forgetting the past
Limits under guise of oxymoronic forced liberty	Expands under aegis of allegiance to nature
Destroys what is not perfect	Perfects what is

Professor Joyce Little on the distinctions between power and authority

That arguments occur over the Bible and its interpretation proves the lack of formal sufficiency for the Bible itself. Catholics believe the Bible to be materially sufficient but tradition as established within the Bible for the Church is needed to decide on controversial issues unclear in the Bible itself. For Protestants, the Bible's alleged sufficiency is actually an impeccability far beyond the Church's infallibility. For Protestants, *sola scriptura* is their own tradition which the Bible itself does not state.

Samuel A. Nigro

If *sola scriptura* is the norm, then why can't Catholics do it their way!

Name Lost

The Church is not something that we make today but something we recognize from the history of those who believe and that we pass on as yet incomplete, only to be fulfilled when the Lord shall come again.

Cardinal Ratzinger

Authority derives its legitimacy from the givenness of the reality to which it bears witness.

Joyce Little

STATUS OF WOMEN

At the time of the founding of the Church and in those early days, the social status of women appeared to be in two extremes: As property owned or as equal to men. That is, subcultures existed of the Jewish mold which relegated the woman's status almost to be property, while other subcultures (more of the Greek and Roman mold) had women equal to men in all things including priesthood, property owners, etc.

The Gospels and writings of the Fathers give evidence to a "command" from Jesus which effectively insisted on distinctive differences between men and women in the Spiritual Order. With bold Loving Truth, Jesus did two things that had not been done before: First, He elevated women above men through Mary as the source of all grace, but second, subordinated women in a mysterious complementary companion analogy (which subtly elevated women again) of husband-wife and Jesus-Church.

The Roman Catholic Church since its inception has reinforced the reality of the incompleteness of males *and* females in human nature, requiring their complementary companionship rather than "equality" in all things.

Gnosticism and many other social-cultural phenomena (existent in the time of the early Church and intermittently appearing throughout history) have regularly promoted "equality," but the Church has always resisted such efforts in the spiritual realm because the Church was founded by Christ in this manner.

"Inferiority" is in the eye of the beholder nowhere more than in the feeling-filled demand that anthropology define theology, which today is the pretension that women and men are equal regardless of clear observations to the contrary.

In the temporal realm, throughout history the Church has sustained benefits and promotions for persons of either sex, provided they were virtuous. Indeed, when Emmanuel Kant was philosophically defining women for evening enhancement only, Pope Benedict XIV and other Popes were installing women into university professorships in mathematics, philosophy, and physics! The Church is just not guilty of a policy of temporal suppression of women. But in the spiritual realm, the Church promotes the command from Jesus (as described in the early Church and throughout the Church) that distinctions should be maintained between men and women which can only be labeled "inferiority" by those who want to force age-bound ideas on that which will never be defined by an age.

A marketplace, the Church will never be (John 2:16). The Church is not a product of any age but brings the same message to every age. Therefore "tensions" will always occur between the Roman Catholic Church and whatever nonsense an age offers. The Church will resist Marcion in 144 and Montanus in 155 (both wanting women priests), Macedonius in 360, McBrien in 1980 and Curran in 1985.

In the midst of social turmoil of the first centuries of the Church where it would have been not necessarily unusual, no women were made apostles, and no women were ordained (allowed to speak, teach, consecrate) even though this was discussed vigorously in those days. Obviously such was decided to be against "the command of the Lord." Jesus could have done otherwise, but He did not. And those who lived then knew it.

One has little basis to second-guess the prohibition of women priests by the Roman Catholic Church. The question is not its rightness or wrongness in our time. The historical fact is that *this is how it was given to us* and not as the product of any age. Indeed, an indepth look at the effects of forced "equality" raises clear concern about the trends in a society that allows this to happen. We cannot reason why this mystery. We can only recognize that consequences are dire when men and women are not seen as different, even if the only tangible difference left in a society is that women are not ordained to be Roman Catholic priests. One must doubt that this alone will be enough symbolism to sustain healthy male/female relationships, family defining, social growth, and salvation.

God obviously has given this ancient secret to the Church: In spite of overlapping characteristics, men and women are different. Men are centrifugal beats of matter with transcendence. Women are centripetal flows of form with immanence. The matter of things is a particular object for males. The form of things is a particular object for females. When these distinctions are flawed, chaos, suffering, and unhappiness abound.

This fact pattern cannot change. Fidelity to the teachings of Jesus did not include women priests.

Summary of Manfred Hauke's *Women in the Priesthood?* by Ignatius Press

Catalolic Campaign For America

Principles Of "Public Catholicism"

I. Public Catholicism calls us to be *faithful* to the Holy Father and Magisterium of the Church.

II. Public Catholicism calls us to be *knowledgeable*, always growing in our understanding of what the Church teaches.

III. Public Catholicism calls us to *engage* the present culture with the liberating power of our faith. It calls us to offer substantive contributions to the public debate.

IV. Public Catholicism calls us to be *humble* when interjecting our perspective into the public conversation and to work with a collaborative spirit with those of other faiths. It calls us to affirm.what Catholics stand for, not just what we stand against.

V. Public Catholicism calls us to be *charitable*, .remembering in essentials unity, in non-essentials diversity and in all things charity — especially toward those who disagree with us.

VI. Public Catholicism calls us to be *responsible,*always sensitive to the appropriate role of the Church.

VII. Public Catholicism calls us to be *consistent,*integrating our faith into every aspect of our lives. It means seeing our faith as the foundational element of our professional,family and public lives.

VIII. Public Catholicism calls us to be *proud* of our Catholic heritage, celebrating the richness and beauty of our faith and the historic, monumental contributions that Catholic Americans have made to the cultural, spiritual, and moral life of our country.

IX. Public Catholicism calls us to be *courageous* in articulating the Church's teaching in the face of potential criticism

X. Public Catholicism calls us to be *optimistic* and confident that our faith is capable of transforming ourselves and the contemporary culture.

The courage that it takes for the Roman Catholic Church to take the stands she has taken in this century alone qualifies her to be the prophetic voice of Christ to the world.

Name Lost

For God, to me, it seems, is a verb, not a noun.

Buckminster Fuller

This hatred (against the Catholic Church) is rooted in the rejection of the order of right living that the Church is bound to uphold against the political enactments of its opposite.

James V. Schall

This is why there should be no national flags on church grounds.

The floor of hell is covered with skulls of bishops.

St. John Chrysostom

A SENSE OF MYSTERY

If I search for a rational, reasonable explanation to why I remain a priest, I find myself both unsatisfied and frustrated. It's similar to a newly engaged person trying to explain why he or she has fallen in love with a certain individual and not another. This dimension of mystery is common to each of our lives. Do we not find that life's major decisions — whom we marry, the career we follow, the values we make our own — often transcend logic and reason?

The answer to the question is more poetry than prose, more intuitive than discursive. In the depths of my soul, I experienced a desire for communion with God that from the start (in my case, early childhood) was interwoven with a life of ministry as priest. This desire indeed was mysterious. From whence did it come? Was it of the Spirit? Was it a divine invitation to priestly ministry? My years as a priest, almost 30 now, suggest that this desire was indeed of the Spirit.

Immediately this movement toward priesthood was in conflict with a powerful desire not unrelated to my desire for God: the desire for closeness to a young woman. I must confess that from the first day of school I wanted to be a priest and from that first day of school I was in love with a lovely and intriguing classmate. My affection for her endured through twelve years of education during which we shared the same homeroom. And my desire to be a priest endured and deepened. There is mystery here.

I am reminded of Edward Schillebeeckx's insight that speaks to the mystery of celibacy: it is simply "an inability to do otherwise." This inability to do otherwise has led me to discover that my truth is not only priestly ministry, but paradoxically, celibate priestly ministry. In spite of the human longing for wife and family, for the joy and pain of a life shared intimately with another, I have discovered through the mercy of grace a communion of spirit with God and friends that remains unspeakable — that remains mystery. Always there were sustaining moments of communion. That's as close as I can come to an answer. These were feasts of grace and communion that happened for the most part at table. Certainly the Lord's table. I felt I was closest to the core of my truth when I was presiding and preaching at Eucharist.

Coaxed by the grace of God, individuals form an assembly, listen with a single ear to the living word, speak a prayer of sacrificial praise, eat and drink from the one table; and in so doing discover they are embraced by the divine presence, the divine mystery. No unbeliever can understand the profound privilege of participating in this feast of grace.

There are other feasts of grace that nourish and sustain me. These, too, are situated at table. Dinner with a dear friend or a married couple, with brother priests or with my family — all, at one time or another, have been sacraments of communion. On occasion, the warmth of God's eucharistic presence transforms a quiet restaurant table into sacred space. And "heart speaks to heart" (John Henry Newman).

Father Donald B. Cozzens

Leave the mess in God's hands after you've done what you can.

John H. Miller

Secular psychologists reject God because of their logic and their science, but because of the "correct" demands of their logic, they have no reason for believing their science either. They have nothing and from this position of leadership proclaim to the world that the most it can have is the knowledge that it has nothing.

Madeline Greenberg

Relativism defeats itself. . .because it makes an absolute statement.

Joseph M. de Torre

Truth is not certainty; it is not happiness; it is not the greatest good; it is not whatever works; it is not whatever flows; and it is not what one believes.

Joseph M. de Torre

The "therapeutic" has failed.

Joseph Vaccaro

OTHER WAYS?

"Outside the Church, there is no salvation." Indeed, since Jesus redeemed all humanity, how can one be saved if not a Roman Catholic?

Try this:

The Church is a figurative "David" (of Loving Truth) facing Goliaths (of evil) of each generation. In this venture, the Church is the only way to God. That is, to be saved, you must be part of "David" (the Church).

The head of "David" (the Church in this paradigm) is Jesus Christ who founded this specific Church with specific ideals historically traceable to the faithful Apostles in Rome.

The body of "David" (the Church) is comprised of people who add little to the defeat of whatever Goliath confronts us. But the better we (the people) follow Jesus (the head of the Church, the head of "David"), the nearer we are to God, so Goliath will never defeat us either collectively or individually. That is, the opportunity for Salvation is open to us regardless of what we do because of the Sacrifice of Jesus. But whether we achieve salvation depends on our free will placing us somehow *in* the Church.

The formal and the most efficient manner of being *in* the Church ("David") and thereby attaining salvation is through grace from the sacraments by orthodoxy in the Roman Catholic Church. This is the most radical, nonconforming, and usually "minority" way to live.

There is, however, a penumbra of behavior and activity (Natural Law) which effectively *duplicates* the salutary functioning of sacramental life, even if such activity is neither formally nor overtly linked to the sacraments. There exists a natural healing by "grace" through Natural Law.

By similarity or imitation within the Natural Law, salvation is possible even if not consciously linked to Roman Catholicism. But it remains true that "outside the Church, there is no salvation," because by similarity or imitation, one can be and is, *in the Church* whether one likes it or not. Supernatural faith and charity can be present wittingly or unwittingly and overtly or covertly in alliance with Rome and a life of grace and good works lead to salvation. It may be that if you follow Natural Law, you are an implicit member of the Roman Catholic Church.

"Good" persons will make it. By one's fruits and acts according to the Natural Law, grace is obtained and thereby we are all known to God — whether we acknowledge Jesus or not — but clearly, the easiest and most pleasing way is to follow openly the Church which was given by God to humanity.

Some of the interesting unique qualities of the Roman Catholic Church are evident when it is perceived as the way for human beings to distinguish themselves as members of the animal kingdom in a different, new, and unique way. That is, there are human beings who remain simply part of the animal kingdom in the biological sense. However, through Roman Catholicism, a spiritual component elevates human beings into the image of God, but it requires some different perceptions and activities.

These activities are actually a rebellion. They are a rebellion that distinguishes a person from the ordinary. The Roman Catholic rebellion is not part of the problem, but is part of the solution. The rebellion is not the "same old thing" which always turns out to be grimy animality. The distinguishing rebellion led by the Roman Catholic Church *is NOT to follow the same impulses that always occur*.

Several questions emphasize the point: What group really rebels? What group really promotes a counterculture to grimy animality? What group says, "We are different and do not do that"? What group says, "I am free of this brutality, of this animality, of the same old things"? What group even says, "We can be and are forgiven" while admitting to sin but also being offered is the means of obtaining forgiveness?

The answer to all those questions is: The Roman Catholic Church. No other group does these things and there is no other way.

Samuel A. Nigro

Jesus is actually the image for all of us of what we were to be before the Fall.

George Maloof

Mohammed preached and insisted upon a whole group of ideas which were peculiar to the Catholic Church and distinguished it from the paganism which it had conquered in the Greek and Roman civilization. Thus, the vary foundation of his teaching was that prime Catholic doctrine, the unity and omnipotence of God. The attributes of God he also took over from Catholic doctrine: The personal nature, the all-goodness, the timelessness, the providence of God, His creative power as the origin of all things, and His sustenance of all things by His power alone. The world of good-spirited angels and of evil spirits in rebellion against God was part of the teaching, with a chief evil spirit, such as Christendom had recognized. Mohammed preached with insistence that prime Catholic doctrine, on the human side — the immortality of the soul and its responsibility for actions in this life, coupled with the consequent doctrine of punishment and reward after death. . .but he advanced a clear affirmation, full and complete, against the whole doctrine of an incarnate God. He taught that Our Lord was the greatest of all the prophets, but still only a prophet: a man like other men. He eliminated the Trinity altogether. . . With that denial of the Incarnation went the whole sacramental structure. He refused to know anything of the Eucharist, with its Real Presence; he stopped the sacrifice of Mass, and therefore the institution of a special priesthood. In other words, he, like so many other lesser heresiarchs, founded his heresy on simplification.

Hilaire Belloc on why Islam is more properly called
Mohammedism, i.e. a heresy rather than a new religion.

The only reason the Church is picked on by liberals is that it is non-violent, which makes liberals to be the biggest cowards ever.

Samuel A. Nigro

If the Great Chief of the Christians is in danger, send him a message from me. We will build him a lodge in the middle of our camp; we will hunt game that he may be fed; and we will be his guards to protect him from the enemy.

Chief Victor of the Flathead Indians in 1840 inviting
the Pope to visit The Man Who Talks to the Great Spirit.
Native Americans' title for Father Peter John De Smet

On the 18th of last September two Catholic Iroquois came to visit us. They had been for twenty-three years among the nation called the Flatheads and Pierced Noses, about a thousand Flemish leagues from where we are. . . By their instructions and examples they have given all that nation a great desire to have themselves Baptized. . . The sole object of these good Iroquois was to obtain a priest to come and finish what they had so happily commenced.

Father Peter John De Smet in 1839

On Sunday, the 5th of July, I had the consolation of celebrating the holy sacrifice of mass *sub dio*. The altar was placed on an elevation, and surrounded with boughs and garlands of flowers; I addressed the congregation in French and in English, and spoke also by an interpreter to the Flatheads and Snake Indians. It was a spectacle truly moving for the heart of a missionary to behold an assembly composed of so many different nations, who all assisted at our holy mysteries with great satisfaction. The Canadians sang hymns in French and Latin, and the Indians in their native tongue. It was truly a Catholic worship.

Father Peter John De Smet in 1840

At last we reach the Great Bend, where the boat came to land opposite a camp of Yanktons, a powerful tribe of the Sioux nation. . . The Indians gave us the sad tidings of the ravages which the small pox was then causing. . . At my request the captain put me ashore, and two hours after I was among the sick. I baptized all the little children who had not yet been fortunate enough to receive that sacrament. I spent the night with them, giving them all the consolation of my power.

Father Peter John De Smet in 1849

We must admire those who suffered martyrdom in their native land, Egypt. For as soon as sentence was pronounced against the first, one after another rushed to the judgment seat and confessed themselves to be Christians. And they received the final sentence of death with joy and laughter and cheerfulness so that they sang and offered up hymns of thanksgiving to the god of the universe til their last breath.

Eusebus

Did we win, Dad?

Michael Nigro, age 4, to his father as he left church the first time taken to mass

We are never free until some institution frees us, and liberty cannot exist till it is declared by authority.

G.K. Chesterton

Troublemakers among you want to change the Good News of Christ. . .if anyone preaches a version of the Good News different from the one you have already heard, he is to be condemned.

Galatians 1:8-10

The fallacy of the age: they have suggested that our task, in ethics, is to choose between competing points of view, when there are no correct answers. But if there is no way of choosing between these alternative moral arguments, then there is, finally, no rational ground for our moral judgments. Acceptors of that reasoning must simply install the premises of relativism and dissolve their problem: after all, if there is no right or wrong answer on moral questions, why is it necessary to strain and reflect and agonize before we decide? Is there a tension between our interests and duties? But so what? On what ground of reason would the commands of obligation take precedence over the commands of self-interest, or the manifold appeals of the things that simply give us pleasure?

Hadley Arkes

I do not believe there is any person who is not primarily dominated by his religion, by his views of the universe, whatever they may be.

G.K. Chesterton

Our town believes in outcome-based morality.

Garrison Keeler

Most Roman Catholics were raised with the intimidating feeling that talking about Jesus and the Church was the sole province of priests and nuns. No way. Learning to speak up has several phases: first is "yep, I believe." Then is "hey, don't talk about my Church like that." Third is "I hear you but here is why Jesus' Church is correct." Then comes "let me tell you something." And finally is "listen to this!"

Name Lost

It takes an incredible inflated arrogance for someone to believe that they could discuss or discover something genuinely new about Christianity. To compete with the Fathers of the Church, or to compete with the scholars of Rome who have been the deposit of Christian writings since the time of the Apostles, or to compete with those who have access to the Vatican libraries, is to set oneself up as a fool. To believe that one could discern a truth not contained within the reach of the Vatican begs rational belief. Yet it is done everyday. . .by individuals who want to believe they know what they are doing but who must be challenged to confront the fact that whatever "truths" they can come to can *never be confirmed* unless authenticated by the Vatican. Such indeed is the nature of the intellectual process of Christianity.

Samuel A. Nigro

Is that Jesus? Is that Jesus?

Two excited preschool boys to their mother as the priest came onto the altar

First, humans seem to have understood from the earliest times that we are all social creatures. Each person is born into a social context that is much greater than his or her own individual existence. And we come to know ourselves by our relationships within this social world. Second, human beings express themselves and understand themselves through symbols. Language itself is a symbol system. What we moderns call psychological concepts have long been explained in symbols such as those in myths. Symbols are vital elements of self-awareness. In a special sense, a human society first comes into existence when it articulates an awareness of itself, usually in terms of the hopes, fears, ambitions and concerns of being alive. Third, every ancient society that we know about, including nonWestern societies such as China, understood itself as the representation of a cosmic order. When we talk about a cosmic order we are saying that the universe is a coherent whole in which every part is related to every other part. To believe in a cosmos is to believe that everything in the world or in one's experience of the world is a part of some greater structure. We might say that the cosmos has a larger meaning or purpose beyond the fate of individual lives. Virtually every religion throughout history has required that its followers submit to something greater than themselves.

Nicholas Capaldi

Our duty and our conscience will not allow us Roman Catholics to give up our role as voice crying in the wilderness.

Cardinal Mindzendy

Submission to a weak man is discipline. Submission to a strong man is only servility.

G.K. Chesterton

Saying that Jesus was a great man is not enough. His message has positive uniqueness and longevity justifying at least the possibility that He was more than human. To reflect on the genuine meaning of His message coupled with the spectacular events of the Gospel mandate the hypothesis that Jesus was extraordinarily special and second to none in human history. Comparable mythological fables have been found to be just that: fables. Coupled with the positiveness of Jesus' messages, the unique intensity of His sacrifice and conquering of death plus the universality of its application and the oneness of its potential end result, all complimented by the singular claim to be God-made-man for man's sake out of self-sacrificing love (an idea so foreign to humanity that it must have been given by God Himself), the composite emerging is that "a great man" is not enough.

Samuel A. Nigro

It is not the creed, but the criticism that is always crumbling away, age after age.

G.K. Chesterton

When I call myself a Catholic with a modern consciousness I don't mean what might be implied in the phrase "modern Catholic", which doesn't make sense. If you're a Catholic you believe what the Church teaches and the climate makes no difference.

Flannery O'Connor

State first of all what Jesus said, not what you think He would have said if He had expressed Himself more clearly.

G.K. Chesterton

There are none so blind as those who would not see.

Old Proverb

Rationalistic efforts against the creed produce a gradual social degradation following on the loss of that direct link between human nature and God which is provided by the Incarnation.

Hilaire Belloc

Proven by the communications technology heresy empire of the last half of the twentieth century.

The real fountain of youth is the living of a 2000 year old message. The real fountain of youth is the Roman Catholic Church.

Name Lost

You cannot really understand any myths till you have found out that one of them is not a myth.

G.K. Chesterton

It is the unique mark of a religion of race that it permits the worshiper to worship himself.

G.K. Chesterton

When Christ at a symbolic moment was establishing His great society, He chose for its cornerstone neither the brilliant Paul or the mystic John, but a shuffler, a snob, a coward — in a word, a man. And upon this rock He has built His Church, and the gates of hell have not prevailed against it.

G.K. Chesterton

Stand up to be counted. Speak out to be heard. Sit down to be remembered.

George Ruttler

There is no knowledge, no ignorance, no destruction of ignorance. There are no four truths. That is to say, there is no pain, no origin of pain, no stoppage of pain, and no path to the stoppage of pain.

Zen Buddhist Sutra recited every morning
and before each meal

Self-contradicting statements if there ever were any.

My Father is at work until now, so I am at work.

John 5:17

For there is one God. There is also one mediator between God and the human race, Christ Jesus, himself human.

1 Timothy 2:5

There is no salvation through. . .any other name.

Acts 4:12

People are saved *through* the Church, they are saved *in* the Church, but they are always saved *by the Grace of Christ.* Besides formal membership in the Church, the *sphere of salvation* can also include *other forms of relation to the Church.*

John Paul II

Despite some common aspects, Christ does not resemble Muhammad or Socrates or Buddha. He is totally original and unique. . . He is the one mediator between God and humanity.

John Paul II

A Marion dimension and Mariology in the Church are simply another aspect of the Christological focus.

John Paul II

God so loved the world that he gave his only Son, so that everyone who believes in him might not perish.

John 3:16

For God did not send his Son into the world to condemn the world, but that the world might be saved through Him.

John 3:17

Why do we celebrate Christmas? Because ever since Jesus was born, the world has never been the same! And, if followed properly, it should have been only for the better!

Name Lost

Reasoned dialogue has a limited ability to withstand an assault by the mythic power of falsehood, especially when that falsehood is rooted in an age-old social and cultural phenomenon.

Deborah Lipstadt

I call you not slaves but my friends.

John 15:15

Our Lady's Fiat — "Let it be unto me according to thy word" —
meant that she gave herself, soul and body, to be made into Christ.
She gave him her eyes to be his eyes, her mind to be his mind,
her heart to be his heart; and before she gave birth to him,
before his human body was fully formed from hers,
she knew the impulses of his love, who lived secretly within her.
She was driven out by his charity to her cousin Elizabeth,
his presence in her lifted her voice in an expression of joy in God
that rings down the ages; through his presence in her
she became conscious of the unborn generations that
would know him, and she exulted in his mercy to them.
"My spirit has found joy in God who is my savior."
She accepted too the suffering that he would inevitably bring
into her life, and that too began before he was born,
in Joseph's misunderstanding, and in the added hardship of
obeying the law and journeying to Bethlehem when he,
her life's sweetness, was also her heavy burden.

Caryll Houselander

The Hindu says "being saved is being nothing." The Buddhist says "whatever it is now, it is saved if it is." The Muslim says "you've been saved or else." The Protestant says "I've been saved no matter what." The Jew says "I don't think anyone is ever going to be saved." And the Catholic says "Jesus saves but you've got to do the Word by the transcendentals, virtue and the sacraments.

Samuel A. Nigro

Angels are dimensions of life required for a coordinated time-bound, coherent universe. If good is to be personal in such existence, more fortitude comes from considering the angels.

Samuel A. Nigro

You can buy everything but time. Once you waste time, it's forever gone. Do not waste time.

Mom

Faith is always at a disadvantage; it is a perpetually defeated thing which survives all its conquerors.

G.K. Chesterton

What tradition enables individuals to develop on their own in most respects??

Name Lost

"Prayer" to be used on public grounds, in schools and everywhere:
It is the duty of all nations to acknowledge the providence of Almighty God, to obey His will, to be grateful for His benefits, and humbly to implore His protection and favor. . . That great and glorious Being who is the beneficent author of all the good that was, that is, or that ever will be, that

SALVATION: HOW IS ONE SAVED? TAKE YOUR PICK.

Protestant	*Catholic*
Faith is essential, completely sufficient and once assented to can never be undone.	Faith is essential, sufficient, cannot be improved upon, but can be lost.
Works are absolutely irrelevant (except the "work" of assent??).	Works are essential if one has free choice.
No self-help is possible (no works and no worries).	Cannot be earned but self-help is important because salvation can be rejected or lost.
Manifest one's true self by forced automatic robotile compliance with true faith (There is no freedom).	Manifest one's true self by willing cooperation with true faith (There is freedom!).
Hold to the word of Jesus Christ by words and nothing else matters.	Hold to the word of Jesus Christ not only in word but in deed.
Trust in Jesus Christ alone means that one needs to do nothing; one can do anything even sin.	Trust in Jesus Christ alone means doing something consistent to manifest oneness with Jesus. One must try even if it is ineffective in the absolute but essential in our individual freedom.
Even sin saves because God does not care as long as you assent so He can forgive.	God is not offended but pleased by one's efforts to do good works. In addition, God is displeased and will rule against one's unforgiven sins.
Faith does not care what you do; the Ten Commandments are irrelevant.	Faith requires compliance with the Word in action as well as words.

we may then unite in rendering unto Him our sincere and humble thanks for His kind care and protection of the people.

President George Washington's proclamation designating a national day of prayer and thanksgiving (the origin of our current legal holiday) as requested by the House of Representatives the day after the First Amendment was adopted on September 24, 1789

I know that my Redeemer liveth.

William F. Buckley, Jr. when asked how he knew his beliefs would not crumble sooner or later

To reject Western Civilization is to be forever outside it and all the benefits it alone can give.

Samuel A. Nigro

A quest is always an education both as to the character of that which is sought and in self-knowledge.

Alasdair McIntyre

Such an inquiry is lived out: It cannot be an armchair adventure.

Pamela M. Hall

Man is basically overwhelmed by information, ideas, data, shouts, pleas, enticements and threats. What to do? What to do: Go Roman Catholic. . . It is for everyone. It uplifts. It advances. It creates a personal and social good life. It is family supporting. It is consistent with the world and nature. It is a universal, simple, comprehensive theory of esteemed longevity. Operationally, it is not past or future but *now* and it discards all that sullies the mind. It makes one relate. It makes one transcendentally sound. It absorbs and assimilates whatever is compatible. It wastes little time on what is ineffectual. It hurries not into mistakes. It gives joy. If there is another answer, it must compete with Roman Catholicism — real Roman Catholicism and not a straw man version.

Samuel A. Nigro

For the body is not one member, but many. If the foot says, "Because I am not a hand, I am not of the body," is it therefore not of the body? And if the eye says, "Because I am not an eye, I am not of the body," is it therefore not of the body? But as it is, God has set the members, each of them, in the body as he willed. Now if they were all one member, where would the body be? But as it is, there are indeed many members, but yet one body.

1 Corinthians 12:14-19

When members of society have a terribly bad case of "look at me," who else do they pander to except members of the press and media.

Name Lost

I am not tortured by the problems that torture a great many other people, because I do very sincerely and very simply believe in God and in the whole of the Christian experience. And there are enough resources in it to show me where to go.

William F. Buckley, Jr.

The Saracens of Tobriz are wicked and treacherous. The law which the prophet Mohammed has given them has laid down that any harm they do to one who does not accept their law and any appropriation of goods is no sin at all, and if they suffer death or injury at the hands of Christians, they are accepted martyrs. For this reason they would be wrongdoers if it were not for the government. And all the other Saracens act on the same principle. When they are on the point of their death, up comes one of their priests and asks if Mohammed was the true messenger of God. If they answer "yes" then he tells them they are saved. . . They are allowed great license to sin, and according to their law, no sin is forbidden. . .

Marco Polo

Imparting information is our weakness.

Isabel Paterson

Words are angels. Make it so!

Samuel A. Nigro

Had no precursor in the years before
And peerless shall remain forevermore,
In whom with joy of motherhood we find
The glory of virginity combined.

Sedulius

PRECEPTS OF THE CHURCH

1. Assist at Mass on Sundays and Holy Days of obligation.
2. Fast and abstain on the days appointed.
3. Confess your sins at least once a year.
4. Receive Holy Communion during the Easter time.
5. Contribute to the support of the Church.
6. Observe the laws of the Church concerning marriage.

Now you know why you can't take women seriously.

Larry Dolan as he watched the jiggling NBA cheerleaders

Okay! Look, we've been waiting two thousand years for the promised savior. If it is not Jesus, who is it? When is he coming? Where is he? Everybody is tired of waiting. . . When *is* he coming, if he hasn't come already?

Samuel A. Nigro

But God has so adjusted the body. . .that there may be no discord in the body, but that the members may have the same care for one another. If one member suffers, all suffer together; if one member is honored, all rejoice together.

1 Corinthians 12:25-27

Christians are so in this together that they can even ask saints for help.

Transcendental analysis and promotion automatically contain reason and proof.

Samuel A. Nigro

The sin and sorrow of despotism is not that it does not love men, but that it loves them too much and trusts them too little.

G.K. Chesterton

Stupid is he who revolts against that vicar who holds the keys of the blood of Christ crucified. Even if he were the devil incarnate, I should not raise my head against him, but always humble myself.

St. Catherine of Siena

This is a religion that will not fail. It has gone underground for many years. It has been overlaid with contemporary concerns many of the latter worthwhile of course, but this kind of religion is bone of my bone and flesh of my flesh. And that is how many people feel about it. . .far more than is allowed for in contemporary philosophy.

Larry Henderson, euphoric elderly convert after attending the Tridentine Latin Mass for the first time

The truth can never hurt the Roman Catholic Church — it *has* the truth.

Michael Davies

There are things that are true and things that are false and it matters!

John Henry Newman's Dogmatic Principle

The first collegial decision for Catholic bishops is described in Matthew's Gospel. It was when, after declaring their unflagging allegiance to Jesus, the Apostles fled led by the soon-to-be Pope. Cowardice of the clergy goes a long way back to those who said "I know not the man. . ."

Michael Davies

Some theologians read the *New York Times* to find out what is happening to God.

William Marra

And if those also who follow heresies venture to avail themselves of the prophetic scripture. . .in the first place, they will not make use of all the scriptures and then they will not quote them entirely nor is the body and texture of prophecy described. But selecting ambiguous expressions, they wrest them to their own opinion gathering a few expressions here and there not looking to the sense but making use in the new words. For in almost all the quotations they make, you will find that they attend to the names alone while they alter the meanings, neither knowing as they affirm nor using the quotations they adduce according to their true nature. But the truth is not found by changing the meanings.

St. Clement of Alexandria, 200 A.D. on the misuse of Scripture

People have fallen into a foolish habit of speaking of orthodoxy as something heavy, humdrum and safe. There never was anything so perilous or so exciting as orthodoxy. It was sanity: And to be sane is more dramatic than being mad.

G.K. Chesterton

Thinking is actually real thinking only if it is transcendentally processed. Genuine thinking is reflecting upon whatever in terms of its matter, form, truth, oneness, goodness and beauty. Reflection upon the transcendentals as it applies to *whatever*, is to make one's thinking processes to be genuinely conscious. Such a mode of thinking has an impact which is readily testable. All one has to do is *try it*.

Samuel A. Nigro

The world within it has been more lucid, more level-headed, more reasonable in its hopes, more healthy in its instincts, more humorous and cheerful in the face of fate and death, than all the world outside. For it was the soul of Christendom that came forth from the incredible Christ; and the soul of it was common sense.

G.K. Chesterton

But I have written to you rather boldly here and there, brethren — as it were to refresh your memory — because of the grace that has been given to me by God, that I should be a minister of Christ Jesus to the gentiles; sanctifying the Gospel of God, that the offering up of the gentiles become acceptable, being sanctified by the Holy Spirit.

Romans 15:15-16

Is anyone among you sick? Let him bring in the presbyters of the Church, and let them pray over him, anointing him with oil in the name of the Lord.

James 5:14-15

"But these people abuse anything they do not understand; and the only things they do understand — merely by nature like unreasoning animals — will turn out to be fact to them. . . alas, for them, because they have followed Cain; they have thrown themselves into the delusion as Balaam for a reward; they have been ruined by the same *rebellion as Korah* — and share the same fate. . . They are mischief makers, grumblers, governed by their own desires, with mouths full of boastful talk, ready to flatter others for gain."

Jude 10-11 and 16 on New Testament
believers not following Church leaders

"The same rebellion as Korah" is told in Numbers 16: Korah and 250 Israelite leaders of the community banded together against Moses and Aaron, proclaiming that the entire community was consecrated and that Moses and Aaron and others should desist from priestly ministries. One reads how Korah and his family were swallowed by the earth and that fire consumed the 250 non-ministerial men offering incense. The bronze censers which had been carried by the men, destroyed by the fire, were hammered into sheets to cover the altar. But on the following day, the whole community of Israelites were muttering against Moses and Aaron, blaming them for the killings. In response, God placed a plague in the community and almost 15,000 died apart from those who died because of Korah. "They are a reminder to the Israelites that no unauthorized person, no one not of Aaron's line, may approach and offer incense before Yahweh, on pain of suffering the fate of Korah and his party, as Yahweh had said through Moses" (Numbers 16:5). In the final analysis, the letter of Jude in the New Testament clearly identifies "the rebellion as Korah" to be a hazard for New Testament believers who do not respect the sacramental priestly ministry of the Church founded by Christ.

James Akin, Protestant Minister
convert to Roman Catholicism

Nay, much rather, those who have seen the more feeble members of the body are more necessary; and those that we think the less honorable members of the body, we surround with more abundant honor, and our uncomely receive a more abundant comeliness, whereas our comely parts have no need of it. But God has so tempered the body together in due portion as to give more abundant honor where it was lacking; that there may be no disunion in the body, but that the members may have care for one another. And if one member suffers anything, all the members suffer with it, or if one member glories, all of the members rejoice with it. Now you are the Body of Christ, member for member. And God indeed has placed some in the Church, first Apostles, secondly prophets, thirdly teachers; after that miracles, then gifts of healing, services of help, power administration, and the speaking of various tongues. Are all Apostles? Are all prophets? Are all teachers? Are all workers of miracles? Do all have the gift of healing? Do all speak with tongues? Do all interpret? Yet strive after the greater gifts.

1 Corinthians 12:22-31

There lives more faith in honest doubt, believe me, than in half the creeds.

Tennyson

If you can do anything you want to do, you cannot have what you really want.

James Schall

The problem with Catholicism is not Catholicism; it is Catholics!

Karl Keating

By invoking the doctrine of Sola Scriptura, we Catholics claim equal right to profess our interpretation.

Name Lost

To abandon the Church and its teaching for the psychology, psychiatry, social work and psychotherapy approaches is self-destructive and detrimental. The proof is forcefully in: Look around for what has happened in the thirty years of "therapy instead of Church." Therapy just has not worked and matters are getting worse and worse without the Church.

Samuel A. Nigro

Genuine liturgies trace their origin right back to the time of the apostles, the exception being the rites composed by the Protestants at the time of the Reformation. That was a complete break with tradition when Protestants started composing their own rites.

Michael Davies

Let's not talk about Jews. . .it will ruin my Sabbath.

Jewish historian Solomon Schecter

I doubt any contemporary Bible-Christian theme has not already been worked through completely in and by the early Roman Catholic Church. So what always *seems* to be a new startling idea and interpretation is almost always rather old and even in the presentation of the Bible, "there is nothing new under the sun."

Samuel A. Nigro

Every Catholic must feel a personal love for those sacred rites when they come to him with all the authority of the centuries. Any rude handling of such forms must cause deep pain to those who know and love them. For they come to them from God through Christ and through the Church. For they would not have such an attraction were they not sanctified by the piety of so many generations who have prayed in the same words and found in them steadiness in joy and consolation in sorrow.

Cardinal Gaskay on the faithful adherence to tradition and suspicion of changes in liturgy

The most pleasant, albeit ignorant, thing about being Protestant is that one can discard the entire history of the Roman Catholic Church and thereby save oneself a lot of reading.

Samuel A. Nigro

When you see a cosmic force you don't like, trick it, my boy.

Basil Grant

If we do not fight with words, we will fight with guns.

Samuel A. Nigro

Every man is dangerous. . .I was once dangerous myself.

Juan del Fuego

The reason other religions bad mouth the Roman Catholic Church especially is to keep themselves and their members from converting to Catholicism.

Name Lost

If you would enter life, keep the Commandments.

Matthew 19:17

Superstition is only the creative side of agnosticism.

G.K. Chesterton

These sects that proclaim the end of the world will be better off proclaiming the end of themselves and those "prophets" who profess new insights will be better off professing the Ten Commandments.

Name Lost

Whoever's crazy idea does the least harm — that is the idea to follow.

Name Lost

Miracles are only the pretty pictures in the Book.

Georges Bernanos

Jesus Christ is the outstanding personality of all time. . . No other teacher — Jewish, Christian, Buddhist, Mohammedian — is still a teacher whose teaching is such a guidepost for the world. . . Other teachers may have something basic for an Oriental, an Arab, or an Occidental; but every act and word of Jesus have value for all of us. He became the Light of the World. Why shouldn't I, a Jew, be proud of that?

Shalom Asch

Why do therapists invariably never ask patients if they pray? Why don't the therapists pray? I always ask the patient, "Do you pray?" The answer, either way, pokes a huge hole both in my pretentions and his defenses. There is a peculiar if not singular power to the question, it does lift a veil, it does reveal a depth, a need. Indeed, the answer to the question, "Do you pray" is diagnostic for it tells us how a man lives with his fear, his dread. Prayer, you know, is not only our converse with God, it is our converse with our own selves.

Joseph Mauceri

The best psychology is a strong theology.

Joseph Mauceri

When Catholics get insulted and protest it, we get lectured on the First Amendment.

Samuel A. Nigro

There is but one religion which can only decorate even its triumphs with the emblem of defeat. There is only one army which carries the image of its own captain not enthroned or riding, but captured and impaled.

G.K. Chesterton

Christians do not differ from other men as to habitat, language or custom. They live among Greeks and barbarians, wherever destiny has put them. They follow local custom in garb and diet and other matters. But their way of life is nonetheless strange and unbelievable to many. They live in their native land, but as sojourners; as citizens they share everything with their fellowmen; yet they are treated as aliens; any alien country is a homeland to them, and every homeland an alien country. They marry as men do and beget children; but they do not practice abortion. They share tables but not beds. They live in the flesh but not according to the flesh. They dwell on earth but regard heaven as their city. They follow established law but in their way of life go beyond what the law requires. They love all, and everybody persecutes them., No one knows them, while all condemn them; they are put to death and still are very much alive.

To put it all briefly: What the soul is to the body, Christians are to the world. The soul is present in all the body's members; so are Christians to the world's cities. The soul dwells in the body, but does not originate from it; Christians live in the world but do not have their origin there. The invisible soul abides in the visible body; Christians are seen as living in the world, but their piety is invisible. On the other hand, the body, though it suffers nothing from the soul, hates it and makes war upon it because it cannot enjoy its pleasures in peace; the world suffers nothing from Christians but hates them because they reject its pleasures.

The soul loves the flesh and members which hate it; so do Christians love those who hate them. The soul is enclosed in the body, but it contains the body; Christians must remain in this world as in a prison, but they contain the world. The immortal soul dwells in a mortal home; Christians are pilgrims in a corruptible world while they look forward to heavenly immortality. God has set them in the world as His sentinels, and they may not leave their posts.

Saint Justin Martyr, Second Century

ANYWAY

People are unreasonable, illogical, and self-centered,
LOVE THEM ANYWAY
If you do good, people will accuse you of selfish, ulterior motives,
DO GOOD ANYWAY
If you are successful,
you win false friends and true enemies,
SUCCEED ANYWAY
The good you do will be forgotten tomorrow,
DO GOOD ANYWAY
Honesty and frankness make you vulnerable,
BE HONEST AND FRANK ANYWAY
What you spent years building may be
destroyed overnight,
BUILD ANYWAY
People really need help
but may attack you if you help them,
HELP PEOPLE ANYWAY
Give the world the best you have
and you'll get kicked in the teeth,
GIVE THE WORLD THE BEST YOU'VE GOT ANYWAY.

Mother Theresa's sign of the wall of Shishu Bhavan,
the children's home in Calcutta

The Christian mysteries are so far democratic that nobody understands them at all.

G.K. Chesterton

The relics of medieval Christendom, often called "the Dark Ages," may make us blush in terms of what we have accomplished today. Medieval Christendom has given us at least the following: Dante, Chaucer, Giotto, Oxford, Cambridge, Paris, Thomist philosophy, trade unions, the printing press, the press itself, parliament, the Magna Carta and science. It is difficult to find anything called "good" today which cannot be traced back to those so-called "dreary" days.

Name lost

There can only be two basic loves. . . the love of God unto the forgetfulness of self or the love of self unto the forgetfulness and denial of God.

St. Augustine

Peace lies in the acceptance of the transcendentals. . . and one will be non-peaceful if something less is accepted.

Samuel A. Nigro

The heart of it is this: to make the Lord in His immense love for you constitutive of your personal worth. Define yourself radically as one beloved by God. God's love for your and His choice of you constitutes your worth. Accept that, and let it become the most important thing in your life.

Name lost

All I want to say to you is, "You are the Beloved," and all I hope is that you can hear these words as spoken to you with all the tenderness and force that love can hold. My only desire is to make these words reverberate in every corner of your being — "You are Beloved."

Henri Jim Nouwin

Ministry was sharing, not dominating; understanding, not theologizing; caring, not fixing.

Brennan Manning

In a revealed religion, silence with God has a value in itself and for its own sake, just because God is God. Failure to recognize the value of mere being with God, as the beloved, without doing anything, is to gouge the heart out of Christianity.

Edward Schilebeeckx

From seat to seat throughout this realm, to all the realm is pleasing. For in his will our hearts have found their peace.

Piccarda, who is on Heaven's lowest level in the Divine Comedy, when asked by Dante if she was not discontented with her lowly place. T.S. Eliot called this the profoundest line in all human literature.

True religion never begins in comfort. It begins in repentance and humility and fear.

Peter Kreeft

That's exactly the point of modern quantum theory. So a thirteenth century theologian discovered one of the basic principles of modern nuclear physics 700 years ago!

Niels Bohr, the great twentieth-century quantum physicist upon hearing how angels move instantly from one place to another without passing through space or time.

In my own small way, I am helping people, if only by leaving most of them alone.

Ashleigh Brilliant

Try to relax and enjoy the crisis.

Ashleigh Brilliant

There is nothing good nor bad but thinking makes it so.

Hamlet

My words fly up; my thoughts remain below. Words without thought never to heaven go.

(Angels are words?) from Hamlet

Jesus is the human face of God.

Karl Rahner

You'll never understand a man 'til you stand in his shoes and look at the world through his eyes.

Atticus Finch

The unaware life is not worth living.

Socrates

Without discipline we can solve nothing. With only some discipline we can solve some problems. With total discipline we can solve all problems.

Scott Peck

We hold a treasure
not made of gold
in earthen vessels
wealth untold.
One treasure only
The Lord, the Christ
in earthen vessels.

Signature song of St. Louis Jesuits

The heart has her reasons about which the mind knows nothing.

Blaise Pascal

For obvious reasons, atheists have to take very good care of themselves.

Ashleigh Brilliant

There are many angels. . . as many as there are words. . . as if there is an angel for each word and/or for each being for which there is a word. Indeed, every word must be a messenger in more ways than phonemes strung together. Every word must have spiritual energy in proportion to the word's transcendental dimensions. The more the spiritual energy of the word, the higher the angel accompanying and surrounding the speaker and hearer and the object itself. . . and the closer to God.

Samuel A. Nigro

Teach us, good Lord, to serve you as you deserve: To give and not to count the cost; to fight and not to heed the wounds; to toil and not to seek for rest; to labor and not ask for any reward save that of knowing that we do your will.

St. Ignatius of Loyola

When you encounter a conflict between science and religion, you're either dealing with a bad scientist or a bad theologian.

Theodore Hesburgh

Religion people are not trying to *impose* their views on anyone. But they will no longer be denied their right to *propose* their views along with everyone else's.

Mary Ann Glendon

Everyone belongs to the Body of Christ, everyone, without a distinction between innocent life and guilty life.

Helen Prejean

When we are deeply committed and unswerving in our commitment to a deep cause of right, Providence begins to work for us and our lives find their way for us.

Goethe

Religion is terrible without a good Pope. . . .

Name lost

There is no bigot like an atheist.

G.K. Chesterton

A lie can be half way around the world before the truth has its boots on.

James Calaghen

There is a greater intensity and quality of existence in the act of dying through faithfulness to duty than in a long contented life preserved through cowardice.

Father Yves de Montcheuil prior to his execution by the Nazis

I commend myself to God, to Our Lady, to St. Alphege and to St. Denis. . . .Into your hands I commend my spirit. . . .For the name of Jesus and for the defense of His Church, I'm ready to die.

St. Thomas Becket as he was being hacked
with swords at his murder by Henry II's men

Oh God, for Whose Church the glorious Bishop Thomas fell by the swords of the wicked, grant we beseech thee that all who implore his help may obtain a salutary answer for their petitions.

Collect for December 29 Feast Mass of the Martyrdom

Imbued with self-righteous cowardice in the guise of lovie dovie better-than-thou liberalism, demasculinized ("feminine" but not "female") priests and bishops proclaim unthinking (irrational) feel-good (gnostic) relationship see-how-better-we-are-nambie pambie equality pablum, until challenged forthrightly at which time they abandon their wimpery to become vicious tyrants suppressing unequally those against them by a nasty self-contradiction of the mealy pap they have been preaching and practicing all along.

2X4 upside the head

The fruit of silence is PRAYER.
The fruit of prayer is FAITH.
The fruit of faith is LOVE.
The fruit of love is SERVICE.
The fruit of service is PEACE.

Mother Theresa

Most likely it (whatever is is) did NOT happen the way they told you. All that really happened is that IT happened to be in the news. So refuse to be suggestible. Refuse to be gullible. Do not believe much of what you hear or read as "news."

Samuel A. Nigro

Liberals are willing to tolerate anyone or anything for the sake of freedom, except those who stick to their high values. Thus liberals are frauds and living self-contradictions whenever challenged.

Name Lost

To claim that Jesus preached nothing new or original but rather the standard teachings of the rabbis flies in the face of what was done to Him and His followers by fellow Jews. Christianity is a branch of Judaism, deviant in its fundamental difference and fulfilling in its Scriptural completing.

Samuel A. Nigro

It is a kind of pride to believe others are happier or more fortunate or more content than we are, just as it is a bit of a perversion to want to live some life other than our own.

James Schall

Peter is named 195 times in the New Testament, 45 times as "Simon Bar Jona" and 150 times as "Peter." The next name most frequently mentioned is that of John the Evangelicst, which occurs 29 times.

Karl Keating

Religion does not conform to us, but we to it.

James Schall

In the temporal order, *dimensions* are space coordinates (length, width, height, or equivalents) and time. So is Holy Orders: poverty, chastity and obedience without time. Fulfill your role.

CHAPTER 9:

MATRIMONY

In the physical order, *uncertainty* is the accuracy of position being inversely related to the accuracy of movement. Your human beingness is an uncertainty.

In the spiritual order, *Matrimony* is *uncertainty* about "person-centered candidness" in that all occurrences are not known when one's own being achieves a one-personness with another. Resultant is *liberty* (personified by the Son) conveying *temperance* — moderation and self-control when facing desirables.

"I thirst."

Matrimony makes you an uncertainty — a point of liberty moderated by temperance.

Live Matrimony — relating into a duality.

To be two in One Flesh
To Enter God's Creating
and to participate in the
Incarnation

In physics, *uncertainty* of the accuracy of position is inversely related to the accuracy of movement. So is Matrimony.

Matrimony is the Sacrament which unites a Christian man and woman in lawful marriage. Matrimony is an *uncertainty*.

Matrimony is the pattern of "person-conscious centered" open relatingness coinciding with *uncertainty* in the physical world meaning that all accuracies are not known. The human principle resultant is that of *liberty* (personified by the Son) resulting in the activity of *temperance* wherein moderation and self-control result enabling two to become one.

C^2CC Centered Candidness. . .

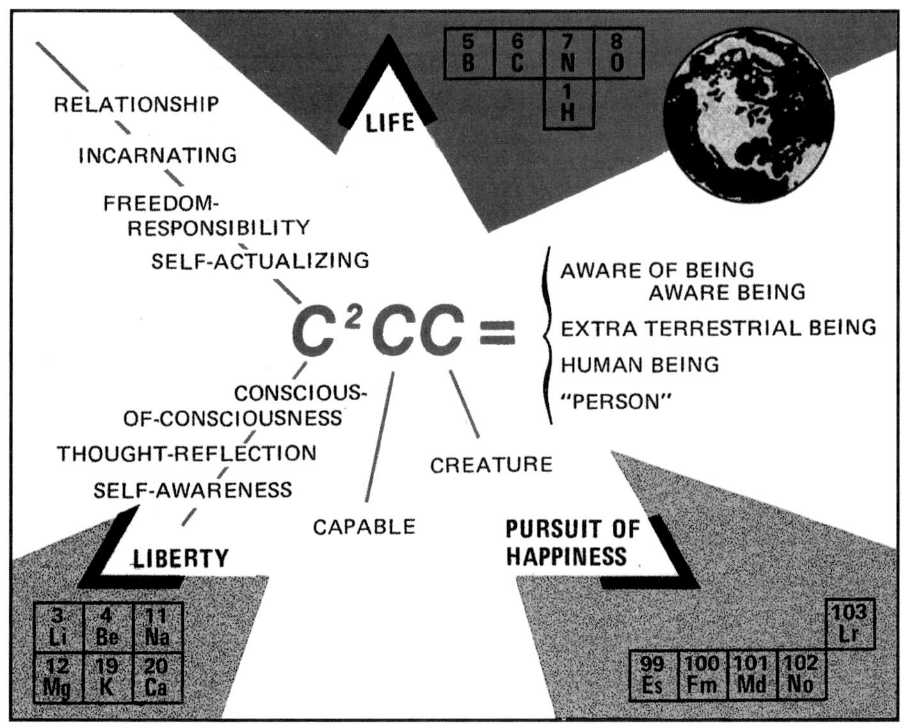

. . . .One way to be a human being. Animals may be conscious but not conscious of consciousness. Human beings, however, reflect (like human cerebra) back on themselves conscious of their own consciousness. This consciousness squared (C^2) gives partial freedom from biological evolution by virtue of reflective thought manipulating matter in the sequential priorities of Life first, Liberty second, and the Pursuit of Happiness third. So candidly center yourself on behalf of C^2CCs. To do so is to acquire not only humanbeingness but is to ascend, expand, and achieve community with any Conscious-of-Consciousness Capable Creature ever anywhere in the Universe.

C^2CC Centered Candidness

One must speak fairly and accurately as to what is seen. Tension needs to be identified, and the need to lighten up must be mentioned by speaking softly and gently: "I can hear you — I see. . . . Think of the consequences — Your actions are speaking louder than your words." All must be on behalf of the person: a Conscious of Consciousness Capable Creature (C^2CC).

* * * * *

Character consists of what you do on the third and fourth tries.

James Michener

The group consisting of mother, father and child is the main educational agency of mankind.

Martin Luther King, Jr.

Don't add to the truth; if you do, you will subtract from it.

Anonymous

Feigning invariably fails.

Malcolm S. Forbes

Basically my wife was immature. I'd be at home in the bath and she'd come in and sink my boats.

Woody Allen

Ninety-nine percent of the failures come from people who have the habit of making excuses.

George Washington Carver

Enthusiasm is at the bottom of all progress. With it, there is accomplishment. Without it, there are only alibis.

Henry Ford

We can all learn something from the parrot, which is content to repeat what it hears without trying to make a good story out of it.

Anonymous

The enthusiastic, to those who are not, are always something of a trial.

Alban Goodier

Pick battles big enough to matter, small enough to win.

Jonathan Kozol

Heroes you have to love. Celebrities are an infatuation — easy come, easy go.

Melvin Maddocks

Unless you are married to it, it is not a real problem.

Evelyn Nigro

Enjoy your age before it's past; don't try to be eighteen so fast. You're only fourteen once, my dears, but you'll be thirty-five for years.

Elinor K. Rose

I'm always on an even keel. You are so lucky.

Sue Nigro

Almost half my life I have been working — since I was 16 — and I want to be a homemaker, a wife, and a mother — and a real one of each for at least a little while. . . .

Depressed woman patient in mid-30's

Perseverance is not a long race; it is many short races one after another.

Walter Elliott

If indeed you must be candid, be candid beautifully.

Kahil Gibran

One does not make friends. One recognizes them.

Garth Henrichs

It was a great day but I hurt all over. No bending. No pulling. No pushing. No twisting. No turning. No tugging.

Sue Nigro at 55th birthday

A lifetime isn't nearly long enough to figure out what it's all about.

Doug Larson

A few kicks in the behind never do any harm. The funny thing is that they are never given you for the real reason. But they wake you up, and that's the important thing.

Pierre Auguste Renoir

A job is like being married. You think you have made a mistake at least once a day.

Samuel A. Nigro

Sam: When you are right you don't need to communicate.
Sue: That's when you need to communicate the most.

Before you are frank with another, ask yourself: "Why?" Is it to diminish the other, to make yourself feel better at his expense? The ethical question is to ask: "Will this foster the relationship?" There is always a way to be honest without being brutal.

Arthur Dobrin

Facing it — always facing it — that's the way to get through. Face it!

Joseph Conrad

It is one thing to show a man that he is in error, and another to put him in possession of the truth.

John Locke

To be liked by others, you at least first have to pretend you like them — such is "testing the waters" and then let "liking" take its course.

Samuel A. Nigro

The Sacrament of Matrimony is the Sacrament which unites a Christian man and woman in lawful marriage.

Baltimore Catechism

The good life is doing things right.

Samuel A. Nigro

You are what you love. So choose well. Drugs? Alcohol? Sex? Satan? Truth? Knowledge? Goodness? Helping others? Family? Respect? Peace? Good goals?

Samuel A. Nigro

Don't talk to victory. Talk to people.

Anonymous

You've got a good head. Use it for something besides a hat rack.

Leon Kranz

The fastest way to ruin a good meal or a good time is to start "problem-solving" in a manner that *demands agreement*.

Samuel A. Nigro

How can anyone so smart be so damn dumb?

Charles C. Nigro

God bless the child who has his own.

Rich Nero

The most difficult self-sacrifices of marriage are two: Pretending that it doesn't bother you when you are sexually frustrated and pretending that you are sexually interested when you are not. Those times are when you find out the genuine meaning of "self-sacrifice of marriage."

Samuel A. Nigro

What's the matter? Are you about to have your period, you dummy?

Sue Nigro (to her cranky husband)

He who speaks the truth cannot be overcome.

St. Thomas

The future isn't what it used to be.

Paul Valery

I don't know. If it comes, it comes. Who knows?

Madam Rose, Fortune Teller

They have invented a new phrase, a phrase that is a black-and-white contradiction in two words — "free love" — as if a lover ever had been, or ever could be, free. It is the nature of love to bind itself, and the institution of marriage merely paid the average man the compliment of taking him at his word.

G.K. Chesterton

The whole aim of marriage is to fight through and survive the instant when incompatibility becomes unquestionable. For a man and a woman, as such, are incompatible.

G.K. Chesterton

Don't you understand that all the crazy things men do and all the "talking about it" they cannot do, is to hide how weak they are?

A man who prefers to be anonymous

If my children are happy and my husband is happy, I am happy.

Sue Nigro, at 27th wedding anniversary

Are you that funny way *again*??!

Sue Nigro, newlywed

It appears to us that of all the fairy tales, none contains so vital a moral truth as the old story, existing in many forms, of Beauty and the Beast. There is written, with all the authority of a human scripture, the eternal and essential truth that until we love a thing in all its ugliness, we cannot make it beautiful.

G.K. Chesterton

A teacher who is not dogmatic is simply a teacher who is not teaching.

G.K. Chesterton

He that spares the rod hates his son.

Proverbs 13:24

But each has his own special gift from God, one of one kind and one of another. . .all these are inspired by one and the same Spirit, who apportions to each one individually as He wills.

1 Corinthians 12:11-13

(Does not sound like "equality," does it?)

For the most dangerous of all forms of ignorance is ignorance of work.

G.K. Chesterton

Truth, of course, must of necessity be stranger than fiction, for we have made fiction to suit ourselves.

G.K. Chesterton

To complain that I could only be married once was like complaining that I had only been born once.

G.K. Chesterton

The man who marries for money will earn it.

Anonymous

Because Moses by reason of the hardness of your heart permitted you to put away your wives: but from the beginning it was not so. And I say to you, that whosoever shall put away his wife, except it be for fornication, and shall marry another, committeth adultery; and he that shall marry her that is put away, committeth adultery.

Matthew 9:4-9

Children need love from a man *and* a woman. If they do not get it during their childhood from their mother *and* father, they *will* get "it" from another, but, sadly in all likelihood, it will *not* be maternal or paternal love.

Samuel A. Nigro

Everything is easy as long as you know how.

Charles C. Nigro

Never, never, never ask your children, especially your daughters, which one loves you the most.

King Lear

Whosoever shall put away his wife and marry another, committeth adultery against her. And if the wife shall put away her husband, and be married to another, she committeth adultery.

Mark 10:10-12

To them that are married, not I but the Lord commandeth, that his wife depart not from her husband. And if she depart, that she remain unmarried, or be reconciled to her husband.

1 Corinthians 7:10-11

The only difference between what tempts you now and what tempted those ten thousand years ago is perfume.

Samuel A. Nigro

You marry a person — you do not just marry a body. . . .

Barbara Willke

There is no more important environment to keep healthy for the next generation than the female uterus.

Donald DeMarco

Feminists may be beyond rational persuasion, and will continue to proclaim their errors with complete assurance. But they are, in the end, asking women to make themselves unattractive to men and to forgo love and children.

Michael Levin

Spouses should take frequent neighborhood walks to solve problems and foster togetherness because you do not fight in front of neighbors or strangers.

Samuel A. Nigro

It takes an Act of God to make a marriage work, which is why marriage is a Sacrament. You also need to pray.

Samuel A. Nigro

Whomever humbles himself will be exalted.

Matthew 23:12

He who is least among you all is the one who is great.

Luke 9:48

We have met the enemy and he is us.

Pogo

What therefore God hath joined together, let not man put asunder.

Matthew 19:6

Things are not what they seem. . . . They are what you make of them!

Samuel A. Nigro

When they shall rise from the dead, they neither marry, nor are given in marriage; but are as the angels which are in heaven.

Mark 12:25

It is better to marry than to burn.

1 Corinthians 7:9

He that is married careth for the things that are of the world, how he may please his wife.

1 Corinthians 7:33

She that is married careth for the things of the world, how she may please her husband.

1 Corinthians 7:34

Sex is a living pathway of connection, an intricate web of desire that begins with lust and ends not with orgasm but with children, families, communities, and nations. That ends, in fact, with love.

Maggie Gallagher

For this cause shall a man leave his father and mother, and shall be joined unto his wife, and the two shall be one flesh.

Ephesians 5:31

Set thine house in order.

Isaiah 38:1

Two important rules exist for parents in dealing with their teenagers:
1. Keep them as busy as possible in discreetly-adult-supervised activities;
2. Make home life such a *pleasant* place to be that, secretly, a teenager would rather be *at home* than with so-called "friends."

Anna Marie O'Hare

The best way to lose weight is to be helpful around the house — very helpful around the house.

Charles C. Nigro

Happiness is obedience to God married to freedom.

Samuel A. Nigro

Sitting home and watching TV all the time, that's terrible.

Dave Winfield, New York Yankee

It is not good that man should be alone.

Genesis 2:18

Ye have heard that it was said by them of old time, thou shalt not commit adultery. But I say unto you, that whosoever looketh on a woman to lust after her, has committed adultery with her already in his heart.

Matthew 5:27-28

Equality may perhaps be a right, but no power on earth can ever turn it into a fact.

Honore de Balzac

Every 18 to 24 months, a kid takes a "turn for the worse" which lasts anywhere from 3 to 6 months. Those times will pass. This pattern continues until age 48, when the durations of "turn for the worse" become 3 weeks or less.

Samuel A. Nigro

Motherhood is proof of the greater capacity of women to love. From a mother's love springs family, culture, civilization and faith. All human beings are monuments to the love, courage and work of mothers through whom God gives all life, all grace and all love. The more women are valued in this way, the greater the civilization. Maternal (and paternal as well as familial to some extent) themes are overwhelmingly present and almost unique to Roman Catholicism, especially when compared to other religions. Unisexist and anti-family feminism are obstructions to women using their greater capacity to love.

Samuel A. Nigro

There are no family crises — just growth steps.

Samuel A. Nigro

Can't you ever say anything trivial?

Sue Nigro to her husband

Everybody gets seven "bad" days a month. Women get theirs all in a bunch. Men get theirs on weekends. And children get their seven "bad" days in half-hour doses scattered throughout each day. You have a real family if you can survive when everyone is having their bad days all at the same time.

Samuel A. Nigro

I apologize for all those lousy things I did. . . . It was not because I am bad. It was because I am weak and stupid and can't be in two places at once.

Universal Marriage Apology

Some day, you gonna go crazy!

Anna Marie or Samuel A. Nigro
(statement from one to the other indicating the argument is over)

Well, I'm sorry too.

Nancy Kranz

Marriage is a 90:10 contract with each trying to do 90 percent of the work and sacrifice.

Sue Nigro

To older couples: Put a little adolescence in your life — just do not get arrested in the parking lot.

Samuel A. Nigro

Marry the one you love, but the Sacrament of Matrimony means you love the one you marry.

Samuel A. Nigro

So they are no longer two, but one. Man must not separate, then, what God had joined together.

Matthew 19:6

No success in life can compensate for failure in the home.

Sven Rydenfelt

Be merciful, just as your Father is merciful.

Luke 6:36

Shirt sleeves to shirt sleeves in three generations. . . .

Italian immigrant lamentation of
the failure to keep family values

TEN COMMANDMENTS OF TEENAGE HAPPINESS

I. Never believe anything on television, in movies or from newspapers (except sport scores) without two independent verifications.

II. Never believe any celebrity about anything.

III. Sex for any reason except to have a baby is stupid.

IV. Books are better than alcohol and drugs.

V. Playing smart is smart. Playing dumb is dumb.

VI. To the gals (guys): guys (gals) are no good until they prove otherwise over and over and over. . . .

VII. Only virtue and transcendentals make you free.

VIII. The best adulthood is when you are true to your best days of childhood, so stay out of adult stuff as long as you can. You are not missing a thing.

IX. Whatever you think is new has already been tried and failed, so read about it first before you try it again.

X. No, you do not know it all.

When you "put on love," none of this is a problem (but read *every* word):
Brethren: Let wives be subject to their husbands as to the Lord; because a husband is head of the wife, just as Christ is head of the Church, being Himself savior of the body. But just as the Church is subject to Christ, so also let wives be to their husbands in all things. Husbands, love your wives, just as Christ also loved the Church, and delivered Himself up for her, that He might sanctify her, cleansing her as in a bath of water by means of the word; in order that He might present to Himself the Church in all her glory, not having spot or wrinkle or any such thing, but that she might be holy and without blemish. Even thus ought husbands also to love their wives as their own bodies. He who loves his own wife, loves himself. For no one ever hated his own flesh; on the contrary he nourishes and cherishes it as Christ does the Church (because we are members of His body, made from His flesh and from His bones).

"For this reason a man shall leave his father and mother,
and shall cleave to his wife;
and the two shall become one flesh."

This is a great mystery — I mean in reference to Christ and to the Church. However, let each one of you also love his wife just as he loves himself; and let the wife respect her husband.

Ephesians 5:22-33

Analysis of Ephesians 5:22-33:

Wife	*Church*	*Husband*	*Jesus*
-be subject	-be the Body -be subject	-head	-head -Savior of the Body
		-love wife	-love church -delivered Himself up for her (Church and Body)
		-love wife in same manner as Jesus did the Church -love wife as own body	-sanctify her -cleanse her present holy and pure her to Himself
		-no hatred of self (includes wife -nourish and cherish own body (includes wife) -leave father and mother -cleave to wife -become one flesh	-Love Church in same manner as His Own Body (includes all members)
-respect husband		-love wife as self	

When you "put on love," this is a solution.

Samuel A. Nigro

Now we will feel no rain,
for each of us will be shelter
for the other.
Now we will feel no cold,
for each of us will be
warmth to the other.
Now there is no more loneliness
Now we are two persons,
but there is only one life before us.
Let us go now to our dwelling
and enter into the days of our
life together.

AND MAY OUR DAYS BE
GOOD AND LONG UPON
THE EARTH.

American Indian Wedding Blessing

For where two or three come together in My name, I am there with them.

Matthew 18:20

To be happy at home is the end of all endeavor.

Samuel Johnson

. . .in all that really matters, in hope and in love and in joy, the child is the teacher of the adult.

John Saward

I just want to be faithful, to the end, to the child I used to be.

Georges Bernanos

The essential function of the family is to rear children.

Russell Kirk

I never had any trouble finding the kids. All I had to do was close the bathroom door for a little privacy and in no time they would be knocking at the door.

Name Lost

Many young women are playing "I can do it" games in acquiescence to peer pressure. The only thing they will miss is a genuine family really their own.

Samuel A. Nigro

ONENESS DINING

For family oneness, a pleasant "main meal" should be shared each day with the following rules:

1. Give thanks to God for the miracle of one's own being and everything else — do not forget God!
2. One or two phrases read from the Bible with a discussion (and explanation preferably from a Navarre Bible).
3. All family members eating slowly.
4. No one can speak twice until everyone has spoken once (except Mom or Dad or designated leader to re-establish order).
5. Tension not allowed and agreement never demanded.
6. Above all: good news and gentle information.
7. One new vocabulary word (vocabulary is the *only* consistent correlation with success, however defined).
8. What was learned today?
9. Problems can be listed and discussed, but solutions will ruin the meal, so solve problems somewhere else.
10. Everyone eagerly shares the work of preparing, serving and clean-up.

For family maintenance, a unifying, gracious dining event should be planned each day with emphasis on relaxed savoring of good food, good uplifting communication, and deliberative dining.

Nothing will ever be fun again.

Janet Heath, age 9, when she heard of her mother's (Aloise Buckley Heath) untimely death

The image of God is common to both sexes since it resides in the mind where there is no distinction of sexes.

St. Thomas Aquinas

The most difficult thing to teach teenagers is that their friends are not the most important things in life. More important things are their families and their books.

Samuel A. Nigro

Because marriage is impossible family people need to go to church and pray for survival as if they have been trapped in an earthquake-collapsed building.

Name Lost

Contraception renders sexuality to be as trivial for the female as it is for the male, to the detriment of all.

Anonymous

Going without dinner is an appropriate, humane, effective, and civilizing punishment for obnoxious and unacceptable misbehavior of children. Like occasional fasting for adults, going without a meal strengthens one's soul.

Samuel A. Nigro

In all nature, male and female complement one another. But some humans, consistent with humanity's violation of nature in every way possible, demand that men and women be the same.

Anonymous

Always marry a gal three or four years younger than you are — that way you can stay on top.

Charles C. Nigro

Awareness of being aware (consciousness squared) produces the transcendentals by which we relate to the world, live our stories, and save our souls.

Anonymous

Matrimony means that two individuals have become one and therefore they look only to each other for everything.

Anonymous

In the animal kingdom, orgasm is the norm for males. . . . For females, the norm is reproduction and a precious guarding of sexuality.

Anonymous

Do I contradict myself?
Very well then, I contradict myself.
(I am large, I contain multitudes).

Walt Whitman

The quarrel with motherhood is simply a quarrel with life.

G.K. Chesterton

Women command the night.

Pina

If subhuman animals treated sex like humans treat sex, one could not go to the zoo, the woods, the pasture, the veldt, the jungle, the desert, or any place else in the environment without observing all animals copulating or performing a variety of sex acts unknown in the subhuman animal kingdom. Humanity is just not in tune with nature when the female of the species disdains the natural role of females in the animal kingdom. In such regards, sex divorced from reproduction for women is out of synchrony with femaleness, with nature, and with the planet as life has evolved.

Samuel A. Nigro

It is a characteristic common to all the (sexual) perversions that in them reproduction as an aim is put aside. This is actually the criterion by which we judge whether an act is perverse — if it departs from reproduction in its aims and pursues the attainment of gratification independently.

Sigmund Freud (Introductory Lectures on Psychoanalysis, Allen and Unwin, 1952, p. 266)

. . . a mother's nightmare — not to be of use. . . .

Barbara Grizzuti Harrison

The sexes are two stubborn pieces of iron; if they are to be welded together, it must be while they are red-hot.

G.K. Chesterton

The man is head of the house while the woman is the heart of the home.

G.K. Chesterton

Let's come off it, ladies and gentlemen: sex is not *that* important.

Harvard Professor George Homans

If you do not think you have made a mistake in your marriage or job at least once a day, you have probably slept through the day.

Samuel A. Nigro

Man embraces woman unless otherwise stated in the text.

Winston Churchill to a feminist carping about his generic use of the word "man".

The military is no place for family people.

Samuel A. Nigro

Nowhere are the differences between men and women more obvious than in the realm of sexuality. For men, it is simplistically little. For women, it seems intensively large. For the male: "How about it?" For the female: "How dare you?" Obviously, genuine compatibility can only occur when each party moves to imitate the other.

Anonymous

The entire concept of "premature" ejaculation is not in nature. In nature, the rule tends to be: the faster the safer the better. Only when humans, consistent with our tendency to deform everything, redefine sexuality as a form of recreation do we arrive at the concept of "premature" ejaculation which is a complete fraud resulting from anti-reproduction education.

Samuel A. Nigro

If parents would only realize how they bore their children.

George Bernard Shaw

The head-of-the-house role is an affectation except in a crisis — and then everyone knows that the man is head of the house.

Anonymous

For genuine happiness and well being, marry well.

Anonymous

be of love (a little) more careful than of anything.

e.e. cummings

Sex education sends the wrong message because it accentuates what is not important to children and therefore deprives them of childhood.

Samuel A. Nigro

If a husband were permitted to abandon his wife, the society of husband and wife would not be an association of equals, but instead a sort of slavery on the part of the wife.

St. Thomas

Males do not communicate well unless good women teach them how.

Anonymous

The New Testament spiritualizes humanity to supernatural life by lifting mankind beyond his animal nature. The pill and other artificial contraception methods do the opposite and remove humanity from having even the standards of the animal kingdom thereby removing humanity from what is truly natural for the planet.

Anonymous

For adequate conscience formation, a delicate threatening event is necessary sometime during one's youth. This must be a stern, fear-inspiring accentuation of one's vulnerability with an unmistakable heightened awareness of consideration-for-others as essential for one's own well being and survival. This threatens the child's very being without damaging, thereby sensitizing one to a healthy, positive dependency on others. Children must learn graphically that they cannot always have their own way. . .and that reasonable consequences dramatically occur with lack of consideration-for-others. It does not have to be brutal but it must be felt as "I don't ever want this to happen again!" Civilization and conscience depends on the acquisition of a fear of offending others. Without this fear (or conscience), people feel they are invulnerable and can get away with anything, an accurate description of individuals who act uncivilized and end up in jail.

Samuel A. Nigro

Love can be a tiny flame, and you must fan it every single day of your lives together. Sometimes there are horrible things that happen and threaten to blow it out; sometimes it almost putters out simply to a steady glow — and you come to realize that, without it, you would be groping in the dark.

Betty Steel's grandmother on her 70th wedding anniversary to "that cranky old wreck of a man."

Every criminal court judge in America is sickeningly aware of the terrible fact that teenagers are replacing adults on the criminal dockets. What Western country has the lowest juvenile delinquency rate? The answer is Italy. I went into Italian homes to see for myself. I found that even in the poorest family, the father is respected by the wife and children as its head. He rules with varying degrees of love and tenderness and firmness. His household has rules to live by, and the child who disobeys them is punished. The American teenager has been raised in a household where "obey" is an outlawed word and where mother has put herself at the head of the family. Every time mother overrules father, undermining his authority and standing in the child's eyes, she knocks a piece off the foundation on which the child stands. In Italy I found the nine word principle that I think can do more for us than all the committees, ordinances, and multi-million-dollar programs combined: PUT FATHER BACK AT THE HEAD OF THE FAMILY.

Hon. Samuel L. Liebowitz, Justice of the Supreme Court of the State of New York

The future of society is in the hands of the mothers. If the world was lost through a woman, she alone can save it.

Louis de Beaufort

The very definition of mental health is the ability to give and receive love.

Patricia Treece

No house is too small for one family and God.

Old Proverb

No house is big enough for two families. . . for very long.

Evelyn Nigro

Sexual license results in no marriages because marriage is the only "sex license."

Anonymous

If you don't put things back where they belong after you use them, it won't be long and all you'll have is a junk yard.

Evelyn Nigro

He's all boy — leave him alone — how else is he going to learn?

Charles C. Nigro defending his son

I am sorry the pill spoiled young people. It's made them more permissive. People will abuse anything.

Dr. Min Chueh Chang (the co-developer of the birth control pill)

After work, the happy home.

1920's business slogan

No man who owns his own house and lot can be a deadbeat. He has too much to do.

Anonymous

Any federal enterprise always works to undermine the government's principle rival, the family, in creating a population of isolated, ignorant, and dependent sheep.

Allan Carlson

The most important decision you will ever make is the picking of your mate. Your mate will provide you with 90% happiness or 90% misery.

Anonymous

Just to give you something to yell about!

Universal response to: "Why on earth did you ever. . .?"

Stop looking at the opposite sex as an enemy.

Abby Hirsch

Haven't you read the scripture that says that in the beginning the Creator made people male and female: And God said, "For this reason, a man will leave his father and mother and unite with his wife and the two will become one." So they are no longer two but one. Man must not separate, then, what God has joined together.

Matthew 11:4-6

Don't spit in the well: you'll be thirsty by and by.

Russian Proverb

I packed for everybody for this vacation. Nobody forgot a thing. Except I forgot my underwear.

Name prohibited from being used

Do you know what? I am actually tired of shopping. I must be getting old.

Name prohibited from being used

I was ever of opinion, that the honest man who married and brought up a large family, did more service than he who continued single and only talked of population.

Oliver Goldsmith

Snarling, swearing, sexually-abused little girls generally do not make good mothers.

Anonymous

If you want a baby, have a new one. Don't baby the old one.

Jessamyn West

Praise the child and you make love to the mother.

American Proverb

Above all, where social and cultural conditions so easily encourage a father to be less concerned with his family or less involved in the work of education, efforts must be made to restore socially the conviction that the place and task of the father in and for the family is of unique and irreplaceable importance.

John Paul II

Being has polarity — male (transcendentals) and female (immanentals) exist in all things. So all being is a marriage.

Samuel A. Nigro

All created being has a masculine side which activates matter with truth and goodness; and a feminine side which molds form with oneness and beauty. All life is a marriage.

Anonymous

Matrimony makes two people to be one creature.

Anonymous

There are three sides to every marital conflict: his side, her side, and the truth.

Norma Nero

Corinthians says not to let the sun down on your anger. In our marriage, sometimes the sun does not set until 11:00 p.m.

Steve Wood

He who has a head of butter must not come near the oven.

Dutch Proverb

The way to go from rags to riches is to start by getting a decent set of rags.

Leonard and Thelma Spinrad

Make yourself all honey and the flowers will devour you.

English Proverb

Give your children the habit of overcoming their besetting sins.

William D. Sprague

The sooner you treat your son a man, the sooner he'll be one.

John Dryden

Every generation stands on the shoulders of the generation that came before. Jealously guard the principles of our heritage. They did not come easy.

Ronald Reagan

And, ye fathers, provoke not your children to wrath.

Ephesians 6:4

It is better to bind your children by a feeling of respect, and by gentleness, than by fear.

Terence

He that does not bring up his son to some honest calling and employment, brings him up to be a thief.

Jewish Maxim

Choose a wife rather by your ear than by your eye.

English Proverb

Be your own palace or the world's your jail.

Anonymous

Let the good times roll.

Cajun Proverb

Never strike your wife, even with the flower.

Hindu Proverb

For God's sake, choose a self and stand by it!

William James

In marriage do thou be wise; prefer the person before money; virtue before beauty; the mind before the body.

William Penn

Sexually easy women disrupt life for all women because easy sex magnifies a male's uncertainty as well as his reluctance to give a complete commitment to the woman of his choice. That sexual behavior is no longer unique to that one person, then that one person's very uniqueness is diminished. Some relationships therefore which could have achieved a solid, stable permanence will never be such because "other women were easy."

Samuel A. Nigro

Healthy mating rituals occur throughout the animal kingdom. They all are ways of bonding male and female in varying degrees to have a family grouping. This is a confirmed natural law as any observer of the planet knows. But humans, hypnotized by the ejaculation reflex, have created a repertoire of non-mating, non-procreative, non-species enhancing ejaculation pathologies that no species could imitate and still survive. There is a message here. . . and it is an environmentally sound message at that.

Samuel A. Nigro

You do not merely "hold" a baby. You "honeyfy" it by pouring yourself over it by gentle, flowing, warm sweetness and then the baby melts in your arms.

Samuel A. Nigro

Marriage is one-fourth God, one-fourth work, one-fourth sacrifice, and one-fourth silliness — and not necessarily in that order. And, there can be no marriage without each of them.

Name Lost

The sign of a healthy marriage is that you keep laughing when your spouse throws crap at you.

Name Lost

Be subject to one another out of reverence for Christ.

Ephesians 5:21

If you want to have sex, get married.

Anonymous

In marriage if you do not complement each other, you fight. If you do not complement, you grow apart. But complementing one another is not automatic. It needs to be consciously attempted by eager sacrifice over and over by both parties.

Name Lost

Make sure that marriage brings out "the best" because it will surely bring out "the worst."

Anonymous

Never strike the head — the head belongs to God.

Anna Maria Nigro on punishing children

What happens at your house is more important than what happens at the White House.

Barbara Bush

Make love at least once a week — it exercises your heart and lungs; it opens your eyes wide; it stretches every muscle; and it bends every joint in your body helping to prevent arthritis.

Advice to married couples

After reading a mid-life crisis book:
Wife: "Gee, at my age, I should have gone back to school, gone back to work, and had an affair."
Husband: "Well, how are you doing?"
Wife: "Two out of three."

Name Lost

Premarital sex can deprive two people of the exhilarating oneness necessary to keep promises and maintain trust.

Anonymous

Whoever wins the battle for the culture gets to teach the children.

William Bennett

The peculiarity of purity is to keep more excellent natures exempt from such as are subordinate.

Proclus

It cannot be that the son of these tears should be lost.

Bishop to St. Monica as she lamented
the misbehavior of her adolescent son
(St. Augustine)

How much was hoped from sex. How little sex can deliver.

Camille Paglia

(I)t is a patriarchal society that freed me as a woman.

Camille Paglia

Some women see some of their rights as rights only because they are women. . . and this is sexism at its worst.

Name Lost

Any man who has made love to more than one woman has told a lot of lies or said a lot of foolish things.

Anonymous

St. Paul admonishes us to avoid fornication because erotic intimacy binds us, willy-nilly, in a permanent union. If one indiscretion brings us into bondage — as it does, at least in the permanent records of our memory and imagination — then cohabitation with or without benefit of : or license, ties up our habits and our imaginings so tightly that, divorce or no, we can never cut ourselves free from what we were, so-and-so's man, the woman of such-and-such.

Thomas Fleming

Children without parents can never grow up to be fully human, neither can men without women nor women without men.

Thomas Fleming

Not in her times alone, but in her for all times, woman would find her glory and her honor. They could not call her Jew nor Greek nor Roman. Not successful nor beautiful. But "blessed," that is, holy. And blessed she is because by giving birth to the God-man she broke down the trammels of nationality and race. Her son was cosmopolitan. He is MAN *par excellence* and she is WOMAN because she is the Mother of God.

Archbishop Fulton Sheen

Intercourse even with one's legitimate wife is unlawful and wicked where the conception of offspring is prevented.

Saint Augustine

The reason the number 40 is so often found in the Bible is that 40 years tends to be the middle point of one's life. Thus, "40" conveys ceremonies, secrets, kingships, challenges, rulings, punishments, adversities, flight, self-denials, death, and resurrection — all applicable to the "mid-life crisis." But routinely in the Bible, with transcendental focusing and sacramental life, the resolution can always be more than satisfactory.

Samuel A. Nigro

In a marriage that succeeds, the husband has to do 90% of all the work, otherwise it isn't going to get done. The same goes for the wife.

Samuel A. Nigro

We are unmistakably shown through Nature that she depends upon ever-acting Creator and Ruler.

Name Lost

Children first make us older than we are. . . young again.

Samuel A. Nigro

The most successful love affairs are conducted entirely by post.

George Bernard Shaw

And the I married. After the sacrament, I learned what hell is.

Anatole France

A sweetheart is a bottle of wine; a wife is a wine bottle.

Ambrose Bierce

The male's need for desirability is almost identical to his sexual driveness. In nature, the female controls whether or not the male's need for desirability is met.

Name Lost

The subordination of females to males is an essential dependency of the male upon the female to bring out the best in both by "building up" rather than "putting down."

Anonymous

In nature, sexual fulfillment is always elusive. Readily available or indiscriminate sexual activity is the most unnatural phenomenon to be observed in nature and when observed, it almost always occurs in man.

Samuel A. Nigro

Every kid between the ages of 7 and 13 ought to be sent to bed hungry twice a year. It teaches them what real hunger is. It teaches them to know who provides them with bread and butter. It teaches that they indeed can be hurt without injury when they misbehave. It increases their awareness that they can make the world a better place by behaving themselves. It teaches that goodness pays. It creates conscience.

Samuel A. Nigro

Hurting your parents — is the rotten killer instinct of the young which also happens to be the life instinct.

Patricia Hampl

Members of a real family never stop trying to bring out the best of themselves and others in the family.

Anonymous

Any community or group which does not reinforce the natural femaleness of its women, will unleash all the unnatural potential of its men. Where the men are consistently "no good," the real cause is that the women are not being naturally female.

Name Lost

Be nice to your children — they will pay you back for whatever they think you have done wrong no matter what good you do them.

Name Lost

One reason we call children"innocent" is that they are too small to hurt us.

St. Augustine

God sends you kids when you are young enough to stand it.

Evelyn Nigro

Never put your best shoes by the toilet if you have little boys.

Name Lost

Okay, all of you kept acting like the youngest, so you all are going to bed at the youngest's bedtime.

Mary Helen O'Hare, mother of 5, ages 2 to 10
("It works," she says)

If you do not supervise children under ten years old, they will get hurt or abused. If you do not supervise youths from ten to eighteen years old, they will become violent sexualized savages.

Name Lost

This gift of self through love is the fruit of the Sacrament of Marriage. It lays each bare, puts a certain self to death, the "old self," to use St. Paul's words.

Ephesians 4:22

Women really are superior to men — at being a woman. And men are really superior to women — at being men.

Peter Kreeft

Is strength to be measured by the standard of the bully?

Peter Kreeft

Humility is the marriage bond of Heaven. Pride is the frigidity of Hell.

Peter Kreeft

The greatest Woman
who ever lived
Never did anything
By the world's standards.
She simply stayed home
For thirty years
and kept house
For God.

Author Unknown

Marriage is a "beauty and the beast" relationship with everybody taking turns playing each role and loving the ugliness of one another. Thus comes the universal motto of marriage: Love even the ugliness.

Samuel A. Nigro

You give your child to be suckled by a sow where he picks up the habits of his nurse. . . . And when he comes home you cry, "I know not whom you are like; this is no son of ours!"

Fr. Bernardino in 1498 to his parishioners
not having women in the home

I really got lucky when I married your mother. . .so if we ever get divorced, go with her.

Charles C. Nigro

If the men of a group are no good, look to the women. Basically, the women in such a group will be weak in the home and sexually easy. In such regards, a close look at Western Civilization reveals that the overt subordinate status of women, while at times excessive but most often not, carries with it a covert power to civilize men (and women as well). It is this hidden empowerment of women, at hearth and in home, which has been the basis for the tremendous power of Western Civilization and all civilized advancement.

Samuel A. Nigro

. . .immanentals sustain transcendentals which operationally means that women sustain men. . .embarrassed, we men call it subordination. . . .

Samuel A. Nigro

We may never be able to balance the scales for goal-oriented career women. But, at the very least, we can reward child rearing, society's most important profession, as handsomely as we reward the practice of law or public relations.

Dante DiFiore

One hug always leads to another.

Anonymous

Our homes are as intimate a part of us as the clothes we wear. If we are not thoroughly acquainted with our homes and aware of their needs, we are out of touch with a vital part of ourselves. If our homes do not arouse our passion, we are not able to fully appreciate our very existence.

Dante DiFiore

Plenty of things go wrong in human relationships because the nobler and more valuable things are, the more fragile they are. Fine china is breakable; plastic dishes are not.

Alice von Hildebrand

Nothing is small for someone who loves.

Alice von Hildebrand

In marriage, synchronization is always more beautiful than two solos without accompaniment.

Alice von Hildebrand

The trick to making a marriage work is not to be asking for help but to be always trying to help one another without anyone asking. If you don't say or need to say "thank you for complementing me" at least once an hour to your spouse, neither of you are doing it right.

Samuel A. Nigro

If I forgot your silly birthday, would you fuss?

Professor Higgins to his male friend Pickering

Men and women are different.

Natural Law

The beauty you see in another garden is a call for you to tend your own with greater love and care.

Alice von Hildebrand

How empty and short-lived is the happiness that purchased things promise.

Alice von Hildebrand

Sex on the brain is a very unhealthy place to have it.

Malcolm Muggeridge

My back hurts. . .no bending.

Sue Nigro

One mind, one soul, and one heart.

Marcel Clement on marriage

You just think you are mad — you're not really mad! (Try saying that to your wife.)

Samuel A. Nigro

I got better. . .why can't you get better?

Sue Nigro, after 30 years of marriage

A marriage is one being.

Name Lost

In true marriage, the "state" (government), is irrelevant, or perhaps secondary and subordinate at most, to the mutual enhancement of each party's Transcendentals.

Name Lost

More than yesterday; less than tomorrow.

Sue Nigro on marital love

The privacy of children and youth is different than privacy for adults. Indeed, to impose death, mental illness, sexuality, and adulthood onto preadolescents is to violate their privacy, integrity, and beingness.

Name Lost

Why do you think so much? Just stop it. Please. Just stop it.

Sue Nigro

Easy women undermine *all* women.

Sister Florence Marie

Children are hard to like. That is why a family should raise them because "like" does not matter. Love is what matters.

Samuel A. Nigro

. . .the most sincere and sensible people were people who earned their own living.

G.K. Chesterton

If you do not give kids meaningful messages, they do not think there is anything to know.

Anonymous

The human house is a paradox, for it is larger inside than out.

G.K. Chesterton

Neither males nor females can consider themselves as fully human without considering the other.

Name Lost

Every Sunday after Mass, I would sit the kids on and around me and read the funnies with vigor. WE had a great time and they learned to read.

A Child Psychiatrist

The school of Rabbi Hillel actually went so far as to declare that a husband might divorce his wife for any fault that displeased him, even if it were no more than burning his dinner.

Warren H. Carroll

Love is when you submissively take each other's crap in reciprocal commitment to bring out the best of each other.

Samuel A. Nigro

I have found it impossible to carry the heavy burden of responsibility. . . without the help and support of the woman I love.

Edward, Duke of Windsor, Farewell Broadcast, 12-11-36

The old rite for Matrimony contained an optional exhortation; its words, so ideal yet so beautifully sensible, deserve to be remembered: "You begin your married life by the voluntary and complete surrender of your individual lives in the interest of that deeper and wider life which you are to have in common. Henceforth you belong entirely to each other; you will be one in mind, one in heart, and one in affections. And whatever sacrifices you are called upon to make to preserve this common life, always make them generously. Sacrifice is usually difficult and irksome. Only love can make it easy; perfect love can make it a joy. We are willing to give in proportion as we love. And when love is perfect the sacrifice is complete. . . . Greater love than this no man has than to lay down his life for his friends."

John H. Miller, CSC

Women don't have sex when they have headaches, but when men have headaches, they need sex.

Name Lost

If you cannot love the ugliness, you should not be married.

Name Lost

The relations of the sexes are mystical, are and ought to be irrational. Every gentleman should take off his head to a lady.

G.K. Chesterton

We share our lives working together.

Aristotle

The world today needs Christian women — women who are God-fearing, committed to Christ, and who possess these particular virtues or characteristics:

Be a woman of LOVE in a selfish and loveless world;
Be a woman of HOPE in a despairing world;
Be a woman of FAITH in an unfaithful world;
Be a woman of INTEGRITY and HONESTY in a dishonest world;
Be a woman of JOY in a gloomy, sad world;
Be a woman of CLASS in a casual, careless world;
Be a woman of STRENGTH in a soft, weak world;
Be a woman of PRAYER - a woman of GOD, in a GODless world.

Be a woman who dares to live; who dares to be informed; who dares to build up rather than tear down; a woman who has developed the art of being as delicate as a flower, yet as strong as a tall oak.

When each of us comes to die, let us hope people will not say of us, "Isn't it too bad she died," but rather, "Isn't it wonderful that she lived."

Sister Kenan, OSV

Fathers must see to their boys. . .no longer can a man rely on mothers to make men out of little boys.

Name Lost

Get a house and a woman and an ox for the plough, and have your tools all ready in the house.

Hesiod 750 B.C.

. . .worthless women make bad wives even if they bring great riches. . . .

Euripides

Family is more important than peace of mind.

Steven Kranz

You both gotta do what you gotta do.

Elderly couple when asked how they did it at their fiftieth wedding anniversary.

Take a moment to listen today
To what your children are trying to say,
Listen today, whatever you do.
Or they won't be there to listen to you.
Listen to their problems, listen for their needs.
Praise their smallest triumphs, praise their
Smallest deeds.
Tolerate their chatter, amplify their laughter
Find out what's the matter, find out what
They're after.
But tell them that you love them
Tell them "Everything's all right. Tomorrow's
Looking bright!"
Take a moment to listen today
To what your children are trying to say,
Listen today, whatever you do.
And they will be there to listen to you.

Name Lost

No, you will not find happiness ever in the elitist, most perfect of marriages either. Remember, marriage is a sacrament which means it is a way to God (who is happiness), but it is not happiness in and of itself. No doubt, happiness occurs to some extent but not all the time. Marriage is a sacrament, a way but not an end in and of itself.

Samuel A. Nigro

Marriage is when a man and woman commit themselves to a permanent process of trying to drive each other crazy.

Samuel A. Nigro

Don't speak to strangers. And never get in a car with a stranger. Act retarded. Jabber with your tongue out. Then run or fight like hell — because once you get in that car you'll never get out.

Universal instruction for all children

Male integrity requires, rightly or wrongly, that women allow men to do what the woman knows she could do better. Quite frankly, men "go bad" when women won't support men in their efforts to lead or whatever.

Name Lost

In marriage, the hearts beat as one.

Tertullian

When the chips are down, when tension is high, when disagreement is massive and you are married, there is only one thing to do: Sacrifice!

Name Lost

THE ELEVEN DIMENSIONS OF FEMINISM

1. The Secret Law of Equal Criticism: Men cannot criticize women; women cannot criticize women; and everyone from animals to angels can criticize men.
2. The Feminist Golden Rule: I am; I feel; I want; gimme; and how dare you.
3. The New First Commandment: Never remind a feminist that she is not a man because she has a lady's sensitivity whenever made to feel unmasculine.
4. The Four Horsewomen of the Apocalypse: Noise, Promiscuity, Pollution, and Power.
5. The Grand Illusion of the Equality Goddess: That any difference between males and females is a subordination indicating a superior/inferior dichotomy.
6. Equality-is-a-Loaded-Gun — furnished by feminists with which women regularly shoot themselves in their egos and men in their brains.
7. The ERA Forever: The Engagement Ring Amendment to the Equal Rights Amendment, i.e. engagement rings will be required even though invidiously discriminatory against men who get nothing in return.
8. No Double Standards Here: Men hold back so women can barge ahead.
9. Schroeder's Spies (any and all military women) proclaiming that Equality is a woman's rank to be lorded over the men.
10. Forget It! Having forgotten what real femaleness is, women are embarrassed by what feminists say it is (so forget it).
11. Combat! is fun for women because more men die when their combat units are weakened.

Samuel A. Nigro

Kids need to know that they "earn their daily bread" by doing their home chores. No chores, no food.

Name Lost

As long as a marriage is founded on a good solid incompatibility, that marriage has a fair chance of continuing to be a happy marriage.

G.K. Chesterton

The mutuality between male and female is incredible. You sense it in relating to your parents, to those with whom you are infatuated as well as to those whom you genuinely love. But those who moan and groan will lose it and mess it up for the other. The wholeness of love sought in fantasy or in partnership will still be incomplete in terms of achieving happiness because happiness is only through God beyond the dimensions of human relationships.

Samuel A. Nigro

Never marry a feminist. . . . Your boys will be no good except for being nice to girls.

Name Lost

I tell you, an ordinary honest man is part of his wife even when he wishes he wasn't. I tell you, an ordinary woman is part of her husband even when she wishes him at the bottom of the sea. I tell you, whether the two people are for the moment friendly or angry, happy or unhappy, the Thing marches on, the great four-footed Thing, the Quadruped of the Home. They are a nation, a society, a machine. I tell you they are one flesh, even when they are not one spirit.

G.K. Chesterton

If ever monogamy is abandoned in practice, it will linger in legend and in literature.

G.K. Chesterton

As unto the bow the cord is
So unto the man is woman.
Though she bends him, she obeys him,
Though she draws him, yet she follows,
Useless each without the other!

Henry Wadsworth Longfellow

YOU'VE COME A LONG WAY, FELLAS. . . DON'T LET THE FEMINISTS DRIVE YOU BACK

Anyone who thinks women have been mistreated by Western Civilization ought to know how men treated women in the Noble Savage Multi-Culture. A few examples:

1. King Shaka Zulu killed all his offspring and many wives out of fear of being overthrown.
2. The "great" Gandhi refused British medical care for his wife but used it for himself.
3. High-ranking military land-owning castes of north India killed almost all female offspring up to the twentieth century to reduce the number who could claim inheritance.
4. Some South Pacific societies gang raped women who were "bad" to their husbands.
5. Female infanticide is over three millennia old and still practiced in China. It is spreading by abortion all over the world today. India has sub-cultures which allow the killing of women who will not abort their female offspring as determined by ultrasound.
6. Islamic fundamentalism, as of this writing, allows polygamy, flogs for indecent dress, stones women to death for adultery, prohibits women

from driving cars, bars them from any travel without their husband's permission, and divorce is the husband saying "I divorce you" three times rapidly.

7. Child brides are for sale in India and the usual buyers are Muslims.
8. Some society's men decided whom women should marry and forced them to remain even if brutalized. Also not uncommon was ceremonial and gang rape in such settings.
9. Wife-beating has appeared as acceptable in every folk society.
10. Some Indian castes have all females raised to be prostitutes.
11. In all history, most women have had impoverished diets as well as less dietary protein than men. Some Papuan women overcame starvation by regularly eating the flesh of deceased relatives while others kept food from the men by hiding it in their vaginas. The food hoarding Somali men of 1992 are typical of non-Western approaches.
12. A not so ancient Jewish prayer began by thanking God "for not making me a woman."
13. One thousand years of crippling footbinding of women in China was only recently stopped, and a deformed foot ("the golden lotus") was as crazily attractive to men then as the female breast (crazily, again) is to men today.
14. Ancient Greeks considered most women secondary to their preferred orgasm experts, i.e. other men, and a persistent commitment to a woman was a foreign bizarre idea until St. Paul.
15. The infibulation technique of some Muslims and others in Africa goes like this: The clitoris and both sets of vaginal labia are slashed off a young girl with the resulting wounds sutured together leaving a two millimeter opening for the passage of urine and menstrual blood. With marriage, the opening is enlarged painfully.
16. The homicide rate for women almost always exceeds men's and was ritualized at times as sati (suttee) in India where the wife is cremated alive with her predeceased husband. The Vikings had a similar rite: The dead chief's colleagues raped his wife who was then strangled by the oldest woman of the tribe and then the dead chief and wife were cremated together in the chief's boat set afire and adrift.
17. Since the collapse of the Russian Empire in the 1990's, the absence of Western civilizing Christian influence became more evident for Russian women because authorities ignored cases of rape and assault of wives by husbands. Furthermore, women became the first to be fired when jobs were reduced, and job advertisements specify women applicants must be "young, blonde, longlegged" and "without inhibitions."
18. Perhaps the most telling description of non-Western (non-Catholic) treatment of women is *Tales of a Thousand Nights and One Night* (now Arabian Nights and Entertainments) wherein Scherzade saved her own life night after night because of her stories which fascinated King Sharizad. . . otherwise she would have joined all his other wives whom he decapitated after spending the night with him.

In addition, women were the primary victims in societies wherein accepted were torture, witchcraft, cannibalism, economic exploitation, and slavery.

In summary, women in the non-West were considered inferior physically, morally and intellectually. They were to be taken advantage of in any way possible. Resultant was misery for both sexes. . .an internecine equality-crazy contest in which everyone loses.

All listed above cannot be honestly rejected by Noble Savage Multi-Culture enthusiasts. All mentioned has adaptive aspects fabricated (?), accepted and expected by the involved men and women alike. All listed was how things were done. No advantage was overlooked nor was there reason to do so.

Interestingly, those who see all listed as tragic have been and usually are espousers of Western Civilization. Others just do not care.

Uncommon outside the West were kindness, caring, sustained affection, keeping of promises, freedom, thought, reason, and any sense of personhood. These are all concepts of Western Civilization and along with "women and children first" are totally at odds with human nature in the non-West. Indeed, feminism would only be tolerated in the West while elsewhere, women's survival (and not equality) is the issue. Feminism only exists where there are patriarchs, make that Western patriarchs.

Feminists appear to have overlooked all this, rendering themselves to be if not ignorant, then selfishly self-destructive, in the long run. "Utterly dishonest and unrealistic" could also be added.

Feminists' persistence in the demand for power, in the demand for male compliance to a degree that feminists themselves do not countenance, and in the demand for flawed equality which is far from equal, carries within it a massive denial of the need for men to be willing to be different from what has been routine as already listed. And men's willingness may be more fragile than recognized when some realize that even the West has too many incidents still unacceptable.

Today's complaining women have forgotten that men need cogent reasons, and Western Civilizing reasons at that, to keep from regressing.

Only when convinced, will men treat women with less than the advantage-taking power available. Only when unprovoked will men artificially, unnaturally and voluntarily suppress their own energies.

Contemporary moaning ignored, Western Civilization found the way to do this. And it is important to understand how this was first done.

Indeed, where did Western Civilization's treatment of women come from? Try Colossians 3:18-19: "you who are wives, be submissive to your husbands. This is your duty in the Lord. Husbands, love your wives. Avoid any bitterness towards them."

These statements, among others, including Ephesians 5:22-33, are reasoned compromises worthy of Solomon and of the wisest of wise negotiators because they provide a male/female truce for the West and a delicate balance convincing males to replace their power with submissive love in exchange for female's reasoned submissive duty. There is a trade-off here and when compared to non-West styles, it is no small advancement. In fact, it was and is a first-rate good life and good news for men and women. Both sexes have benefitted and even blossomed, especially when the selfish power urges of males and the selfish poor-me surges of females are foregone.

Indeed, the Roman Catholic Church's "Holy Family" themes undergird all positive male/female relationships in the West. Therein is gentleness, support, complimentarity, balance, fairness, and a commitment to self-sacrifice on the part of everyone. Such themes do not exist firmly anywhere else and their absence has many alternatives, many of them listed at the beginning of this article.

Have you ever seen the Holy Family symbolism outside a Roman Catholic Church or book? This not only tamed men but women too and enabled a genuine synthesis of the two sexes not notably found elsewhere.

A final reflection is that feminists are to all men what non-Western males have been to all women.

Samuel A. Nigro

When it comes to communication, men are *slow learners* while women are quick demanders. This is an incontrovertible incompatibility between men and women. Thanks to the patient effort of gentle women, the men finally catch on — at which time, the women generally wish that the men would shut up. Sex is just the opposite.

Samuel A. Nigro

The elaborate courtships and preliminaries in the animal kingdom for the attentions of the female of the species *mean something*! For nature, they mean something more than consummated orgasmic infertile interactions.

Name Lost

Never tell a child to go to sleep. They don't know how to do that. You tell a child to close his eyes, shut his mouth, and make no noise. That is how you tell a child to "go to sleep."

Samuel A. Nigro

With consciousness-squared (C^2), entropy becomes knowable and voluntary. But with original sin, entropy became unconscious and involuntary in spite of consciousness-squared (C^2). This means that an uncertainty will always be present in human relationships. Even though humans are conscious of consciousness (C^2), it is no longer enough as it was prior to the Fall.

Samuel A. Nigro

It seems interesting to notice that the tradition of abstaining from conjugal intercourse on the first or more nights of the wedding is described not only in the Old Testament, but also in other religious traditions. For example, *triratravrata* (abstaining for the first three nights) is the tradition cited in the Hindu holy scriptures. Folklore scientists report similar behavior still in use in our days in some remote parts of Northern Europe. See R. Bali Pandey *Hindu Samskaras* Motilal Banarsidass, Delhi 1976, p. 195 and D.M. Balashov *The Russian Wedding* Moscow 1985, p. 296. These examples help us to realize how highly the virtue of chastity is respected universally in human experience.

Gintautas Vaitoska

In the middle of an argument:
Sam: You love me, and there isn't anything you can do about it.
Sue: You're only half right. Would you care to guess which half?

When women badger men to "talk about it," the men must understand that the women do not really want to know what is on your mind but just that you will tell them something they can agree with. Understanding that, men must be prepared to help women not to take personally whatever else men tell them.

Samuel A. Nigro

Money, always money, that is the nerve of democracy.

Proudhon

I don't know what happens. My billfold is empty again. Do you have any money?

Sue Nigro

If you didn't have that sense of humor, you'd be worthless.

Sue Nigro to her husband

Man will never have his pleasure unless he shares it with his woman.

Lysistra

. . .no one who has seen a baby sinking back satiated at the breast and falling asleep with flushed cheeks and a blissful smile can escape the reflection that this picture persists as a prototype of the expression of sexual satisfaction in later life.

Sigmund Freud

No doubt he wrote that while taking cocaine.

Lovers get old but love does not.

Old woman defending her elderly husband and herself against an aggressive television interviewer

. . . wrestling for hours with gigantic angels and devils.

G.K. Chesterton on playing with children

MOMILIES — CIVILIZING GRACEFUL MESSAGES FROM MARY GLEPKO, MOM OF FATHER ROBERT GLEPKO

Ask your father.
Wait until your father gets home!
"Robert Joseph" instead of Bob.
Eat it — it's good.
If I told you once, I told you a 1000 times.
A stitch in time saves 9.
Don't cry over spilt milk, it already has enough water in it.
Always put on clean underwear in case you're in an accident.
It'll never get better if you pick at it.
Don't sit so close to the TV — you'll wreck your eyes.
I'm only doing this for your own good.
This hurts me more than it hurts you.
As long as I'm around I'll be your mother.
The best sleep is the sleep you get before midnight.
A bored person is a boring person.
I'm not asking you — I'm telling you.
I don't care if Jesus is tap dancing on TV — turn if off and do your chores!
Don't ask me why — the answer is no.
Oh, so it's the egg teaching the chicken!
If you can't say anything nice, don't say anything at all.
You can go out in the rain — you won't melt.
Why do you think I have gray hairs.
Always put toilet paper on the seat.
Put that down! You don't know where it's been.
A dog always knows when you're afraid of it!
Don't cross your eyes or they'll stay that way.
Never try anyone else's glasses or you'll go blind.
Don't hit your mother or your hand will come out of the grave.
Is that a threat or a promise?
Good, I'll pack your lunch.
Excuse me for living.
If it's worth doing, it's worth doing well.
Never say "never."
I didn't buy all these clothes just to decorate the closet.
It's not what you wear; it's who you are.
Sit up straight.
How come you always offer to do the dishes at other people's houses?
Sleep tight and don't let the bed bugs bite and if they do, take a shoe and beat them 'til they're black and blue.
Eat the carrots — they're good for your eyesight.
Think of all the starving in China.
You can't start out the day on an empty stomach.

If it didn't taste bad, it wouldn't be medicine.
Don't marry anyone until you've seen them drunk.
You can choose your friends but you can't choose your relatives.
The apple doesn't fall far from the tree.
Water seeks its own level.
You can't make a silk purse out of a sow's ear.
A beer pocketbook with champagne taste. . . .
You're not going anywhere dressed like that.
Let me kiss it and make it better.
Don't talk with your mouth full.
I don't care what their mothers let them do.
Turn that noise down.
Look at me when I'm talking to you.
If you get separated from me in the crowd. . .write.
I'm going to teach you how to pray.
Say after me — father, son,. . .
"Silence is Golden."

> This ecstacy doth unperplex,
> We said, "And tell us what we love;
> We see by this it was not sex,
> We see we saw not what did move.

John Donne

Kisses make me good.

3-year-old boy when his mother asked, "What can we do to make you be a good boy?"

Being "one flesh" is such a being-filled reality. . .it is so real that nine months later you may have to give it a name.

Kimberly Hahn

Mind your mother!

Dad

Woman was not taken from man's head for she was never meant to rule, nor from his feet to be his slave, but from his side to walk beside him, from beneath his arm to be protected by him, from near his heart that he might love and cherish her.

Hugh of Saint Victor, 12th Century theologian

Sex is a twenty year or more warm-up.

Helen Trobisch

I was macho but now I'm a man.

Mexican husband after learning natural family planning with his wife

When you have to discipline yourself, you learn to discipline your children wisely.

African husband after learning natural family planning with his wife

This method is love.

African woman on natural family planning

Unnatural forms of birth control are a form of homicide.

John Calvin

I would like to thank my mother and father. You wouldn't think much of either of them alone, but they have been a wonderful combination.

Australian lad at his 21st birthday celebration

The Church's stand on birth control is the most absolutely spiritual of all her stands and with all of us being materialists at heart, there is little wonder that it causes unease. . . . Either practice restraint or be prepared for crowding.

Flannery O'Connor

"What God hath put together, let no man put asunder" refers to not only a man and woman in marriage but to procreation and unition.

John Kippley

Unnatural birth control is a form of sodomy.

Martin Luther

No. I love most, the one who most needs love.

Dr. Elizabeth Anscom, mother of 8, to the question,
"Do you have the same love for each of your children?"

Parents should enlist their children in every project around the house or apartment of a construction, repair or clean up nature. While often they are more interference than actual help, what the children will learn from the parent is (1) to understand how things work; (2) to muster energy to assume responsibility; (3) to try courageously to problem solve; (4) to outsmart material objects; and (5) to organize and deal with people in a helpful prosocial way. Always, always, always get the kids to "help" in completing tasks making it a game-like learning experience.

Samuel A. Nigro

Only when women assume responsibility ensuring that sexuality is reproductively oriented, will the males of the species be socialized, tamed, and civilized. The negative consequences of females not assuming such responsibility becomes obvious when sexual activity becomes other than reproduction oriented.

Samuel A. Nigro

If you do not put things back where you got them from, you'll never find them again. Put things back where you got 'em.

Mom

Any genuinely loving relationship is one of mutual psychotherapy.

Name Lost

The experiences of children impact on them forever. This is why children need extraordinarily gentle and instructive messages and comfort with good music from the ages of two through eighteen. The best place for that is at Mass, at home, in the neighborhood and in school — in that order of importance. What is experienced will be influential and savored in memory forever.

Samuel A. Nigro

There is no analogy between sex and anything else in this world: it is entirely unique. It is a separation which results in an attraction. . . . Marriage is not a hammer, but a magnet. The family does not rest on force, but on sex. The upshot of it is that most of the ancient customs of the sexes are conveniences; not things imposed by one party, but things equally desired by both.

G.K. Chesterton

I hate it when you think you're right. . . . I even hate it when you are right.

Sue Nigro

Humanity's place is in the home.

John Peterson

Most marriages are happy marriages; but there is no such thing as a contented marriage. The whole pleasure of marriage is that it is a perpetual crisis.

G.K. Chesterton

If perfection is sought, if biological intactness is to be secure, if ecstacy approximates the Divine, if the amusing geometry of sex is to be sanctified, if minds and bodies genuinely become one, if power and self-control become love, if society is to be salutary and life is to be holy, *then in the matter of sex, marriage is the form.*

The wisdom of the Roman Catholic approach is psychologically sound. To this extent, a brief commentary about virginity is appropriate.

Essentially, the nonvirginal partner(s) has already "sacrificed" himself/herself to a pseudocommitment — which renders less-than-complete any subsequent mutual sacrifice on behalf of a marriage relationship.

Essentially, pre-marital and extra-marital sex will be a violation of marriage vows and any other promise of commitment *to be made*. Pre-marital and extra-marital sex are before-the-fact violations of mutual betrothal.

This creates a nagging, subliminal at least, *doubt* automatic with the awareness that *this* spouse has already betrayed the commitment vows. At a minimum, an unconscious sense exists that "this person gave-in already" — she/he "can be had" because she/he has already "been had." An ominous psychological premonition that she/he will "fail again" is almost automatic. Attendant to the lack of mutual virginity at the time of marriage is a lack of complete trust and a lack of complete capacity for genuine commitment. These lacks result in a more difficult time for a couple to remain faithful and to believe in the partner's capacity for fidelity. This is a troubling self-fulfilling aspect which, gratefully, can be overcome. Nevertheless, engaged nonvirginal couples have a strike against them before they marry. They know they have betrayed themselves and their spouse already. Only hard work, self-sacrifice, and the Grace of God can keep them together. Roman

Catholic sex would have made it easier.

Samuel A. Nigro

It takes more than one parent to raise a child. It takes more than two parents to raise a child. It takes a whole church.

Sister Thea Bowman

A choking child should be propped on one's lap face down or across a table or chair face down and then slapped on the back four times. Then a quick check to see if breathing. This could be repeated three more times in an increasingly "upside down" posture if possible. If after the fourth effort of doing this, the child is still not breathing, a finger-wave into the back of the child's throat deep and gently pulling forward should be done, the child then checked to see if breathing, and then back-slapping operations repeated.

Samuel A. Nigro

If the possibility of parenthood is deliberately excluded from marital relations, the character of relationship between the partners automatically changes. The change is away from unification in love and in the direction of mutual, or rather, bilateral, "enjoyment". . . . Their relationship is transformed to the point at which it becomes incompatible with the personalistic norm. When a man and a woman entirely reject the idea that he may become a father and she a mother. . .the danger arises that objectively speaking there will be nothing left except "utilization for pleasure," of which the object will be a person.

Karol Wojtyla

The person is a being for whom the only suitable dimension is love.

John Paul II

With family living comes a universal phenomenon: fighting. Family members often get more angry and enraged at other family members than they do at anyone else. Why? What does it mean? First, it means that one can take the other party for granted — an occurrence which is proof of the family commitment because one cannot take the other party for granted unless that deep commitment is there. Second, it means that one has regressed to an immature degree of dyscontrol negatively experienced in one's own childhood, meaning that one overtly acts out against current family members what was done to oneself in earlier family experiences. Third, one *knows* the family member to whom one's ire is expressed, and with that intimate knowledge is the confidence that retaliatory response will be acceptable. Fourth, fighting within a family occurs because other family members are also so affected and react in the same way triggering a response as if in a mirror. The end result of all four points is a repetitive habit pattern of stimulus-response fighting almost compulsive in nature at times. So what can be done? The only way to offset this is to discuss these four points with family members over and over with the developing of approaches other than the irate, abusive raging one rarely experiences anywhere but in the family setting.

Samuel A. Nigro

Every family should have a plan for fire, invader, other crises — as to general procedures and what to do, how to spread the alarm, how to escape, how to call help, and where to meet and how to communicate. This should be gone over at least twice a year in a disaster plan mode. Such planning could not only prepare for after effects of an event but helps prevent the events by sensitizing family members to what all can go wrong.

Samuel A. Nigro

Sue: Do you like these cards?
Sam: No.
Sue: Don't give me that psychiatric mumbo jumbo. . . .

???

Evelyn: Did I ever get a bargain today!
Charlie: Yeah, we're going broke with your saving money.

During all the wild wedding preparations and the hecticness of it all, when things got too bad, I stopped for a moment to remember what all this was really about.

Bernadette Veider Nigro

Angels are uncertainties of the freedom between movement and position. If self-control and motion are sought to co-exist, more temperance comes from considering the angels.

Samuel A. Nigro

Take care. When someone defies me to do a thing, it is soon done.

Carmen

Contraception renders sexual behavior to be only recreational. . .and such non-reproductive sexuality is against the planet because it is nowhere else to be found in the entire animal kingdom. One can't be more anti-planet (anti-environmental) than by contraception.

Name Lost

Marriage is an alliance against the world!

Steve Petti

Lips say no, no, no but eyes say yes, yes, yes.

Name Lost

I will tell you what I think the Church has been trying to say to us all these years — and maybe it hasn't done a good job [of conveying its message]: We have to learn to be bigger than ourselves; we have to try to go beyond our comforts, our pleasures. It is so easy and tempting to wrap ourselves in our desires — and defend ourselves [as we do so] for being compassionate toward these *favelados*! To connect our sexual life to children, to the gift of life to the world — that is a noble idea, a high ideal. To ask people to sacrifice on behalf of the next generation, to deny themselves some pleasures and conveniences so that another child and another child come here [on earth] to live — that is also a noble idea, a high ideal. A lot of people — I believe it, I observe it — want to control our "population": It is a principle, an abstraction, they are upholding. In their own lives they care mightily [hugely] for themselves, and they don't want "a lot of children" because they don't want to exert themselves in that direction, only in other directions, for [toward] themselves. Is not selfishness, plenty of selfishness, a part of this story — as well as ignorance?

Roman Catholic nun running a soup kitchen in a Rio de Janeiro *favela* when asked if a birth control education program should be set up there

GOOD KID TOOLS

Teens need the following 30 "assets" in their lives to succeed according to a book based on a Search Institute study of more than 270,000 students in grades six through *twelve*.

External assets kids need:
1. Warm, caring family home.
2. Approachable parents.
3. Communicative parents.
4. Other approachable adults.
5. Other communicative adults.
6. Parental involvement in school.
7. Positive school climate.
8. Parental standards.
9. Parental discipline.
10. Parental monitoring.
11. Limits on away-from-home socializing
12. Positive peer influences.
13. Music lessons.
14. Organized extracurricular activities.
15. Community activities.
16. Involvement with a faith community.

Internal assets kids need:
17. Desire to achieve.
18. Desire to advance educationally.
19. Desire for above average grades.
20. Self-discipline to do 6-plus hours of homework a week.
21. Desire to help people.
22. Global concern.
23. Empathy.
24. Sexual restraint.
25. Assertiveness.
26. Decision-making skills.
27. Friendship-making skills.
28. Planning skills.
29. Self-esteem.
30. Hope.

How many assets do most teens have?

The Search Institute found that teens on average had 16 of the 30 assets. Well adjusted teens should have a minimum of 25 assets.

Grade	*Average number of assets*
6	17.8
7	17.1
8	16.6
9	16.1
10	16.0
11	15.9
12	16.0

How do assets make a difference?

Teens with the most "assets" seldom engage in risky behaviors.

No. of assets involved in:	Alcohol use	Sexual activity	School failure	Depression/ suicide	Antisocial behavior and violence
0-10	44%	52%	31%	42%	51%
11-20	23%	34%	13%	25%	29%
21-25	9%	17%	4%	11%	13%
26-30	3%	7%	1%	5%	6%

Source: "What Kids Need To Succeed: Proven, Practical Ways to Raise Good Kids," by Peter L. Benson, Judy Galbraith and Pamela Espeland

Here and there is born a St. Theresa, foundress of nothing, whose loving heart beats and sobs after unattained goodnesses tremble off and are dispersed among high instances of centering on some recognizable deed. Yet, these small, quiet goodnesses performed in silence and without attention have the most profound effects of all. And so the sincere idealists though they may be thwarted in their most ambitious plans and hopes, can never truly be defeated as long as they continue to live their idealism in the daily practical affairs of life.

George Elliott

The growing of good in the world is partly dependent on unhistoric acts.

George Elliott

A child more than any of the gifts offered to declining man bring with it hope and forward looking thoughts.

Wordsworth

Hope is knowing that salvation will come even as you sit in the darkness.

Christopher de Vinck

The fine print of any wedding contract clearly states: "husband gets the bat" (A flying bat, that is, when loose in the house).

Christopher de Vinck

I came into the world for this; to bear witness to the truth; and all who are on the side of truth listen to my voice.

John 18:37

EIGHT BEATITUDES FOR THE HOME

Blessed is the home where father, mother and children go to Confession regularly, receive Holy Communion frequently, and pray much; for the Lord abides in such a home.

Blessed is the home in which the Sundays and holy days are properly observed, for the members will one day meet again at the festival of Heaven.

Blessed is the home which no one leaves to go to sinful amusements, for in it the joy of Christ shall reign.

Blessed is the home where evil speech does not enter, nor blasphemy, nor bad literature, nor intemperance, for on that home will be heaped the blessings of peace.

Blessed is the home where father and mother are conscious of the sacred dignity of bringing children into the world and educating them in the service of God, where they faithfully fulfill the obligations they have towards each other and their children, and detest the sins sometimes committed in the married state, for they will merit favor and abundant blessings of God.

Blessed is the home where the children are baptized promptly after they are born, for they will grow up from the first as children of God: and blessed is the home to which a priest is called in time to attend the sick, for their illness will have its consolation and death will be happy.

Blessed is the home where Christian doctrine is properly appreciated and learned from the catechism and good books, for in that home the Faith will be kept firm and active.

Blessed is the home where the parents find their consolation in children that are dutiful and obedient, and where the children find in their parents the example of the fear and love of God, for that home will be the abode of just people, the haven of virtues and the ark of salvation.

Name Lost

Whatever, put your kids in a school where they can get an education.

Name Lost

People who do not like children. . . they have forgotten that they were young once too.

Evelyn Nigro

To those co-habitating:

So you are living together and wish to be married in our faith community. Well, you must hear this: We want you both to be with us. We want you to join our commitment to the Apostles Creed together so we are all in concert with the messages of the apostles. We want you to take the Lord worthily with us, to live the Gospels with us and to relish the sacraments with us in all aspects of our daily lives.

But your co-habitating cannot be *approved* because it is against our beliefs. And your co-habitating cannot be *supported* because you have not yet formally become one creature by marriage.

However, you both are accepted as individuals but not *as if* a married couple. We accept and welcome you based on the following:

(1) That you separately reflect and pray for help to overcome any future problems and mistrusts potentially caused by pre-marital unfaithfulness even though with one another.

(2) That you understand that for marriage, chastity optimally means virginity before and fidelity during and after, which emphasizes a rejection of selfish-

ness — a rejection necessary to become the one creature you will be in your married life. In other words, we want you to learn self-sacrifice now because you are going to need it later for the unitive dimensions of establishing and maintaining a family in the eyes of God.

(3) That you understand that God, the Church and this faith community are also aware of the physical, psychological, economic, peer pressuring and culturally-stimulating factors involved in your decision to co-habitate. We understand but nevertheless pray, like you would pray for your own children in the same circumstance, that you will reestablish and maintain your individual identity, integrity and oneness even though living together until formally married.

While tolerance and love are offered to you from us, we pray that your individual procreative and unitive gifts are kept special and sacred until sanctified by your actual marriage.

The God-given freedom to love also is accompanied by the freedom to sin. The answer is God. The judgment is God's. So please put God in your lives through our faith community committed to Jesus and His Church.

You can for the love of your Church and yourselves overcome the violating of your marriage vows before your marriage. We welcome you to join our community to this end and to obtain further Joy and Suffering in the Body of Christ."

Samuel A. Nigro

Repetitive, persistent, vigorous disagreements between parents in front of their children is extremely detrimental. These put-down disagreements deforms their childrens' perception of maleness and femaleness and diminish the targeted parent's rightful authority. They also reduce the targeted parents believability and create a sexist stereotyping with one being a target and the other an abuser. When parents disagree, it should be away from the children. One can always postpone the arguement by a: Let your mother and I talk about this later and then we will give you an answer.

Samuel A. Nigro

Thou goest with women, forget not thy whip.

Friedrich Nietzsche

Another example of how celebrities treat women.

Funny how my headache goes away when I go shopping. . . .

Sue Nigro

No one should be taught anything about artificial contraception unless they have done all their chores and kept their room completely clean without reminders for an entire week.

Samuel A. Nigro

And having fulfilled the days, when they returned, the Child Jesus remained in Jerusalem; and His parents knew it not. And thinking that He was in the company, they came a day's journey; and sought Him among their kinfolks and acquaintances. And not finding Him, they returned to Jerusalem seeking Him.

Luke 2:43-45
(having a teenager)

I sought Him Whom my soul loveth; I sought Him and found Him not. I will rise and go about the city; in the streets and broadways will I seek Him Whom my soul loveth. I sought Him, and found Him not! The watchmen who keep the city discovered me: Have you seen Him Whom my soul loveth?

Song of Songs 3:1-3
(having a teenager?)

Men and women deal with most things differently especially in family life. This is why men and women are essentially incompatible except in the mutual ability to keep promises like marriage vows. Still what he considers important and worthy of note almost always differs from what she considers important and worthy of note. And he will usually keep it to himself while she will usually be vocal. He will usually shrug it off while she will want to talk it out. Both approaches are usually fine unless they are reversed at which time both parties will recognize that they had better get whatever over with and return to familiar and more tolerable habits.

Samuel A. Nigro

The most important reason that men must(?) assume leadership roles more often than women has less to do with male strength, assertiveness, brainpower, or metaphysical traits (although all these are important factors) than the fact that men have an intense psychological NEED to be in that role because such is an essential component to their own intrinsic self-actualization and self-worth. Wise women will know this and help their men to be men because the alternative is a one-way track to male sociopathy: aggression, sexualization and/or anergic capitulation. Unlike women, men are sort of useless unless they are doing something imagined to be necessary, responsible, worthwhile or important! Unwise women who do not know this or who do not care are called "feminists."

Samuel A. Nigro

Adultery is when grown-ups begin to lie about their age.

6 year old little girl

If you sleep in it. . .make it up.
If you wear it. . .hang it up.
If you drop it. . .pick it up.
If you eat out of it. . .put it in the sink.
If you step on it. . .wipe it off.
If you open it. . .close it.
If you empty it. . .fill it up.
If it rings. . .answer it.
If it howls. . .feed it.

If it cries. . .love it.

Rules of the House of Nancy and Bob Lally
(parents of 16 children)

Love is one human being standing beside another, exchanging mutual gifts of our bodies, songs, dreams — perhaps madness, but in such madness we return to the next morning whole and complete, until the emptiness begins to return and we seek once again what is beautiful or what is ugly. Both will fill up the void, but only one will keep us alive.

Christopher de Vinck

Pregnancy means that something is there. More precisely, pregnancy means that someone is there like you or me were once there and, as was evident then and now for us, that each moment of existence is sacred.

Name Lost

Some of the strangest people in the world are married to each other.

Ashleigh Brilliant

Women fall when there is no strength in men.

from Romeo & Juliet

Knavish speech sleeps in a foolish ear.

from Hamlet

I have known many happy marriages, but never a compatible one. The whole aim of marriage is to fight through and survive the incident when incompatibility becomes unquestionable.

G.K. Chesterton

Men speak to a motion. They talk to a topic. Women talk to each other.

G.K. Chesterton

A child who gets his own way brings shame to his mother.

Proverbs 29:15

There are more women than men in Heaven. . . because women will stop and ask directions.

Joan Orndoff

Marriage is no place to hold a grudge.

Name lost

A man and a woman cannot live together without having against each other a kind of everlasting joke. Each has discovered that the other is a fool, but a great fool. This largeness, this grossness and gorgeousness of folly is the thing which we all find about those with whom we are in intimate contact; and it is the one enduring basis of affection, and even respect.

G.K. Chesterton

I too have known joy sadness and, on the whole, I prefer joy.

Ashleigh Brilliant

Who is in command of this bed?

Ashleigh Brilliant

I'm so glad you told me what I didn't want to hear.

Ashleigh Brilliant

It's always good to see a friendly face — could you make yours a little friendlier?

Ashleigh Brilliant

Mealtime will, of course, be enhanced by common prayer. The grace before meals can be the time to remember a sick relative or neighbor or a dearly departed person on the anniversary of his death. At mealtime or at bedtime prayers of petition are multiplied, and each member of the family can be convinced that no petition is unimportant and no wished outcome too trivial to share with an omnipotent God. In a large family the age differential may result in an admission to a graduate school, a date for the prom and the return of a missing puppy all being placed before God solemnly and equivalently in a shared prayer of petition.

Eugene F. Diamond

Every child has the right to undertake without presuming and to persevere without succeeding. Some parents, in their misguided indulgences, deprive their children of a basic and essential lesson — how to endure adversity and failure. It is not necessary that one endure privation or squalor. Every child must learn the social limits of what can be done and what must be done. He must learn to tolerate frustration and to endure loss and defeat. No child should be allowed to believe that everything costs nothing or that the world around him exists for the purpose of indulging him or sparing him pain.

Eugene Diamond

When we have a babysitter, my children know if they fight or misbehave they will have to pay the sitter out of their own allowances. We have had no problem getting sitters since implementing this rule — the children are always well-behaved.

Julie Noble

Tired of constantly separating my children because of arguing, I decided that each time I heard them battling, or whenever they came to me to tattle, I would make each of them write five reasons why the other child was special. This stopped the arguing, and it made them use their writing skills.

Kristen Chambers

Instruction Before Marriage in the Traditional Nuptial Mass

Dear friends in Christ: As you know, you are about to enter into a union which was established by God Himself. By it, He gave to man a share in the greatest work of creation, the work of the continuation of the human race. And in this way He sanctified human love and enabled man and woman to help each other live as children of God, by sharing a common life under His fatherly care.

Because God Himself is thus its author, marriage is of its very nature a holy institution, requiring of those who enter into it a complete and unreserved giving of self. But Christ our Lord added to the holiness of marriage an even deeper meaning and a higher beauty. He referred to the love of marriage to describe His own love for His Church, that is, for the people of God whom He redeemed by His own blood. And so He gave to Christians a new vision of what married life ought to be, a life of self-sacrificing love like His own. It is for this reason that His Apostle, St. Paul, clearly states that marriage is now and for all time to be considered a great mystery, intimately bound up with the supernatural union of Christ and Church, which union is also to be its pattern.

This union then is most serious, because it will bind you together for life in a relationship so close and so intimate, that it will profoundly influence your whole future. That future, with its hopes and disappointments, its successes and its failures, its pleasures and its pains, its joys and its sorrows, is hidden from your eyes. You know that these elements are mingled in every life, and are to be expected in your own. And so, not knowing what is before you, you take each other for better or for worse, for richer or for poorer, in sickness and in health, until death.

Truly, then, these words are most serious. It is a beautiful tribute to your undoubted faith in each other, that, recognizing their full import, you are nevertheless so willing and read to pronounce them. And because these words involve such solemn obligations, it is most fitting that you rest the security of your wedded life upon the great principle of self-sacrifice. And so you begin your married life by the voluntary and complete surrender of your individual lives in the interest of that deeper and wider life which you are to have in common. Henceforth, you belong entirely to each other; you will be one in mind, one in heart, and one in affections. And whatever sacrifices you may hereafter be required to make to preserve this common life, always make them generously. Sacrifice is usually difficult and irksome. Only love can make it easy; and perfect love can make it a joy. We are willing to give in proportion as we love. And when love is perfect, the sacrifice is complete. God so loved the world that He gave His only begotten Son; and the Son so loved us that He gave Himself for our salvation. "Greater love than this no man hath, that a man lay down his life for his friends."

No greater blessing can come to your married life than pure conjugal love, loyal and true to the end. May, then, this love with which you join your hands and hearts today, never fail, but grow deeper and stronger as the years go on. And if true love and the unselfish spirit of perfect sacrifice guide your every action, you can expect the greatest measure of earthly happiness that may be allotted to man in this vale of tears. The rest is in the hands of God. Nor will God be wanting to your needs; He will pledge you the life-long support of His graces in the Holy Sacrament which you are now going to receive.

Learning to live with the rhythms of life is important for a married couple. One of those rhythms is the time of fertility and infertility in a woman's menstrual cycle. Married couples who use Natural Family Planning (NFP) to monitor their cycles will be aware of those times. By sharing these times with each other they are able to give of themselves totally and to make shared decisions of their intentions. When the NFP couple experiences their fertile time, they realize the awesomeness of that time in that they have the potential to create new human life. This power is best exercised in the context of love between two married individuals in a co-creative relationship with God.

Artificial contraception disrupts the rhythms of a woman's menstrual cycle. Fertility no longer becomes a time for the creation of new life but something to be avoided. Couples on artificial contraception forego the rhythms of fertility and sterility and, because of this, they lose a sense of holiness and sense of the creative hand of God.

Richard J. Fehring

. . .birth control by contraceptives and the like is a profound error.

Gandhi

First, I make the bed while I am still in it. You have to figure out how to do it but you also get to move every joint in all sorts of ways. It sounds kind of strange but don't laugh. Then I slither out of bed and dress laying on the floor trying to put all my clothes on while flat on my back. Your legs are in the air a lot. Your arms are in the air a lot. You roll in all sorts of ways. It sounds kind of strange but don't laugh. Of course, D.J., my husband, has already left for work. . . . It really works and I feel great!

Anna Marie O'Hare on early morning exercise

The family asserts its primacy in all human activities not only from the role of procreation but in the role of teacher and conserver of the truths, values and morals of the community. Among the three monotheistic religions, Judaism, Islam and Christianity, the family is the primary and longest standing social unit into which each society places all its future hopes while still remembering its past.

Joseph Mauceri

God's faith is given in the language of fatherhood. . .and what we are in danger of losing is not family but fatherhood.

Rabbi Jonathan Sachs

Psychoanalysis made parents feel self-conscious and terrified of inflicting neuroses on children. They (parents) acquired a phobia for discipline and subscribed to the now exposed fallacy that an undirected child knows best what is good for him. Among these many cases there was no lessening of sexual neuroses.

Abram Kardiner

The disruption of Western Civilization and the Church after World War II is a function of communication technology and moreso by the missing men, killed or disturbed by the war. We miss those good men and fathers. We still miss them fifty years later.

Samuel A. Nigro

Sex is important only when it is important, otherwise, the hell with it.

Name Lost

Why cannot we grant that children chose to be the way they are? Why do we always have to blame good parents? We have to realize that children are free. They can be much, much worse than their parents. The goodness of wisdom of parents is not necessarily disproved by the children's vices.

James V. Schall

In the temporal order, uncertainty of the accuracy of position is inversely related to the accuracy of movement. So is Matrimony. Really: Do the BEST you can.

CHAPTER 10:

GRACE

In the physical order, *force* is that which affects matter particles. Your human beingness is a force.

In the spiritual order, *Grace* is force of "relationships and allegiance to mankind through Jesus and his Church" in confluence with the *pursuit of happiness* (personified by the Holy Spirit) resulting in *holiness* as a dedication and consecration to God's service.

"Graces are strings between God, people and one another."

Grace makes you a force pursuing happiness through the Holy Spirit in relationship to all others.

Live Grace — relating with the sound of God calling your name.

To be Free.
To Enter the World of Loving Truth and to participate in the Incarnation.

In physics, *force* is that which affects matter particles.

Grace means a supernatural gift of God bestowed on us through the merits of Jesus Christ, for our salvation. Grace is *force*.

Grace are patterns of the "strings" between human particles manifest in the physical world by *force* affecting matter particles. The human principle resulting is that of *pursuit of happiness* (personified by the Holy Spirit). The activity resultant is that of *holiness* by dedication to the service of God.

Pax

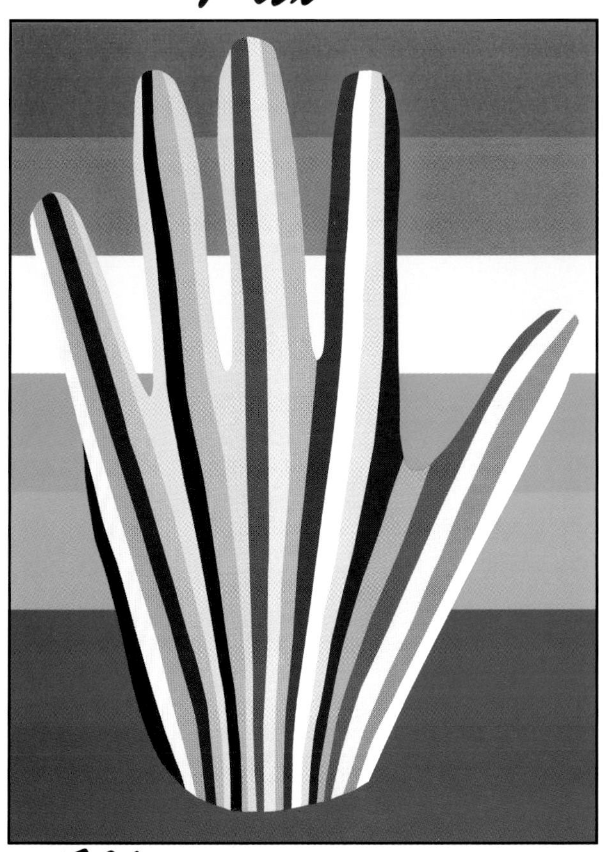

Misericordia

The FLAG of HUMANITY. . . The FLAG of MANKIND

THE HAND OF PEACE AND MERCY

The color spectrum background represents the unorganized energy of the Universe. The hand represents Man, the most organized energy form yet evolved. The 21 different skin colors indicate the variations of the color triad black-yellow-white repeated seven times, once for each continent.

PLEDGE OF ALLEGIANCE

I pledge allegiance to Mankind and to its flag, for which no one should die; and to evolving life on this planet, for living things are precious. I pledge to treat all humanely by caring for and respecting others' bodies; by understanding others' minds but being true to myself without disrespect; and by accepting the emotions of others as I control my own. I will have mercy on others with gentle liberty and empathic justice for all.

PERSONAL DECLARATION OF INDEPENDENCE

I hold these truths to be self-evident:

That everyone and their posterity are created equal regardless of age, sex, religion, or creed, race, language, color or appearance, political or other opinion, national or social origin, property, personal value system, birth, size, or other status.

That everyone and their posterity are endowed by their Creator at their creation with certain unalienable rights; that primary among these are life, liberty, and the pursuit of happiness.

That if any government does not acknowledge these rights or violates them, it not only fails in duty but its orders completely lose juridical force.

That authority ceases to be authority when it is used against the order of Life, Liberty, and the Pursuit of Happiness.

That whenever any form of government becomes destructive of these unalienable rights, it is the duty of the people to alter or to abolish it, and to institute a new government, laying its foundation on the principles of life first, liberty second, and then the pursuit of happiness; and to organize the new government's power in such form as shall seem likely to promote life, liberty, and the pursuit of happiness in that order.

Therefore, appealing to the Ultimate Triune Personification(s) of Life, Liberty, and the Pursuit of Happiness for the rectitude of my intentions, I do, in my name and by the authority of myself as a human being, solemnly publish and declare:

That I am, and of right ought to be, a free and independent being.

That I am a citizen of the World Community in accordance with the encyclical *Pacem in Terris*.

That I am absolved from all allegiance of any country in consonance with the religious freedom guaranteed by the United Nation's Universal Declaration of Human Rights.

That I disassociate myself from all political connections with any government that does not have as its foundation the principles of Life first, Liberty second, and the Pursuit of Happiness third with all else subordinate to those Divine Principles.

And, for the support of this declaration, with a firm reliance on the protection of the Trinity by Divine Providence, I personally pledge my life, my liberty, and my pursuit of happiness.

Freedom is the ability to choose the good.

William R. Luckey

I believe in the supreme worth of the individual and his right to life, liberty and the pursuit of happiness.

I believe that every right implies a responsibility; every opporunity an obligation; every possession a duty.

I believe that the law was made for man and not man for the law; that government is the servant of the people and not the master.

I believe in the dignity of labor, whether with head or hand; that the world owes no man a living, but that it owes every man an opportunity to make a living.

I believe that thrift is essential to well-ordered living and that economy is a prime requisite of a sound financial structure whether in government, business, or personal affairs.

I believe that truth and justice are fundamental to an enduring social order.

I believe in the sacredness of a promise, and that a man's word should be as good as his bond; that character — not wealth or power or position is of supreme worth.

I believe that the rendering of useful service is the common duty of mankind and that only in the purifying fire of sacrifice is the dross of selfishness consumed and the greatness of the human soul set free.

I believe in an all-wise and all-loving God, named by whatever name, and that the individual's highest fulfillment, greatest happiness, and widest usefulness are to be found in living in harmony with His will.

I believe that love is the greatest thing in the world; that it alone can overcome hate; that right can and will triumph over might.

The Creed of John D. Rockefeller, Jr.

. . . without deviation, without exception, without any ifs, buts, or whereases, freedom of speech means that you shall not do something to people either for their views they have or their views they express or the words they speak or write.

Justice Hugo Black

Poor Ireland and poor Scotland. They will never be free. They are the only way England can keep its empire. . . by what has turned out to be geography's most cruel joke.

Samuel A. Nigro

Stupidity won't kill you, but it can make you sweat.

English proverb

To be conscious that you are ignorant is a great step to knowledge.

Benjamin Disraeli

To be a champ, you have to believe in yourself when nobody else will.

Sugar Ray Robinson

Morality is its own advocate; it is never necessary to apologize for it.

Edith L. Harrell

Law is an ordinance of right reason for the common good promulgated by one who has care of the community.

St. Thomas Aquinas

In my friend, I find a second self.

Isabel Norton

Never hesitate to hold out your hand; never hesitate to accept the outstretched hand of another.

Pope John XXIII

If you don't want anyone to know, don't do it.

Chinese Proverb

Do what you can with what you got and do it now!

George Washington Carver

There is a time to let things happen and a time to make things happen.

Hugh Prather

People must be judged only by the content of their character.

Martin Luther King, Jr.

Losers sleep in.

Samuel A. Nigro

There are two classes of people in the world — those who take the best and enjoy it and those who wish for something better and try to create it. The world needs the appreciation of the first and the discontent of the second.

Florence Nightingale

Everything but God is time-bound.

William Smith

The most solid stone in the structure is the lowest one in the foundation.

Kahil Gibran

One man cannot hold another man down in the ditch without remaining down in the ditch with him.

Booker T. Washington

People judge you by your actions, not your intentions. You may have a heart of gold, but so has a hard-boiled egg.

Good Reading

The overwhelming majority of us are not racists or xenophobes or anything else — so it is wrong to condemn all or act as if all are, because of the few who actually are.

Samuel A. Nigro

People need to be self-determining, accountable, and absorbed in stretching their capabilities, just as they need food and shelter.

Charles Murray

Grace does not come from an "entertainment-church." Grace comes from a church of Loving Truth.

Samuel A. Nigro

Injustice anywhere is a threat to justice everywhere.

Martin Luther King, Jr.

Justice must be swayed by pity, valor tempered by discretion and determination softened by kindness.

Donald DeMarco

The world needs you doing things right!

Samuel A. Nigro

Government is not reason; it is not eloquence; it is force! Like fire, it is a dangerous servant and a fearful master.

George Washington

When you can't solve the problem, manage it.

Rev. Robert H. Schuller

Ideals are like the stars. We never reach them but, like the mariners on the sea, we chart our course by them.

Carl Schurz

Whenever you are to do a thing, though it can never be known but to yourself, ask yourself how you would act were all the world looking at you, and act accordingly.

Thomas Jefferson

It is my purpose as one who lived and acted in these days (of World War II) to show how the malice of the wicked was reinforced by the weakness of the virtuous, how the councils of prudence and restraint may become the prime agents of mortal danger. . .and how the middle course, adopted from desires for safety and a quiet life, may be found to lead direct to the bull's-eye of disaster.

Winston Churchill

The human consensus, from Homer to Patton, is that the army's job is to stomp the bejesus out of the enemy.

William Murchison

Disaster is only 1/2 a second away — always.

Samuel A. Nigro

Sometimes a majority simply means that all the fools are on the same side.

Claude McDonald

There is no happiness if the things we believe in are different from the things we do.

Freya Stark

Some men storm imaginary Alps all their lives, and die in the foothills cursing difficulties that do not exist.

E.W. Howe

I think it would be a good idea.

Mahatma Gandhi on Western Civilization

What if they gave a war and no one came?
Then the war will come to you!
He who stays home when the fight begins,
And lets others fight for his cause
Should take care:
He who does not take part,
In the battle will share in the defeat.
Even avoiding battle does not avoid,
Battle, since not to fight for your own cause
Really means,
Fighting on behalf of your enemy's cause.

Bertold Brecht

In a consumer society, there are inevitably two kinds of slaves: The prisoners of addiction and the prisoners of envy.

Ivan Illich

All that is necessary for the triumph of evil is that good men do nothing.

Edmund Burke

God will not help with what you can do yourself.

Name Lost

Free enterprise works when you work!

Samuel A. Nigro

Social conditioning is incapable of initiating an impulse.

Donald DeMarco

We have had enough government — enough state — enough sociology and laws. And science has given us A-bombs, nerve gas, biological warfare, pollution, dehumanizing television, and abortion. Look to the Church.

Samuel A. Nigro

Five hundred years from now, people will look back in amazement at our abuse of sex: women trying to be men; sex as recreation; abortion on demand, and contraception a necessity. They will either laugh or be appalled at our antics and wonder how human beings could be so primitive, barbaric and pagan.

Samuel A. Nigro

Leaders are totalitarians at heart — *all* leaders, from student groups to the throne, from a world event to "what's for dinner."

Samuel A. Nigro

The state is for man, not man for the state.

Jacques Maritain

The challenge of education is not to prepare a person for success, but to prepare him for failure. It is in disaster, not success, that the heroes and the bums really get sorted out.

James Bond Stockdale

Socrates was right when he cursed, as he often did, the man who first separated utility from Justice; for this separation, he complained, is the source of all mischief.

Marcus Tullius Cicero

Only the winners decide what were war crimes.

Garry Wills

A sacrament is an outward sign instituted by Christ to give grace.

Baltimore Catechism

. . .a regime which denies the spiritual nature and eternal destiny of man can offer no coherent security for rights, including the right to live.

Charles E. Rice

The first formal documented declaration against slavery was the Papal Bull of 1537 by Pope Paul III.

Name Lost

Every question you answer correctly in school is earning power worth $1 a year income for the rest of your life (more with inflation):
Grade School - 8,000 questions - $8,000 per year
High School - 16,000 questions - $16,000 per year
College - 32,000 questions - $32,000 per year
Graduate School - 75,000+ - $75,000+ income per year

Samuel A. Nigro

When a man's willing and eager, the gods join in.

Aeschylus

Work is what works — school work, home work, house work, job work, and peace work.

Samuel A. Nigro

Democracy is like a raft. It won't sink, but you'll always have your feet wet.

Russell Long

Finally, let us not forget the religious character of our origin. Our fathers were brought hither by their high veneration for the Christian religion. They journeyed by its light, and labored by its hope. They sought to incorporate its principles with the elements of their society, and to diffuse its influence through all the institutions, civil, political, or literary. Let us cherish these sentiments, and extend this influence still more widely; in the full conviction, that that is the happiest society, which partakes in the highest degree of the mild and peaceful spirit of Christianity.

Daniel Webster

Democracy evolves to socialism and then to dictatorship.

Plato

Man creates culture and through culture creates himself.

Pope John Paul II

Take your work seriously but yourself lightly.

C.W. Metcalf

Political authority is a sacred trust.

Edmund Burke

Democracy, like any noncoercive relationship, rests on a shared understanding of limits.

Elizabeth Drew

Do good and avoid evil.

St. Thomas

Who is this? We? Or our Lord?

Saint Frances Cabrini

The morality of a great writer is not the morality he teaches, but the morality he takes for granted.

G.K. Chesterton

We do not want, as the newspapers say, a Church that will move with the world. We want a Church that will move the world.

G.K. Chesterton

A person is an individual substance of rational nature.

Boethius

Christianity has died many times and risen again; for it had a God who knew the way out of the grave.

G.K. Chesterton

I Never let your business standards fall below your personal ones.
II The business must observe the law.
III Be loyal.
IV Give employees equality of opportunity.
V Always improve education.
VI Stress creativity.
VII Seek to excel.
VIII Always think in terms of commercial cause and social effect.
IX Business has a specific duty to the environment beyond the call of legal obligation.
X Promote beauty.

Paul Johnson's Capitalist Decalogue

Power corrupts. Absolute power corrupts absolutely.

Lord Acton

Don't bleed in public. Stand your ground.

William Bennett

There was never a democracy yet that did not commit suicide.

John Adams

Whenever you find yourself on the side of the majority, it is time to pause and reflect.

Mark Twain

The Christian ideal has not been tried and found wanting. It has been found difficult; and left untried.

G.K. Chesterton

We lose our bearings entirely by speaking of the "lower classes" when we mean humanity minus ourselves.

G.K. Chesterton

You cannot bring about prosperity by discouraging thrift. You cannot strengthen the weak by weakening the strong. You cannot help the wage earner by pulling down the wage payer. You cannot further the brotherhood of man by encouraging class hatred. You cannot keep out of trouble by spending more than you earn. You cannot build character and courage by taking away man's initiative and independence. You cannot help men permanently by doing for them what they could and should do for themselves.

Abraham Lincoln

State education is simply Conscription applied to culture, or to the destruction of culture.

G.K. Chesterton

You see then, that it takes deeds as well as faith if a man is to be justified.

James 2:24

Natural Law is rejected not because other philosophies are deeper, better, or more correct, but because Natural Law will not let people do what is wrong.

Samuel A. Nigro

Oh Liberty, what crimes are committed in thy name.

Madam Roland dela Matiere

I hold that a little rebellion now and then is a good thing. . . . It is a medicine necessary for the sound health of government.

Thomas Jefferson

Liberty gives the opportunity to do wrong but not the right to do wrong.

Name Lost

If there is no God, everything is permitted.

Dostoyevsky

I would give my right hand for your faith in Jesus.

Thomas Huxley, biologist and atheist,
to a man of simple, deep faith

Man's capacity for justice makes democracy possible; but man's inclination to injustice makes democracy necessary.

Reinhold Niebuhr

God forbid that we should ever go twenty years without a rebellion.

Thomas Jefferson

Pacifism? Who needs it? Some things are not worth defending. When the people are no good, military service is stupid. If we cannot stand the vices or the cures, it is over.

Samuel A. Nigro

Do you like cherries?

One question I.Q. test for admission to the submarine service in World War II. (If you laughed, you were in.)

. . .Grace does not replace but transfigures nature.

Dietrich von Hildebrand

The term "democracy" as I have said again and again, does not contain enough positive content to stand alone against the forces you dislike — it can be easily transformed by them. If you will not have God. . ., you should pay your respects to Hitler and Stalin.

T.S. Eliott

The marvelous civilization of antiquity perished because it did not adapt its moral code and its legal system to the vagaries of the market economy. The social order is doomed if the actions, which its normal functioning requires, are rejected by the standards of morality, are declared illegal by the laws of the country, and are prosecuted as criminal by the courts and the police.

Ludwig Von Mises

This means that the initial state of the universe must have been very carefully chosen indeed if the hot, big bang model was correct right back to the beginning of time. It would be very difficult to explain why the universe should have begun in just this way, except as the act of a God who intended to create beings like us.

Stephen W. Hawking

The Anthropic Principle: "We see the universe the way it is because we exist."

Stephen W. Hawking

After all calculations, the earth is found not to be the center of the solar system, but in fact to be the very center of the universe, with all the universe rotating around it.

Samuel A. Nigro

Roman Catholicism is environmentalism for the soul, mind, family, and society. Environmentalism is Roman Catholicism for nature.

Samuel A. Nigro

Men are qualified for civil liberty in exact proportion to their disposition to put moral chains upon their appetites, in proportion as their love of justice is above their rapacity, in proportion as their own soundness and sobriety of understanding is above their vanity and presumption, in proportion as they are disposed to listen to the counsels of the wise and good, in preference to the flattery of knaves.

Edmund Burke

Freedom cannot endure unless we are willing to nurture that religious understanding which is its sanction; unless we maintain the springs of ordered liberty.

Russell Kirk

The (Berlin) wall will fall for it cannot withstand faith; it cannot withstand truth; the wall cannot withstand freedom.

Ronald Reagan (In June 1987, two years before the wall was opened)

I am the light of the world.

John 8:12

Politics is the interacting of symbols of Truth between people.

Samuel A. Nigro

To begin with unlimited freedom is to end with unlimited despotism.

Dostoevski

The truth will make you free.

John 8:32; Psalm 1

Verily, I say unto you, before Abraham was, I am.

John 8:58

A right is a moral power, ability, or duty which allows us to keep the moral law or restrain others from interfering with our keeping of that law.

William R. Luckey

Don't you understand? The world will end if you do not do right.

Samuel A. Nigro

For after all, what is man in nature? A nothing in relation to all? An all in relation to nothing? The end of things and their beginning are hidden from him in an impenetrable secret. He is likewise incapable of seeing the nothing from which he has come and the all in which he is engulfed.

Blaise Paschal

Love is a fire. . .it must spend itself in service.

Catherine de Hueck Doherty

For God so loved the world that he gave his only Son, so that every one that believes in him may not die but have eternal life.

John 3:16

Power is the capacity to influence events and subject the events to moral scrutiny.

John East

It is terribly difficult to be wise, as Socrates, the father of moral philosophy, never tired of pointing out, where it is incomparably easier to seem to be wise. Wisdom requires a long apprenticeship and suffering; being a "wiseguy" demands little more than listening to gossip.

Donald DeMarco

(Or listening to the press and media which is the same thing.)

Never allow yourself to be a glazed, blurry-eyed, zombied man debrained to the diarrhea of insignificant morphemes and desensitizing photons from television, movies or newspapers, all of which are most accurately called *psychochezia* (mind defecation.) This *is* our press and media today.

Samuel A. Nigro

But what is liberty without wisdom and without virtue? It is the greatest of all possible evils.

Edmund Burke

Democracy is degenerate without the leaven of virtue.

St. Augustine

My commandment is this: Love one another, just as I love you.

John 15:12

I have come into the world as light, that everyone who believes in me should not remain in the darkness.

John 12:46

In the absence of virtue a void existence into which sweeps, without any real resistance, a hoard of harmful vices. . . . The best way to keep vices out is not to tell them to stay away, but to crowd them out by the presence of strong virtues.

Donald DeMarco

Is not Life wonderful?
Is not Life strange?
To breath. . .and know it.
To like. . .to love. . .to suffer. . . .
To reflect on who what where when how we are. . . .
To grasp our uniqueness. . .our experiences
To savor all under which we go
As an amazing gift from God. . . .
Is not Life strange?
Is not Life wonderful?

Samuel A. Nigro

Every epoch which is in the process of retrogression and disintegration is subjective, but all progressive epochs have an objective trend.

Geothe

Corraggio! (Have courage about it all!)

Pope John XXIII

Six mistakes of man:

(1) The delusion that individual advancement is made by crushing others;
(2) The tendency to worry about things that cannot be changed or corrected;
(3) Insisting that a thing is impossible because we cannot accomplish it;
(4) Refusing to set aside trivial preferences;

(5) Neglecting development and refinement of the mind, and not acquiring the habit of reading and study;

(6) Attempting to compel other persons to believe and live as we do.

Cicero

I am only a public entertainer who has understood his times and exploited as best he could the imbecility, the vanity, the cupidity of his contemporaries.

Picasso

A bigot is a person who relies excessively on one of his own attributes to the degree of losing his humanity.

Samuel A. Nigro

The worst tyrant is not the man who rules by fear; the worst tyrant is he who rules by love and plays on it as on a harp.

G.K. Chesterton

"I've got a new idea" is a tyranny unless this "new" idea has been researched in history. It is the "making the same mistake" which is so detrimental when people think their ideas are "new" when they are old, been tried and found wanting. History keeps repeating itself because of "new ideas" not deeply researched.

Samuel A. Nigro

All that we call spirit and art and ecstasy only means for one awful instant we remember that we forget.

G.K. Chesterton

It is easy to be perfectly just about trivial things.

G.K. Chesterton

The perversion of science lies in elevating empiricism to a moral principle.

Barbara Grizzuti Harrison

The function of art is to promote growth, harmony and community.

John Dewey

The voice of the people is the voice of God.

Nello the bartender

The "free press" which does not care about truth becomes a tyrant because it is "free lying." Such a press places everyone "on trial" day in and day out. The press is practicing law without a license. The press, when not governed by truth, usurps democratic constitutional government by its influence and unregulated power. Without the truth, the press is criminal and traitorous, and the system will not work.

Samuel A. Nigro

One of the things that make this country great is the right to be offended.

Bruce Iglauer

I admire the exaggerated way you tell the truth.

Balfor to Winston Churchill

All reality is Sacramental.

Peter M.J. Stravinskas

Fiction legitimizes nothing. Legal fiction only engenders disrespect for the legal institutions that employ it, the judges who invoke it, and the law proclaimed as a consequence of adherence to it.

Robert L. Cord

People who really "care" have virtue, exude transcendentals, and live Sacramentally.

Name Lost

Angels are all around. Call on them. Use their names. . . all the words ever. Call out for energy, support, ideas, relief. . . anywhere for the asking. . . everywhere for the same! Properly called, angels will respond but only for transcendental purposes. So know your transcendentals. Samples: *Moral* angel help me. *Intellect* angel help me. *Car* angel keep it moving. *Road* angel stay smooth. *Dry* angel, dry us out. *Rain* angel, water the plants. In other words, invoke the angels in all things about all things.

Samuel A. Nigro

. . .to compel a man to furnish funds for the propagation of ideas he disbelieves and abhors is sinful and tyrannical.

Thomas Jefferson

Virtue is an infinite regress within the extremes of "for me/for you" that leads to the ultimate infinity of ultimate eternity with God. The Beatitudes range within those extremes.

Samuel A. Nigro

Language skills are necessary to be developed in the right language because not all language can cope with a complicated civilization.

Anonymous

Freedom that is in flight from responsibility or virtue is not freedom.

Name Lost

The victors become the vanquished by feckless incontinent descending into a decadence made possible by victory not remaining true to the standards required to be victorious in the first place.

Samuel A. Nigro

The same civilization which asserted free will in the 13th century, produced the thing called "fiction" in the 18th. When Thomas Aquinas asserted the spiritual liberty of man, he created all the bad novels in the circulating libraries.

G.K. Chesterton

Civilization is not to be judged by the rapidity of communication, but by what is communicated.

G.K. Chesterton

The part of journalism that I would feel tempted to suppress would be the serious part: The leading articles and the learned reviews and the authoritative and infallible communications from special foreign correspondents. . . . Jokes are generally honest. Complete solemnity is almost always dishonest. . . . The writer of the leading article has to write about a fact that he has known for twenty minutes as if it were a fact that he has studied for twenty years.

G.K. Chesterton

All is a procession. The universe is a procession with measured and perfect motion.

Walt Whitman

George Washington said you could not maintain a free republic without virtuous people. Thomas Jefferson said you could not maintain one with ignorant people. They were both right.

Charlie Reese

And there is nothing worse than ignorance of virtue.

Our duty to human government is either to make it work swiftly or to stop it working.

G.K. Chesterton

The Inquisition was nothing compared to the deaths given us by science, to the poverty created by socialism and to the mental injury caused by the untruths from the press and media.

Samuel A. Nigro

Number is the dust that settles when something goes by so fast that no one can make out what it is. It is the abstract residue, the ghostly remains of a life we did not take the time to know or to experience. It is the language employed by occupants of a hollow universe who can count but cannot comprehend. It is the dates that mark the tombstone and omit everything that happened between birth and death.

Donald DeMarco on statistics

Birds of prey have no song.

Monsignor Ronald Knox

If a war is not a holy war, it is an unholy one — a massacre.

G.K. Chesterton

Rights depend upon Western civilizing attitudes guarded by laws which reinforce those attitudes more than reinforce the rights.

Samuel A. Nigro

But by the Grace of God I am what I am, and His grace toward me was not in vain.

1 Corinthians 15:10

Her ways are beautiful ways and all her paths are peaceful.

Proverbs 3:17

Every virtue causes its possessors to be in good state and to perform their functions well.

Aristotle

Virtue is a state that decides in a mean, the mean relative to us, which is defined by reference to reason, i.e. to the reason by reference to which the intelligent person would define it.

Aristotle

Arrogance makes scientists stupid!

Samuel A. Nigro

Doctrine once sown strikes deep its root, and respect for antiquity influences all men. Still, the dye is cast, and my trust is in my love of truth and the candor of cultivated minds.

William Harvey, preamble to his treatise on the circulation of blood

If fatalism and nausea are always possible views and experiences, so, too, are theism and joy, God and Grace.

G.K. Chesterton

Why is it that when you go into a newspaper building, the bathrooms have signs in them asking individuals to "flush the toilet twice"?

Name Lost

In general, people tend to behave like they are expected to behave. And the press and media convey expectations of behavior. This is why it is important to diminish the impact of the press and media by a continuous belittling of them.

Anonymous

Entertainment celebrities deal with fiction, with pretend, with fantasy. Entertainment celebrities deserve nothing but a hoot. They deal with nothing. They are nothing but hoopla. Enjoy without belief.

Samuel A. Nigro

Imperialism is learning how to get along with one's social inferiors.

English schoolboy in the 19th century

The people, sir, your people is a great beast.

Alexander Hamilton to George Washington

To friends, everything; to enemies, the law.

Spanish Proverb

Everyone must say "I'm sorry" at least three times a day for civilization to work.

Samuel A. Nigro

After studying all the constitutions of the world, the only possible conclusion is that none of them work, but it is the people who make them work, a people with a critical mass of individuals who are committed, whether they know it or not, to traditional virtue and to the transcendentals with which everything is possible and without which nothing works not even the U.S. Constitution.

Samuel A. Nigro

Imitate Jesus and Socrates.

Benjamin Franklin

The final objection to what is called "peace at any price" is simply that we should pay the price and not get the peace.

G.K. Chesterton

Art, like morality, consists of drawing the line somewhere.

G.K. Chesterton

The intrinsic danger of government help is that it tricks people into believing that they are beholden only to the government which in turn conveys the message that people can behave anyway they want unless the government prevents them (which subliminally means that "anything goes" unless the government says "no"). Thus the psychological message of government help is: No conscience is necessary unless government imposed.

Samuel A. Nigro

Anyone in a position of power does not deserve to be there intrinsically because they have arrived there through some Machiavellian means, and therefore people in power should not be trusted or even respected except by their following Natural Law.

Name Lost

Do what you ought, and let what will come of it.

Italian Proverb

Grace is the projection and interaction of transcendentals.

Anonymous

Genuine freedom can only be manifest in the ability to choose the good in the face of pain and danger.

Name Lost

All being is polarized into male or female by the balance of transcendentals versus immanentals.

Samuel A. Nigro

The greatest evil is for good men to do nothing.

Edmund Burke

The trouble with Socialism is that it is an attempt to design a system so perfect that no one will have to be good.

T.S. Eliott

Above all, gentlemen, no zeal.

Diplomatic advice from Talleyrand

In World War II, we had landed on the Pacific Island, the Japanese withdrawing without much of a fight. The remaining natives, however, were terrified of the Americans, having been told how cruel and violent we would be. We had landed and established our control of the island, generally ignoring the natives who were wide-eyed and terrified, huddling all over in large groups of cowed people. Noticing rosary beads around the necks of several natives in one group, I pulled out my own rosary and held it up and began to say it. The natives began to murmur. A sense of relief and composure rolled over the multitudes. Tears of joy and nervous laughter flickered throughout as suddenly the strains of the recited rosary started up around the island. The natives gradually went back to their lives with composure and we Marines finished our business.

An American Marine reminiscing about his
most memorable World War II experience

Freedom is choosing good over inviting evil; it is choosing truth over enticing emotions; and it is choosing love over justifiable hate.

Samuel A. Nigro

God is always at work in you to make you willing and able to obey His own purpose.

Philippians 2:13

To believe in something that is not true, is actually to believe in nothing.

Name Lost

What you can't get out of, get in wholeheartedly.

Mignon McLaughlin

If you kick nature, it will kick right back.

French saying

Against virtue, there can be no laws.

Name Lost

A right (to do something) automatically requires that it be "right" (in virtue and transcendentals). Rights without being "right" do not exist except as a force for evil.

Name Lost

. . .the idea that more than half the people are right more than half the time. . . .

E.B. White's definition of democracy

Socialist scheming is appealing to people because it gives a false sense of control ("here is the solution"), but the only sustainable solution for any problem is based on a summation of individual virtue with the projecting of one's transcendentals.

Samuel A. Nigro

The rosary is a spiritual bombshelter protecting from everything wrong which is why we say it every day.

Father John Sweeney

Freedom without virtue is no right. The so-called "Rights of Man" do not exist without virtue.

Name Lost

Good fences make good neighbors.

Anonymous

(and mind your own business)

My grace is all you need, for my power is greatest when you are weak.

2 Corinthians 12:9

When danger approaches, sing to it.

Arab Proverb

What is called the economic independence of women is the same as what is called the economic wage-slavery of men.

G.K. Chesterton

There is nothing the matter with the human body; what is the matter is the human soul. It needs grace.

G.K. Chesterton

The secular ideals of humanity fossilize very fast.

G.K. Chesterton

You can't use tact with a Congressman. A Congressman is a hog. You must take a stick and hit him on the snout.

Henry Adams

Whereas God always forgives and man sometimes forgives, Nature never forgives — when one thwarts Nature, Nature rebukes, retaliates, strikes back.

Anonymous

There are times when, unless we are willing to do what seems humanly ridiculous, God will not do the miraculous.

Mother Angelica

The real Rites of Man: Baptism, Penance, Holy Communion, Confirmation, Extreme Unction, Holy Orders, and Matrimony.

Anonymous

The market was not something invented by Adam Smith; it is the automatic and inevitable tool devised by human nature to satisfy natural needs.

Thomas Fleming

Law can only kill until the gospel comes to transcend it; the king's head on coins is a death's head unless economic life is ruled by the spirit.

C.S. Lewis

If you want peace, understand war.

B.H. Liddell Hart

Wealth is not physical, but metaphysical, it is to be found not in matter, but in mind.

Warren Brookes

What the law permits, it encourages.

Plato

The difference between freedom and psychopathy is Western Civilization.

Samuel A. Nigro

The one word which most accurately, appropriately, and consistently describes those in the press and media is PSYCHOPATH.

Anonymous

Lawyers are important in direct proportion to the dishonesty of the people.

Name Lost

Both the rebel and the subservicent are reactors, neither living in Christian freedom.

Nancy M. Cross

The problem with most lawsuits for injuries is not that most of all the money will go to the lawyers but it is that the lawyers have turned you into an invalid during the process.

Samuel A. Nigro

Property is merely the art of democracy. It means that every man should have something that he can shape to his image, as he is shaped in the image of Heaven.

G.K. Chesterton

Being *free* means:

1) You can find humor in hurting;
2) You can find persistence against overwhelming odds;
3) You can find and assert your own transcendentals.

Samuel A. Nigro

Ruleless and purposeless freedom is psychopathy.

Name Lost

Grace is how the transcendentals sustain us and all created being. The Father is with all by matter and form. The Son is with all by truth and oneness. The Holy Spirit is with all by good and beauty. All created being is thus sustained by God in such manner.

Samuel A. Nigro

Etienne Tempier and his council declared that in order to remain subject to the teaching of the Church and not to impose limits to God's omnipotence, one had to reject Peripatetic physics. By that move, they implicitly called for the creation of a new physics which the reason of Christians could accept. We shall see the University of Paris try to construct this new physics during the 14th century; by its efforts it laid the foundations of modern science. The latter was born, so to speak, on March 7, 1277, from the decree issued by Monseigneur Etienne, Bishop of Paris.

Pierre Duhem

The end of history is the realization of a common conscience of humanity and that Christianity is the form of that universal conscience.

Albert Dufourcq

A teaching which pretends to have established the irreducible antagonism between the scientific spirit and the spirit of Christianity is the most colossal lie and also the most audacious which has ever been attempted to dupe the people.

Pierre Duhem

Moral restraint gives birth to all freedom.

George Bush

If one wants to separate by an exact line the domain of ancient science from that of modern science, it has to be drawn, we believe, at the moment when Jean Buridan conceived that theory, at the very moment when one ceased to see the stars as if moved by divine beings, at the moment when one admitted that celestial motions and the sublunary motions rested on the same mechanics.

Pierre Duhem

I am creating new heavens and a new earth — so wonderful that no one will even think about the old ones anymore.

Isaiah 65:17

When a psychiatrist does not understand you, he will make a diagnosis. When a psychoanalyst does not understand you, he will talk gibberish about gibberish.

Name Lost

Our society has been bankrupted by giving borrowed money to those whose status is divorced from creative social function.

E. Christian Kopff

(If) you take power and independence from a municipality, you may have docile subjects, but you will not have citizens.

Alexis de Tocqueville

Measure wealth not by the things you have, but by the things you have for which you would not take money.

author unknown

1. Whom the gods would destroy, they first make mad with power.
2. The mills of God grind slowly but they grind exceedingly small.
3. The bee fertilizes the flower it robs.
4. When it is dark enough, you can see the stars.

Charles A. Beard summarizing history in four sentences

Civilization is the affirmation of one's nature by the transcendentals.

Name Lost

Culture is the effort to make beautiful that which is basically ugly.

Anonymous

I told him it was law logic, an artificial system of reasoning, exclusively used in courts of justice, but good for nothing anywhere else.

John Quincy Adams

We see the judges looking like giants, but we do not see who moves them.

John Selden

Only a fool judges the Past with ideas of the Present.

Lord Acton

Faith in the possibility of science is *a most conscious* derivative from the tenets of medieval theology on the Maker of Heaven and Earth.

S.L. Jaki

The contingency of the universe originates in *a priori* discourse about it, while its rationality makes it accessible to the mind though only in *a posteriori* manner.

S.L. Jaki

Faith in the possibility of science, generated antecedently to the development of modern scientific theory, is an unconscious derivative from medieval theology.

Alfred North Whitehead

To the construction of that system (pagan eternalism), all disciplines of Hellenic philosophy — Peripatetics, stoics, Neoplatonists — contributed; to that system Abu Masar offered the homage of the Arabs; the most illustrious rabbis from Philo of Alexandria to Maimonides, accepted it. To condemn it and to throw it overboard as a monstrous superstition, Christianity had to come.

Pierre Duhem

The circle is a stamp on the scientific sterility of all great ancient cultures, all under the spell of the treadmill of eternal recurrences. The arrow, as a symbol of linearity, is expressive of a beginning which is a move in the forward direction. It is a beginning that put Western culture on the move and secured for it a pre-eminent global position.

S.L. Jaki

Nothing can be so spectacularly effective as vanquishing the enemy on a battle-ground of the enemy's choice.

S.L. Jaki

When even the rats leave the sinking ship, Catholics rush aboard.

Pierre Duhem concerning French Socialism

None of the things I have bought, and I mean none of them, have ever really made me happy.

Thomas Monaghan, founder of multi-billion dollar enterprise Domino's Pizza as he sold off and gave away his prized possessions.

From its birth, Greek science is all impregnated with theology, but with a pagan theology. That theology teaches that the heavens and the stars are gods. It teaches that they cannot have other motion than circular and uniform motion which is the perfect motion. It curses the impiety that would dare to attribute a motion to the earth, sacred foyer of the divinity. If these theological doctrines have furnished some postulates, provisionally useful for the science of nature, they quickly became for physics what harnesses become for children: fetters. Had the human spirit not broken those fetters, it would not have been able to surpass Aristotle in physics and Ptolemy in astronomy.
Now, what has broken those fetters? Christianity. Who, above all, profited by the liberty so acquired for pushing on for the discovery of a new science? The scholastics. Who, in the middle of the 14th century, dared to declare that the heavens were not at all moved by divine or angelic intelligences but by an indestructible impulsion received from God at the moment of creation? A Master of Arts in Paris, Jean Buridan. Who in 1377 has

declared the diurnal motion of the earth, a motion more simple and satisfactory for the mind than the diurnal motion of the heavens? Who has neatly refuted all the objections raised against the former of these movements? Another Master in Paris, later the bishop of Lisieux, Nicole Oresme. Who has founded the dynamics, discovered the law of the fall of bodies, posed the foundations of geology? The Parisian scholastic and in times when the Catholic orthodoxy of the Sorbonne was proverbial all over the world. Which role was played in the formation of modern science by those free, much vaunted minds of the Renaissance? In their superstitious and routine admiration of Antiquity, they ignored and disdained all the fertile ideas formulated by the scholasticism of the 14th century, so that they might espouse the least defensible theories of Platonic or peripatetic physics. What was, at the end of the 16th century and in the beginning of the 17th century, that grand intellectual movement which produced doctrines admitted from then on? A pure and simple return to the teaching which, during the Middle Ages, the Scholastic of Paris presented, so that Copernicus and Galileo are the continuators and disciples of Nicole Oresme and Jean Buridan. If therefore that science, of which we are rightly proud, could be born, it was because the Catholic Church served as a midwife.

Pierre Duhem

The Right stands for liberty, a free, unprejudiced form of thinking; a readiness to preserve traditional values (provided they are true values); a balanced view of the nature of man, seeing in him neither beast nor angel, insisting on the uniqueness as human beings which cannot be transformed into or treated as mere numbers or ciphers. The Left (however) is the advocate of the opposite principles; it is the enemy of diversity and the fanatical promoter of identity. Uniformity is stressed in all leftist Utopias, paradises in which everybody is the same, envy is dead, and the enemy is either dead, lives outside the gates, or is utterly humiliated. Leftism loathes differences, deviations, and stratifications. . . . The word "one" is its symbol: one language, one race, one class, one ideology, one ritual, one type of symbol, one law for everybody, one flag, one coat of arms, one centralized world state.

Erik von Kuehnelt-Leddihn

Why burn a flag when you can burn a newspaper?

Samuel A. Nigro

If I am what I have and what I have is lost, who then am I?

Eric Fromm

Culture may be defined as that which makes life worth living.

T.S. Eliott

When words lose their meaning, people lose their identity.

Confucius

That's what you get for talking to psychiatrists: they are the master mold of conventional thinking in the very glass of superficiality.

Florence King

Our disease is democracy. Democracy is a troubled spirit, fated never to rest, and whose dreams, if it sleeps, present only visions of hell.

Fisher Ames

Democracy is not founded on pity for the common man; democracy is founded on reverence for the common man.

G.K. Chesterton

. . .and on reverence for our common origin, too.

One can only speak one:one by transcendentals; one can only relate as *individuals* by transcendentals; and one can only acquire meaning by transcendentals.

Samuel A. Nigro

All men are created equal, but differ greatly in the sequel.

Fisher Ames

Culture is the aggregate of those transcendentals of a group which help everybody. Culture is not a lifestyle, but it is that which makes lifestyles work well. You can tell the culture by the symbols which represent it.

Anonymous

What experience and history teach is this — that people in governments never have learned anything from history, or acted on principles deducted from it.

George Wilhelm Hegel

There is no natural right in opposition to social duty.

Thomas Jefferson

That's what you think.

Louis Pasteur, as he said the rosary during a train ride,
to a young man mocking the rosary as nonsense

Freedom is submission to the will of God.

Russell Kirk

Virtue is the worthiness to be happy.

George Rutler

Objective being is essential to achieving one's true self-actualization.

Name Lost

Virtue neutralizes emotion.

Samuel A. Nigro

Virtue is simply health of soul.

Peter Kreeft

Rights are state impositions that restrict real freedom.

Name Lost

The Sacraments are changes of human beingness like shellfish or animals put on new exoskeletons or skins to grow and cope with the world.

Samuel A. Nigro

It's *all* grace.

St. Theresa

There but for the grace of God go I.

St. Phillip Neri upon seeing a beggar

Humility, humility, humility, and humility.

St. Bernard of Clairvaux, when asked what the four cardinal virtues were

Equality in numbers has nothing to do with equality of attainment.

Frederick Douglas

Unless a *process of opportunity*, equality is a selfish fantasy.

Name Lost

Ethics without virtue is illusion.

Peter Kreeft

Democracy is simply the majority vote of those in a nation who can lick all the others.

Oliver Wendell Holmes

A tyrannical law, through not being according to reason, is not a law, absolutely speaking, but rather a perversion of law.

St. Thomas Aquinas

The common good of the state cannot flourish unless the citizens be virtuous.

St. Thomas Aquinas

To send light into the darkness of men's hearts — such is the duty of the artist.

Schumann

"We the people" has been replaced by "I the Self."

Robert P. Hunt

We attain Heaven by God's grace, but we attain our place or level in Heaven (our degree of ability to participate in grace) but by merit, by works of love, which dig in us a deeper place for more of God to fill.

Peter Kreeft

Virtue is to the soul as health is to the body.

Peter Kreeft

Art is right reason (rational knowledge) of things to be made; whereas prudence is the right reason of things to be done.

St. Thomas Aquinas

There are no manners in this world that do not have a moral substance.

St. Eusebius

Intellect must always precede will (which is "rational appetite") but will does not always precede intellect.

Peter Kreeft

The only thing inferior in Western Civilization to all others is the current press, media, and education establishment.

Samuel A. Nigro

Man longs for the transcendentals.

Max Weber

The simple but startling historical fact that the medieval mind typically assumed that man is by nature happy, while the modern mind typically assumes that unhappiness is our natural condition (see Freud, *Civilization and its Discontents*) speaks volumes about "progress."

Peter Kreeft

Our progenitors were the most impressive assembly of castoffs, renegades, adventurers, refugees, and slaves to converge on this earth. Together, they built a great nation. Surely we, their children, can find a way to preserve it.

Dante DiFiore

Christianity presupposes the Natural, redeems and sublimates it.

Ralph McInerny

Grace builds on nature but does not destroy it.

St. Thomas Aquinas

Truth is the equation of thought and thing.

St. Thomas Aquinas

When the body has alot, the other Transcendentals tend to be lived with great difficulty. . . . When the body suffers, the other Transcendentals tend to be more easily lived.

Samuel A. Nigro

The body (res) is the conscious dimension of our soul while the remaining Transcendentals tend, since Original Sin, to be unconscious if we allow them to remain so.

Samuel A. Nigro

Transcendentals enable you to see all things differently.

Name Lost

That people with strange ideas and activities are tolerated in a society is a principle uniquely confined to Western Civilization.

Name Lost

The only problem with non-Western civilizations is that they do not work except in stagnation.

Name Lost

Christianity is never old; it is always new.

Name Lost

The only candidate I ever wanted to vote for was a man who based his appeal on the fact that, having been confined in a lunatic asylum, he had a certificate of sanity.

Malcolm Muggeridge

Americans are the only people who became decadent without ever being civilized.

Malcolm Muggeridge

I am a human being first and foremost, and as such I am for whoever and whatever benefits humanity *as a whole*.

Malcolm X

You gotta learn a lot that ain't so, before you really figure it out.

Homer Hill

Only when you choose to behave with virtue while you are suffering are you truly free.

Samuel A. Nigro

What a memorable day for the entire world, because it signals the first recognition of the respect due to the dignity and liberty of all men no matter how primitive and uncivilized they may be — a principle that had never been proclaimed before in any legislation, let alone practiced in any country.

Rafael Altimari about Ferdinand & Isabella's
1503 decree granting liberty to the Indians

The Spanish were the first to denounce atrocities by their own compatriots.

Historian, J.H. Elliott

No one is more conservative than a liberal who will not change his or her mind.

Samuel A. Nigro

The enthusiasm with which "feelings" are promoted and embraced needs to be repeated for each of the Transcendentals. Not only one's identity as presented by "feelings," but one's matter, one's truth, one's oneness, one's good and one's beauty, all need co-equality with "feelings."

Samuel A. Nigro

Ill fares the land, the hast'ning ills us prey
Where wealth accumulates and men decay.

Oliver Goldsmith

Don't vote? Don't complain!

Betty Howard

In politics, the nose is more important than the eyes.

Samuel A. Nigro

In a republic, one should never have to vote for any candidate one has not met.

Thomas Fleming

The simple and at times amusing components of the Roman Catholic Church (the Bible, the Mass, the Sacraments, and Grace) and the Apostles and the Saints individually and collectively enhance the Transcendentals. Thusly, one is set free.

Samuel A. Nigro

THE SOUL is the personification of one's Transcendentals. It is the personification of the *permanent* things of our existence. That is, all being at the human level needs Transcendental awareness and projection. Only by such do we "save" our souls. All else, *all else*, is impermanent.

The soul contains six discernible components: the material substance (*res*), forming identity (*aliquid*), truth (*verum*), oneness (*unum*), goodness (*bonum*) and beauty (*bella*).

To relate in tune with the universe and all Nature, to be Catholic encompassing all possible, to be genuinely free, and to "save one's soul," each of the six dimensions listed of the soul need to be enthusiastically promoted and projected at all times.

The material substance (*res*) of one's being must be fostered, cared for, and engaged in and with the world. *Res* is our body. It must be used. It is our matter and our activating fathering capacity.

One's forming identity (*aliquid*) must be established and allowed full and free expression in confluence with the essence of humanity. *Aliquid* is the forming gentle mothering capacity, giving identity and essence to all.

The truth (*verum*) of one's being must be kept consistent, conforming, and in confluence with reality as reality is and not as one wishes it to be. *Verum* is our active orienting of self to reality and to society.

The oneness (*unum*) of one's being must be engaged consistent, conforming and in confluence with one's self, one's family, one's community, one's species, the planet and the universe. *Unum* is the forming of a totality of being from oneself to the universe as a complete family orientation.

The goodness (*bonum*) of one's being must be projected in confluence with natural law. That is, natural law as it is perceived and understood must be followed for goodness. One must be environmentally sound not only in terms of the environment but in terms of one's own personal beingness as part of that environment. Human beings as individuals must be environmentally and behaviorally real and consistent with nature. *Bonum* is activating work.

One's beauty (*bella*) must be projected in confluence with the uplifting dimension of being. That is, the best must be brought out in one's self and in those capable of being influenced. *Bella* is elevating and ascending of self and others.

These six components of our soul, these Transcendentals: material substance, identity, truth, oneness, goodness, and beauty are how each human being, to be part of the third millennium, needs to grasp the awareness of and to project in consciousness embracing all that one deals with. In total, these six Transcendentals personified are one's soul. The soul contains not only our body but in equal proportion an identity, a truth, a oneness, a goodness, and a beauty, all of which need equal attention and expression. When one starts treating all of them as our body is treated, the whole universe changes.

Recognizing this will be the new world, the new age, the new millennium, the new man, consistent with the projection of one's Transcendentals, and there will be a bursting forth of peace on earth.

Samuel A. Nigro

Sacraments are outward signs of inward Grace which increase one's Grace. Everything can have sacramental value. That's what this book is all about.

Name Lost

No matter what anyone says, you are not *free* if you are at the mercy of forces other than choosing to do what is transcendentally true, good, one, and beautiful.

Name Lost

Candid civilized debate is incompatible with political correctness, sensitivity demands, threats of ostracism, or even professing dislike.

Anonymous

Terrorism is autopropaganda — which seeks to demonstrate to the terrorists themselves the power of their own violence and ideology.

Maxwell Taylor

Secular approaches to life usually take Western Civilization (and the Roman Catholic Church) for granted. This is most commonly manifest in those societies where Western Civilization (whether the people realize it or not) allow different ideas to be discussed, debated, argued about, and even harshly presented. This is why "liberals" are hardly existent in any society where Western Civilization (and the Roman Catholic Church) have not been influential. See what happens to the dissent in those countries who do not have Western Civilization traditions.

Samuel A. Nigro

"Feelings" — and just about everything else, but especially feelings — are unworthy of having power unless sacramentally analyzed and synthesized.

1. By being baptized as a dignified event and giving faith.
2. By being confessed into a unified energy spectrum and giving hope.
3. By being transubstantiated into an integrated field and giving charity.
4. By being confirmed as an identifiable quanta and giving prudence.
5. By being spiritually singular and giving justice.
6. By being in ordered dimensions and giving courage.
7. By accepting the liberty of uncertainty and giving temperance.

By such sacramental living, Grace is obtained with the pursuing-happiness force of Holiness and one is free of all less. . . . This is the full use of one's soul. Neither "feeling" nor anything else should be given any power except by sacramental living!

Samuel A. Nigro

The three intellectual virtues are: wisdom — the speculating on highest causes; understanding — the habit of principles seeking truth; and science — the knowledge of knowable matter.

Name Lost

Victory is the only meaning of war. . . . Peace without victory is a dead thing. . . .

G.K. Chesterton

Those who leave the tradition of truth do not escape into something we call Freedom. They only escape into something else which we call fashion.

G.K. Chesterton

Transcendentals and Virtues ("the T's and V's") render humans to be unflappably free of intellectual, emotional, political, social and press media disturbances. The T's and V's place humans in the Statimuum with total functioning, resignation, and peace.

Name Lost

Narrowness is anything less than the transcendentals and virtues.

Samuel A. Nigro

Most crises of mental health — excepting biologically-based ones — can be focused on within the perspective of God and one's own total being in the universe by mechanisms of: (1) Sacramental Living, (2) Transcendentals and (3) Virtues which shrink to solution/resolution the conflictual problem(s) causing the crisis in the first place. Seeing all in the context of God, the universe, Sacramental Life, the Transcendentals, and Virtue is nothing than less than Sanity in it's purest form.

Samuel A. Nigro

Every revolution is a revolution against the last revolution.

G.K. Chesterton

. . .practically all revolutions in human history have consisted entirely of turning back.

G.K. Chesterton

Endless denunciations of distant vices, endless defiance of distant dangers; endless exploiting of people who know nothing by people who know too much; endless entanglements between the worst indecency of rabbles and the worst secrecy of oligarchies; the poor rioting for what they do not know, and the rich scheming for what they dare not say; all the facts fourth-hand and all the principles fourth-rate — these palpable and visible before us, are the actual fruits of Union of the large, highly organized modern State.

G.K. Chesterton

In the city where we work, there is little or no community anymore. There is aggregation — the forming of groups. And the difference is profound. Communities have consciences. Aggregations have programs. Communities work by civility. Aggregations get their way by stridency. . . . The fundamental difference between a community and an aggregation is really the difference between what is in one's *interest* and what one *desires* — between one's hopes and one's appetites.

Irene Impellizzeri

A constitution which can be restored only by its own violation is moribund.

Warren H. Carroll

The nature of law must be founded on the nature of man.

Cicero

In the course of history, the *form* of the government is never so important as its *substance*. . . . Almost any reasonable system of government will work if conducted by men of generally good moral character in a society valuing such character.

Warren H. Carroll

Knowing the secret of happiness to be freedom and the secret of freedom a brave heart, do not idly stand aside from the enemy's onset.

Pericles' funeral oration

No Christian can feel at home with any country. . .but should support their country out of duty; fill all they can with virtue; and then leave it with joy. No country can compare with the personal evolution of a Christian into the Universe.

Samuel A. Nigro

The Complaint of Peace: We must look for peace by purging the very sources of war — false ambitions and evil desires. As long as individuals serve their own personal interests, the common good will suffer. Let them examine the self-evident fact that this world of ours is the Fatherland of the entire human race.

Desiderius Erasmus, 1517 A.D.

In this world, this demented inn, in which there is absolutely no room for Him at all, Christ has come uninvited. But because He cannot be at home in it, His place is with those others for whom there is no room. His place is with those who do not belong, who are rejected by power because they are regarded as weak, those who are discredited, who are denied the status of persons, who are tortured, bombed, and exterminated. With those for whom there is no room, Christ is present in the world. He is mysteriously present in those for whom there seems to be nothing but the world at its worst. . . . It is in these that He hides Himself, for whom there is no room.

Thomas Merton

We are not things to be used by you, but free people with inalienable rights. In the market, it does not matter how we came into the world but what we make of ourselves. We join in cooperative effort for the good of all. If you interfere, you harm all people. If you oppress us, you will lose all that we have to offer and become poor. Throw away your chains and your barbed wire; they are useless now.

The 1992 message to every would-be tyrant by
post-Communist newcomers to the free marketplace

-There is no employment, but no one works.
-No one works, but everyone gets paid.
-Everyone gets paid, but there is nothing to buy.
-No one can buy anything, but everyone owns everything.
-Everyone owns everything, but no one is satisfied.
-No one is satisfied, but 99% of the people voted for the system.

The Six Miracles of Socialism
(by an ex-communist in 1992)

Law is reason without passion.

Fulton Sheen

Unless people are near in soul they had better not be near in neighborhood.

G.K. Chesterton

Man does not live by technology alone. . . .

Name Lost

Demands for equality are always found in people who feel or are inferior. The entire concept of equality is a mental state without substance in nature, because nature abhors equality as much as it abhors a vacuum. Equality is just not a real entity to be grasped in the real world. It is a mental state which does more harm than good because it cannot be achieved in fact. Equality as a fact is not the same as equal opportunity or justice because equality implies a totality which is impossible in that we are always "not equal" in some things. As a mental state, to seek it is to be unequal and to be inferior at least in the frustration of seeking that which is impossible to achieve. Another problem of equality is that it forces people to be less than they can be out of consideration for those "demanding equality." In these regards, equality is the antithesis of liberty.

Samuel A. Nigro

The money that goes to support hospitals, schools, civic organizations, the poor, and the disabled does not, as the saying goes, grow on trees. It can't be willed into existence by good intentions. It is generated by people who are working to produce goods and provide services. Until you create wealth, you can't give it away. Until you have capitalism, you can't have charity.

Kimberly O. Dennis

There is another important thing to remember about capitalism: Failure is not a stigma or a permanent obstacle. It is a spur to learn to try again. Edison invented the light bulb on, roughly, his ten-thousandth attempt. If we had depended on central planners to direct his experiment, we would all be sitting around in the dark today.

Malcolm S. Forbes, Jr.

We live in a Culture of Disgust of the Age of Anathema characterized by labial linguistics, proctological exuberance, flirtation with feces, and phallic abuse. . . . In other words, the Mortuary Life, and the West has fallen.
So stand aside to protect your own but vigorously challenge all that you see wrong, taking comfort in your loneliness, because the rain Baptizes, the wind gives Penance, the bright warm sunlight gives Holy Communion, the chills give Confirmation, the heat gives Extreme Unction, the lightning gives Holy Orders, and the thunder Matrimonyizes. The Sacraments are still everywhere. The Incarnation is completed. Redemption is in hand. Resurrection is just around the corner. Never fear. Easter is coming.

Samuel A. Nigro

Sacramental Weather
Rain — It's Baptizing outside.
Wind — It's Penancying outside.
Bright, comfortable sunlight — It's Holy Communioning outside.
Chilly cold — It's Confirmationing outside.
Sweaty heat — It's Extreme Unctioning outside.
Lightening — It's Holy Ordering outside.
Thunder — It's Matrimonying outside.

Samuel A. Nigro

I don't know much about painting and sculpture, but I have gained a great experience of fortification.

Michelangelo as military engineer in 1545

Wearing all that African garb makes you no more African than my wearing Italian ethnic clothes makes me Italian.

Samuel A. Nigro

. . .I refer to my family as Negroes. This is the term I grew up with, and I still think it's the best description. As a look at any of the Madden family will tell, we're no more "black" than we are "white." And I think that we're too far from Africa, and of mixed blood for too many generations, to be Afro-(or African-) American.

"Negro," "colored," and "person of color" were the terms of respect in my time and the times of my ancestors, and I have used them as such in this book. As a boy, growing up in the era of Jim Crow, I can't begin to tell you what an insult it was to call a Negro, especially by another Negro, "black." We all knew what it was short for: "black nigger." There wasn't a worse thing you could say.

T.O. Madden, Jr.

Those who "disprove Western Civilization" ultimately do it by syllogistic reasoning which is Western Civilization.

Name Lost

Writing badly is the definition of journalism.

G.K. Chesterton

There used to be lessons at home. . .now there is television and it cannot teach anything because it is either incorrect or incomplete.

Samuel A. Nigro

Christianity is the religion of a civilized freedom.

G.K. Chesterton

Oneness means you embrace the world in your mind by a transcendental reaching out, excluding no one and omitting nothing desirable.

Samuel A. Nigro

The foundation of all freedom is self-control.

Samuel A. Nigro

Reality hardly seems related to anything else.

G.K. Chesterton

Of references cited by the Founding Fathers from 1760 to 1805, 3154 in total, 34% came from the Bible. Nine percent were from classical authors like Cicero, Plutarch, Livy, and Plato. . . . Eighteen percent were from Whig writers, 11% derived from English common law, and 18% from so-called Enlightenment thinkers. Significantly, Montesquieu, the author of *The Spirit of the Laws*, was most frequented cited, three times as often as John Locke.

Robert R. Reilly

Neither error nor evil can be the object of a right, only what is true and good.

John Courtney Murray

Society must have a morality before it can have a censor.

G.K. Chesterton

Journalism as a picture of life must be consistently and systematically false.

G.K. Chesterton

The test of a democracy is not whether the people vote, but whether the people rule.

G.K. Chesterton

The difference between a normal and an abnormal person is that the normal person always works toward a goal or a purpose, while the abnormal person looks for escape mechanisms, excuses and rationalizations in order to avoid discovering the meaning and purpose of life.

Fulton Sheen

During World War II, the following events occurred: Colin Kelly was a selfless pilot who sank the first Japanese ship and in doing so lost his life. Edward O'Hare shot down the first Japanese plane. Dick Fleming made himself the first human torpedo in a military action. Daniel Callahan became the first Admiral to go down fighting. Mike Moran was the first Naval Officer to sink six Japanese ships in single combat. And Commander John Shea was the first fighting man whose last letter to his son became a famous American testament on patriotism. Upon reflecting on this, the first question is: What on earth is the Church doing? Why are we sending the cream of our men off to die for the national crazies who sit at home writing and printing newspapers when these young men ought to be going into the priesthood? What sort of education are they getting anyway? It has to stop. No question about it — *this has to stop*!

Samuel A. Nigro

The freedom of the press and media give slavery and tyranny.

Samuel A. Nigro

A government which governs least, governs best.

Thomas Jefferson

In other words: Government destroys its people.

In order to be a respectable man, one must be a good son, a good husband, and a good father; in other words, one must combine all the public and private virtues. . . . Therein lies the true definition of the word "patriotism."

The French Republican to the citizen of Philadelphia

Human Traditions have developed so that most follow them. But there always is a "we-know-it-better" group pointing out that since it (whatever "it" is) has never been done differently (or so they believe), "it" should be done differently. So, some try it differently. . .and proclaim themselves to be "truly free" since they no longer follow Tradition. However, suddenly, this group finds its members behaving as violent savages, dying of weird diseases, and many more becoming ignorant, unmanageable and uncivilized. In the final analysis, what they have not only discovered but have proved, is that Tradition was right.

Samuel A. Nigro

May God's peace, mercy and blessings be with you.

Muslim Greeting

In all the world, there is nothing better to do than to live savoring the fullness of total Being by conscious reflecting on the miracle of one's own being, reaching out by virtue emanating from one's physical, psychological, spiritual, and Transcendental dimensions. Such is genuine freedom. It is genuine living. And it enables a metamorphosis such that it will never end.

Samuel A. Nigro

As long as we pay the poor to continue doing the very things that help make them poor in the first place, then poor they shall remain.

Michael Bauman

Only the saint — that is, the person accepting death and poverty — is free at all times.

Erik von Kuehnelt-Leddihn

When press and media determine morality, morality is depersonalized. And depersonalized morality is not only negative in its impact on people's behavior, but it is immoral itself and sociopathic.

Samuel A. Nigro

One can maintain as a general principle that no authority is strong enough to govern millions of men unless it is aided by religion or slavery or both.

Joseph de Maistre

Don't trust writers. They pretend to have a keener sense about what is going on in the world than most other people. A writer's conclusions are not scientific. A writer's conclusions are, at best, notes on the universe, sketches, scratches really upon the smooth surface of existence.

Christopher de Vinck

Genuine freedom means painless and sinless. If we choose to be anything less, we will be found on deeper analysis to be something other than genuinely "free." Pain is intrinsic to the deformation of the Immanentals (form/

identity/essence, oneness, beauty). Sin is intrinsic to the deformation of the Transcendentals (matter, truth, good). Thus, the female has more pain because the Immanentals are the female dimension of being. And men have more sin because the Transcendentals are the male aspect of being. Therefore, to be painless is to engage and project one's Immanentals, and to be sinless is to engage and project one's Transcendentals. This struggle to engage and project as described is called suffering because struggle is now natural to human beingness ever since Original Sin. Thus, there is a conjoint existence of suffering and freedom together in a semi-mystical convergence of being and existence. Once you figure this out, you will always choose the good, the true, the beautiful, and the oneness, because only then are you free even though you are suffering — but the freedom renders the suffering benign, painless and sinless.

Samuel A. Nigro

History has a way of mocking the complacent.

Peter Rodman

No civil war ends in a coalition of government.

Name Lost

The central conservative truth is that it is culture, not politics, that determines the success of a society. The central liberal truth is that politics can change a culture and save it from itself.

Daniel Patrick Moynihan

In the Society of Status nobody has any rights. The individual is not recognized; a man is defined by his relation to the group, and is presumed to exist only by permission. The system of status is privilege and subjection. By the ultimate logic of the Society of Status, a member of the group who has committed not even a minor offense might be put to death for "the good of society."

Isabel Paterson

And thus we have affirmative action quotas and abortion as two extremes in a Society of Status.

Samuel A. Nigro

The humanitarian puts himself in place of God.

Isabel Paterson

Pity would be no more
If we did not make somebody poor.

William Blake about humanism

Always and everywhere, progress has been made solely by private invention, enterprise, labor and savings, and in inverse ratio to the extent of government.

Isabel Paterson

Just as it is wrong to withdraw from the individual and commit to a group what private enterprise and industry can accomplish, so too, it is an injustice, a grave evil, and a disturbance of right order for a larger and higher association to arrogate to itself functions which can be performed efficiently by smaller and lower societies. By its very nature the true aim of all social activity should be to help members of the social body but never to destroy or absorb them.

The Principle of Subsidiarity of Pope Pius XI

But in the long run, the consequences of the impact of the Christian West upon the world were good — at least until the West largely ceased to be Christian. No honest and reflective Oriental or African really wishes for a return to the society, economy, government and way of life of his people before the West made contact with them, or anything that could reasonably be expected to have developed from those cultures on their own. For the most part, non-Western societies — even when highly civilized, as in China and India and Japan — respected few if any rights of the individual person and offered no political freedom. They confined economic enterprise within their limits. Their religions aroused fear of angry spirits or offered spiritual escape from an evil world, but provided little moral guidance and no hope for perfecting souls or improving the world in which they dwelt.

Warren H. Carroll

Losing kindness, they turn to justness.

Lao-tzu

Who authorized my admiral to treat my subjects in this manner?

Queen Isabel of Spain striking off the chains of enslaved Indians brought to her ports by Columbus

You out there from the West: Stop dumping your garbage on us. We have something to teach you, namely the respect for life, the respect for elders and respect for the family.

African Cardinal

A wall is like a rule; and the gates are like exceptions that prove the rule. The man making it cannot have a city that is all gates anymore than a house that is all windows. Nor is it possible to have a law that consists entirely of liberties.

G.K. Chesterton

Because justice cannot happen, litigation only prolongs itself.

Wendell Berry

If there be any among us who would wish to dissolve this Union or to change its republican form, let them stand undisturbed as monuments of the safety with which error of opinion may be tolerated where reason is left free to combat it.

Thomas Jefferson

A society that does not know the meaning of the transcendentals, cannot know the meaning of anything.

Samuel A. Nigro

As a Christian physician, I have to care as much about your soul as I do your body, and I could not encourage you into a lifestyle that separates you from God forever. . . .

Beverly A. McMillan, M.D.

A society which does not know the meaning of honor cannot know the meaning of disgrace.

G.K. Chesterton

When you are a liberal, be sure you are not loose.

Shakespeare, *Henry VIII*

The worst bigots are those who are afraid to criticize because they might be called "bigots."

Samuel A. Nigro

At the heart of liberty is the right to define one's own concept of existence, or meaning, of the universe, and of the mystery of human life.

Planned Parenthood v. Casey (1992) by
Justices O'Connor, Kennedy and Sauters

> This is the ultimate self-serving, nonsensical definition of liberty. Never before have such intelligent people abandoned reason. Never with more confidence could I say that three Justices of the U.S. Supreme Court are absolute fools. They deserve contempt.

What is true in the reciprocal interaction between the quality of human person and that of institutions is all the more fruitful when we are able to recognize the priority of the ethical and spiritual dimensions, human transcendents. . . . The development of the moral and ethical life, however, seems unfortunately always to be left behind. This gives rise to the practical urgency, the permanent and fundamental necessity to *strengthen the human person from within*. This is the proper task of the Church whose "social doctrine" takes on life only when it is presented by morally and spiritually mature consciences.

Roger Heckel

No matter how poor you are, soap and water are cheap.

Florence Hill

You can sell anything to anybody; you just have to package it right.

Leonard Chretien, former Jehovah Witness

Culture is primarily the art of growing things.

G.K. Chesterton

The biggest puzzle ever in the entire world is: When it is raining, how do the waterdrops get on the insides of one's glasses?

Name Lost

The Formation of Conscience

When a society does not assist in conscience formation, all hell breaks lose. Conscience is (1) an expectation of a negative, painful consequence when not acting with positive, pleasant behavior and later (2) an expectation of positive, pleasant consequence (even if merely a "good feeling" about it) when acting with positive, pleasant behavior.

No conscience can form in a person therefore unless there is an *experience* of negative, "painful" (emotional if not physical but certainly not injurious!) consequence to negative, unsocial activity. Indeed, a person will always remain an unsocialized child (and should be treated as one) if he or she has never learned that unsocial behavior has negative consequences.

Thus, society must provide guidelines and supports for "hurting-without-injury" to reinforce negative consequences for negative behavior. Once that first step, shaming, is achieved, salutary guilt can be developed which is the *sine qua non* for conscience. Conscience operates on guilt, and woe to the individual who does not have guilt as a reminder that "it hurts to do social wrong."

Currently, guilt is ignorantly held in poor stead, but, nevertheless, guilt is the essential second developmental step after shaming for effective conscience formation. Guilt means the person has internalized the hurt for negative behaviors such that he or she is aware of anti-family or anti-social actions and the person automatically feels "bad" about it. Guilt should help inhibit and prevent the person's unsocial impulses.

But effective guilt often still requires environmental reinforcers as demonstrated by the stronger negative urges and lessened inhibitions of people getting into trouble when they leave home to go away to school or to take a trip. Finding themselves in a different town without the accustomed inhibitory forces, some individuals act out in ways they would never do in their own hometown later to their great embarrassment or even worse.

Truly: No guilt, no conscience. And, while guilt as obsessional or excessive is not desired, the only genuinely bad "guilt" is guilt about guilt.

Once a guilt capacity is created, shaming is no longer needed from without because the individual internally carries the pro-family and pro-social messages within.

Hopefully, positive reinforcements (in contrast to negative shaming) can then occur in the individual's life such that the third step for conscience formation occurs: Positive, pleasant experiences gratify and reinforce positive, pleasant behavior, i.e. "virtue becomes its own reward," which is the final step for conscience formation.

Personal conscience formation is a complicated process which can be simplified into these three stages: First, external shaming never omitted by society which is explicit, forceful, hurting without injury, and immediately consequential to misdeeds. Second, guilt of internalized self-punishment for anti-family and anti-social behavior. And third, positive self-enhancement reinforcing positive, pro-family and pro-social behavior.

When a society does not assist in these stages of conscience formation, all hell breaks lose.

Samuel A. Nigro

Hardest servitude has he
That is jailed in arrogant liberty.
Freedom spacious and unflawed
Who is walled about with God.

Francis Thompson

The case for the poor, in much religious rhetoric, had come to embrace the methods of those socialist systems that cannot produce. Hence, the poor will always be with us. . . .

James V. Schall

The worst wage-system is one with only one employer.

G.K. Chesterton

Truth is not determined by a show of hands.

Name Lost

There are three freedoms: (1) the freedom to do what one wants — or anarchy; (2) the freedom to do what we must — or tyranny; and (3) the freedom to do what we ought — which is genuine liberty.

Fulton Sheen

The meanest man is immortal, and the mightiest movement is temporal.

G.K. Chesterton

While there are a glut of self-help books to guide people through their lives, all anyone really needs to know is how to manage in a civilized and decent way the following: pride, covetousness, lust, anger, gluttony, envy, and sloth. Anyone who has civilized mechanisms for dealing with those seven capital sins will find that self-help books are not needed.

Samuel A. Nigro

. . .government (is) a practical thing made for the happiness of mankind, and not to furnish out a spectacle of uniformity to gratify the schemes of visionary politicians.

Edmund Burke

Everybody's strategy depends on everybody else's.

Name Lost

What is owned by everyone is cared for by none!

St. Thomas Aquinas

Not only are we all in the same boat, but we are all seasick.

G.K. Chesterton

Is he then, too, nothing more than an ordinary human being? Now he, too, will trample on all the rights of man and indulge only in ambition. He will exalt himself above all others to become a tyrant!

Ludwig Von Beethoven upon hearing that Napoleon Bonaparte
had proclaimed himself emperor, and immediately
Beethoven tore the title page from Symphony No. 3
retitling it "Eroica" instead of "Bonaparte"

Government by force is a contradiction in terms and an impossibility in physics. Force is what is governed. Government originates in the moral faculty.

Isabel Paterson

[T]he only civil right is the right to live in a nation where persons are judged by the quality of their character, not the color of their skin.

Dr. Martin Luther King, Jr.

. . .so far as face is concerned, any state-sponsored preference to one race over another. . .is in my view invidious and violative of the Equal Protection Clause.

Justice William O. Douglas

. . .that Jewish science from Vienna. . . .

Woody Allen on psychoanalysis

Watankanga Waokia — Literally means "The man who shows his love for the Great Spirit."

How the Sioux honored Peter John De Smet at the initial Great Smoke in 1851

If we are realistic, we will admit that we are not autonomous at all; we are dependent on the good faith (and conduct) of others.

Robert A. Destro

A page of history is worth a volume of logic.

Oliver Wendell Holmes

The life of the law has not been logic but experience.

Oliver Wendell Holmes

How can a man of honor take a newspaper in his hands without a shutter of disgust. . . .

Baudelaire

Christ said it. Buddha said it, Martin Luther King said it: We must live together as brothers or die together as fools.

Dave Brubeck

I'm tired of being dignified all the time. . .sometimes being dignified is shit!

84 year old Lillian Smith

It is unjust to judge any country by its politicians.

G.K. Chesterton

One way that poverty could be abolished is by slavery.

G.K. Chesterton

A multi-culture society, like a universal nation, is a contradiction in terms. A society without a common culture is not a society at all.

John O'Sullivan

Literature is whatever we will read again.

C.S. Lewis

The first opinion poll in history was conducted by Pontius Pilate.

George Rutler

There is a symbiosis of suffering and freedom. Following emotion is not freedom but impulse. Following sex drive is not freedom but bodily reflex. Following whatever is easy is not freedom but conditioned reinforcement. Freedom is choosing the transcendentals in the face of diversity or conflict. One suffers to be free because one's real choices are not impulses, reflexes, or Skinnerian reinforcements. Real freedom is choosing the transcendentals and suffering about it otherwise there is no real choosing. Thus, freedom and suffering are symbiotic. But therein is synergism too: *joy* occurs when one consciously knows that one is doing the above. It's called Catholic joy.

Samuel A. Nigro

To make us love our country, our country ought to be lovely.

Edmund Burke

The history of salvation is very simple. And it is a history that unfolds within the earthly history of humanity, beginning with the first Adam, through the revelation of the second Adam, Jesus Christ (Corinthians 15:45), and ending with the ultimate fulfillment of the history of the world and God, when he will be "all in all" (1 Corinthians 15:28).

John Paul II

Disasters prove that evil is the absence of good. One of the most profound, traditional, ancient, intellectually sound, philosophically tenable, and effective means of Good being in the world are through the hierarchy of angels. Angels exist. Mankind is losing out by not invoking them rationally. Without angels, one is left with the solipsistic silliness of emotive fantasies and paganistic gnostic foolishness that do not really make one transcendentally at one again with the universe. With one's own individual guardian angel, one can ask all the questions; one can plea for all the help; and one can rest assured that guidance and protection will be forthcoming with whatever occurs. The salubrious mental mechanisms which link with the relating to angels are second to none. For, whatever happens to you, one is assured that one's own spirit, one's own soul is in good hands.

Samuel A. Nigro

In our legal method there is too much lawyer and too little law. For we must never forget one fact, which we tend to forget nevertheless: that fixed rule is the only protection of ordinary humanity against clever men — who are the natural enemies of humanity. A dogma is the only safeguard of democracy. The law is our only barrier against lawyers. In the same way, the Prayer-Book is our only defense against clergymen.

G.K. Chesterton

No good man would ever go into politics.

Samuel A. Nigro

Those who trade some liberty for security will soon end up having neither.

Benjamin Franklin

It's no accident that capitalism has brought with it progress, not merely in production but also in knowledge. Egoism and competition are, alas, stronger forces than public spirit and sense of duty. . . . Perhaps I'm overpessimistic concerning state and other forms of communal enterprise, but I expect little good from them. Bureaucracy is the death of any achievement. . . . I'm inclined to view that the state can only be of use to industry as a limiting and regulative force.

Albert Einstein

Above all, don't lie to yourself. A man who lies to himself and listens to his own lies comes to such a path that he cannot distinguish the truth within him or around him and so loses all respect for himself and others. And having no respect, he ceases to love and in order to occupy and distance himself without love, he gives way to passion and coarse pleasures, and threatens to bestiality in his vices. . . all from continual lying to other men and himself.

Father Zossina

No one is more vindictive than a free speech liberal who doesn't like what you say.

Samuel A. Nigro

Conservatives believe it when they see it. Liberals see it when they believe it.

Dick Armey

When the word "leader" or "leadership" returns to current use, it connotes a relapse into barbarism. For a civilized people, it is the most ominous word in a language.

Isabel Paterson

In judging a society, the following questions must be answered: Is man seen as an entity? As a person with an immortal soul? What is the impact of the moral order affirmed? How are the transcendentals implemented and preserved? What are the energy associations? What are the energy conversion modes? Is the law dependable? Who and what are dependable? Who and what have the highest potential energy? How are the virtues promoted and reinforced in individuals?

Samuel A. Nigro

There is no collective good. Strictly speaking, there is not even any common good. There are in the natural order conditions and materials through which the individual, by virtue of his receptive and creative facilities and volition, is capable of experiencing good.

Isabel Paterson

"The greatest good of the greatest number" is a vicious phrase. . . . For if "good" is quantitative and makes up a sum by majority, there can be no judge of what is good except the majority. This rule is, in fact, the justification alleged by the Nazis for the extermination of the Jews, as of the Russian communists for the beastly murder of the most productive members of the population. Both have acted on the same theory.

Isabel Paterson

As a conservative, I want the freedom and power to live my life an obedient man, but obedient to God, subservient to the wisdom of my ancestry; never to the authority of political truths arrived at yesterday at the voting booth.

William F. Buckley, Jr.

It (force) is an instrument of negation, and nothing more. When government begins to rely upon force or intimidation, if the various factors involved could be discovered exactly, and expressed in a mathematical equation with the ratio of the increase of force, the sum would give the length of time remaining before either the government or the nation, or both, must collapse.

Isabel Paterson

Let anyone who does not recognize the connection of these principles (the Christian doctrine of the individual soul, born to immortality, with the faculty of free-will, which includes the possibility of sin or error, yet equally enables us to strive towards its heritage of salvation) try to rewrite the Declaration of Independence without reference to a divine source of human rights. It cannot be done; the axiom is missing.

Isabel Paterson

Civilization is self-control. Savagery is self-mutilation.

Dale Ahlquist

The lust for power is most easily disguised under humanitarian or philanthropic motives.

Isabel Paterson

. . .force cannot compel obedience in the social order. What it can effect is death, whether of subject or king. . . . When the assassin is otherwise sane, and acting from a strictly political grievance, assassination is a symptom of a grave imperfection in the mechanism, a relatively weak connection, or a point of disproportionate stress, where a break occurs. In terms of mechanism, it stops the machine until the broken part has been replaced; but it does not and cannot institute a better type of mechanism. . . . Where force is the arbiter, government ceases.

Isabel Paterson

Almighty God: Our sons, pride of our nation, this day have set upon a mighty endeavor. . . . They will need Thy blessings. . . . We know that by Thy grace, and by the righteousness of our cause, our sons will triumph. . . . Thy will be done, Almighty God.

President Franklin D. Roosevelt announcing to the American people that the D-Day invasion against Hitler had begun

Men enslave themselves, forging the chains link by link, usually by demanding protection as a group. When businessmen ask for government credit, they surrender control of their business. When labor asks for enforced "collective bargaining" it has yielded its own freedom. When racial groups are recognized in law, they can be discriminated against by law.

Isabel Paterson

You are the fairest of the sons of men; grace is poured upon your lips; therefore God has blessed you forever.

Psalm 45:2

For the palace will be forsaken. . .until the Spirit is poured upon us from on high, and the wilderness becomes a fruitful field, and the fruitful field is deemed a forest.

Isaiah 32:14-15

And in the last days it shall be, God declares, that I will pour out my Spirit upon all flesh, and your sons and your daughters shall prophesy, and your young men shall see visions, and your old men shall dream dreams; yea, and on my menservants and my maidservants in those days I will pour out my Spirit; and they shall prophesy.

Acts 2:17-18

And Stephen, full of grace and power, did great wonders and signs among the people.

Acts 6:8

And when they had prayed, the place in which they were gathered together was shaken; and they were all filled with the Holy Spirit and spoke the word of God with boldness.

Acts 4:31

And the believers from among the circumcised who came with Peter were amazed, because the gift of the Holy Spirit had been poured out even on the Gentiles.

Acts 10:45

When he came and saw the grace of God, he was glad; and he exhorted them all to remain faithful to the Lord with steadfast purpose; for he was a good man, full of the Holy Spirit and of faith.

Acts 11:23-24

And hope does not disappoint us, because God's love has been poured into our hearts through the Holy Spirit which has been given to us.

Romans 5:5

And do not get drunk with wine, for that is debauchery; but be filled with the Spirit.

Ephesians 5:18

Angels, angels everywhere clean
And wherever there is a word
Are rarely ever, ever seen
But they always can be heard.

Samuel A. Nigro

He saved us, not because of deeds done by us in righteousness, but in virtue of his own mercy, by the washing of regeneration and renewal in the Holy Spirit, which he poured out upon us richly through Jesus Christ our Savior, so that we might be justified by his grace and become heirs in hope of eternal life.

Titus 3:5-7

Governments pirate the property of people while religions based on anything other than love and reason pirate people's minds.

Name Lost

You can mock Western Civilization all you want. . .except you will want it for yourself. . . .

Name Lost

Equality in itself signifies nothing, implies no values; two zeros are equal.

Isabel Paterson

. . .the proper organization of society must be that of free individuals. And their equality is posited on the plain fact that the qualities and attributes of a human being are ultimately not subject to measure at all; a man equals a spirit entity.

Isabel Paterson

A journalist is an expert in imaginary novella writing about tragedies, problems or messes, but becomes an idiot when confronted with Good News.

Samuel A. Nigro

It takes a real politician to say that politics do not matter.

G.K. Chesterton

The Greeks were never able to validate their hypothesis for democracy because it is a materialistic concept, and materialism will not admit human equality, nor any other principle of human association.

Isabel Paterson

Every atrocity has been defended at one time or another by an obsequious, ignorant, self-righteous murder of cackling journalists.

Samuel A. Nigro

The business of the poet and novelist is to show the sorriness underlying the grandest things and the grandeur underlying the sorriest things.

Thomas Hardy

The greatest improvement in the productive powers of labor seems to be the effect of the division of labor.

Adam Smith

The real price of everything is the toil and trouble of acquiring it.

Adam Smith

Man is born free but everywhere is in chains.

Jean Jacques Rousseau

And is only made free by the transcendentals.

. . .when men really understand that they are brothers they instantly begin to fight.

G.K. Chesterton

If one cannot empathize about justice, one can never be just to others and one should never receive justice for oneself.

Samuel A. Nigro

Union, in peace for prosperity, in war for defense.

Tammany — 17th century Chief of Delaware Indian nations

As a human being, I should feel a longing for a little human justice after all that inhuman mercy.

G.K. Chesterton

Rain is a thing of the past.

Andrew Carnegie

When a rich man thinks he knows it all.

The trouble with professional victims is that they cannot overcome their differences with others to be fully human.

Name Lost

BREAK THE HYPNOTISM. ANALYZE THE ACTING. WHEN WATCHING TELEVISION OR MOVIES SAY OR DO THE FOLLOWING:

— "Look at his/her expression. . . that is good acting!"

—"Wow. . . what wide-eyed alarm. . . he/she must have practiced in a mirror for hours to look like that."

— That was the most realistic and artistic *grunt** I have ever heard! What great acting!"

(*The following may also be used instead of "grunt": pause, stare, glance, glare, stand still, hesitate, stammer, laugh, cry, whimper, moan, scream, shout, jump, walk, run, crawl, roll over, fall, sneeze, belch, cough, sleep, snore, breathe, writhe, grimace, arm-move, foot-move, hand-move, head-move, tongue-move, eye-move, breast-move, butt-move, penis-move, stomach-move, chest-move, shoulder-move,. . .and more.)

—"The guy who thought this up must be wacko. . . hateful. . . stupid. . . disturbed. . . . I wonder what he/she does for a living.

—"How people can lie like that with a straight face is amazing!"

—"That evening news reporter does a great job of reading the script without looking like he/she is reading."

—"I have heard that when people run around naked like that, they cannot help but be a little nervous so they gulp air and then they fart a lot. Such actors and actresses can't stop it either. And the more they do it, the worse it gets. If you look close at the background, you might be able to see the special ventilation fans hidden on the set otherwise the smell is terrible."

—"Listen to the music. . .it is neat how it fits with the scene. . . . Wonder how this scene would keep our attention if the music were `chop sticks'."

There is nothing new in the world except the history you did not know.

Harry S. Truman

It is only the secure who are humble.

G.K. Chesterton

The contents pages of *Miracles of Mary: Apparitions, Legends, and Miraculous Works of the Blessed Virgin Mary* by Michael S. Durbin
The Virgin Mary has appeared more than 21,000 times in the past ten centuries the contents pages list a few of them. *Vis Mediatrix Naturae*

Since television and movies basically have no standards of decency or morality, it is obvious that anyone who pays any attention to television and movies will unwittingly acquire the same pagan immoral attitudes of no standards and no decency.

Samuel A. Nigro

The American Founding was a prophetic and messianic movement, drawing from the depths of the Christian experience of God, as well as a "Proposition." These are the truths we hold. It is here that our true identity as a nation lies.

Donald J. D'Elia

AMAZING GRACE

Amazing grace! How sweet the sound That saved and set me free!
I once was lost, but now am found. Was blind, but now I see!
Twas grace that taught my heart to fear, and grace my fears relieved.
How precious did that grace-appear, The hour I first believed!
The Lord has promised good to me, His Word my hope secures,
He will my shield and portion be, As long as life endures.
Thru many dangers, tolls and snares, I have already come,
His grace has brought me safe thus far, His grace will lead me home.
Yes, when this flesh and heart shall fail, and mortal life shall cease,
Amazing grace shall then prevail, in heaven's joy and peace.
When we've been there ten thousand years, Bright shining as the sun,
We've no less days to sing God's praise, Than when we first begun.

(American Frontier Song)

Locke, like Jefferson, was living off the moral capital and ensuing political principles of the Catholic Middle Ages, although he was oblivious to this fact. So were our other Founding Fathers.

Stephen M. Krason

The earth belongs in usufruct to the living.

Jefferson

Victimhood makes you think that you deserve special treatment. With that automatically comes an unwillingness to deal aggressively with the real problem. Therefore it cripples you and deprives you of any real success you may have had. In a real sense, victimhood makes one an unnecessary failure and unspeakably inferior. The only exception can be when charity is appropriately needed. . .which almost always ought to be a temporary condition.

Samuel A. Nigro

A cult is any group which uses a mind-control process of persuading and influencing by untruthful excitement to destructive ends involving prevarication, deceptive recruitment, intimidating group pressure, and a prohibition of leaving.

Stephen Hassan

We are quickly learning what it means to be non-Christian — modern, mean, and morbid.

Samuel A. Nigro

The purposes of freedom must define its nature and its limits.

Francis Canavan

Social justice also imposes on each of us a personal responsibility to work with others to design and continually perfect our institutions as tools for personal and social development. . . . The ultimate purpose of economic justice is to free each person to engage creatively in the unlimited work beyond economics, that of the mind and the spirit.

Norman G. Kurland

Colin Powell's Rules

1. It ain't as bad as you think. It will look better in the morning.
2. Get mad, then get over it.
3. Avoid having your ego so close to your position that when your position falls, your ego goes with it.
4. It can be done!
5. Be careful what you chose. You may get it.
6. Don't let adverse facts stand in the way of a good decision.
7. You can't make someone else's choices. You shouldn't let someone else make yours.
8. Check small things.
9. Share credit.
10. Remain calm. Be kind.
11. Have a vision. Be demanding.
12. Don't take counsel of your fears or naysayers.
13. Perpetual optimism is a force multiplier.

In extreme necessity, all goods are common.

Old Roman Catholic Dogma

A Authoritative ambassadors
N natural neighbors
G Gracious Guardians and graceful guides
E examples of executive enforcement and encouragement to God's Law
l luminous lights and lovers of god, listeners to his word and leaders to the lord of life
S SERVANTS AS TRUE SONS OF GOD

"Angels" according to Scott Hahn

The press as conceived in the First Amendment is ONLY important in direct proportion to the dishonesty of politicians. Whatever else "the press" does is secondary.

Name lost

It is the duty of the Press to expound; occasionally it is duty to expose. Rarely, very rarely, it is its duty to suppress, though this is almost the only duty which it still performs with gusto.

G.K. Chesterton

The first task of any journalist is to make himself important. This is done by raising questions because of some fact; in order to find out the truth; or by fabricating something. It is usually the last.

Name lost

The liberal capacity to whitewash what is genuinely evil in some instances and then to be able to find problems when there are none in other instances both serve one purpose: to present the liberal as a wonderful, deep-thinking, problem-solving rescuer who controls all for the benefit of all. One is hard-pressed to be more arrogant and ignorant than that.

Name lost

In the battle that goes on for life,
I ask for a field that is fair
A chance that is equal in strife
the courage to do and to dare.
If I should win, let it be by the code
My faith and my honor held high
If I should lose, let me stand by the road,
And cheer as the winner rides by.

Knutz Rockne

Cast down your bucket where you are — cast it down in making friends in every manly way of the people of all races by whom you are surrounded.

Booker T. Washington

I wish the quality of your product were as good as the quality of your advertising.

Ashleigh Brilliant

The ignorant pronounce it Frood,
The caval and applaud.
The Well-informed pronounce it Froyd,
But I pronounce it Fraud.

G.K. Chesterton on Sigmund Freud

On television or in movies, it is good acting or bad acting. Regardless, *it is acting*. . . which should tell you something about the significance and importance of television and movies.

Samuel A. Nigro

With all those who feel powerless to influence events please signify by maintaining their usual silence.

Ashleigh Brilliant

And now I will indulge in a quiet think.

Scarecrow

"Infallibility" has acquired a new meaning: Today, the press, media and educators are so unreliable and dishonest, that nothing is worth believing unless said by the Vatican.

Samuel A. Nigro

From all that terror teaches, from lies of tongue and pen,
From all the easy speeches that comfort cruel men,
From sale and profanation of honor and the sword,
From sleep and from damnation, deliver us, good Lord.

G.K. Chesterton

If a person has no strong conviction as to what is right and what is wrong, if he does not believe in any God or absolute moral values, if he no longer respects contractual obligations, and, finally, if his hunger for pleasures and sensory values is paramount, what can guide and control his conduct towards other men? Nothing but his desires and lusts.

Pitirim A. Sorokin

Man is the measure of all things.

Protagoras

I treat. God heals.

Universal Medical Dictum

Law is found, not made.

Roman Proverb

The press says this. The evening news says that. The polls are in. The voters are out. There is no government. Democracy has failed. Liberals have taken over the country.

Samuel A. Nigro

All that is left is startle.

Name lost (about entertainment)

The typical journalist is really saying "look at me because of what I wrote" — when he should just be writing the facts.

Samuel A. Nigro

Just as one cannot really BE an American without *being* an American, neither can one really be a full human being without trying to be a *full* human being. In both cases, it means going beyond one's own specific particular constricting background.

Samuel A. Nigro

One can only transcend by knowing and using the transcendentals.

Samuel A. Nigro

When I was growing up, my family refused to speak Italian around us kids. And they were always running to the English dictionary or the Bible to look up words or something. By the time I was 7, I thought those books contained everything worth knowing. Now, much older, I realize they do. . . and are the reasons for my own successes. But every once in a while I just wish I could speak a little Italian. . . but I also know that if I could, I would not be where I am today.

anonymous physician

God, saints and angels are *always* with you.

Name lost

Making a judgment about man being a "creature of habit" depends on the habit. That man is more so a "creature of suggestion" is much more problematical.

Samuel A. Nigro

Consequentialist conclusions are always equally correct. . . and therefore equally meaningless.

John Miller

Open your heart to grace and it will be there.

Rev. Edward Krause

The number of votes in a democracy should equal the numbers of individuals in an intact family.

Raphael Waters

Virtue itself escapes not calumnious strokes.

Hamlet

Like a scurvy politician seems to see what thou dost not.

from King Lear

they ain't got no kulture.

Ezra Pound

"Black" as fad or fetish or bully club is as wrong-headed if not as damaging as "white" was when the latter was used in the same way.

Name lost

One will never learn the cruelty or the dishonesty of the press from the press.

Samuel A. Nigro

Fiction means the common things as seen by uncommon people. Fairy tales mean the uncommon things as seen by the common people.

G.K. Chesterton

Proof of non- or anti-therapeutic effects of "talking about" problems is demonstrated daily by the television talk shows wherein bright, glib, "how did you feel?" and "tell me how you felt" confrontation fantasizing show hosts pretend somber pseudo-insightful pretentious therapy. Just as bad are the attempts to present as reality all sorts of criminal, social and family pathologies in cop shows, hospital shows, etc. *It is all unreal* — therefore causes rather than relieves pain unless reminded that it is fantasy. Remember: almost everything seen on television or in movies is planned, scripted and produced *fantasy*. Remember that everything on television and in movies has been *produced* — it is *acting* — it is someone faking something! Never let your children forget all that.

Samuel A. Nigro

The culture of death assumes there is not enough to go around. But the proper creation of distributed wealth makes plenty to go around.

Samuel A. Nigro

A celebrity is someone who makes money by being a fake.

Samuel A. Nigro

There is manifestly much more emancipation in giving a beggar a schilling to spend, than in sending an official after him to spend it for him.

G.K. Chesterton

The Negro has been formed by this nation, for better or for worse, and does not belong to any other — not to Africa and certainly not to Islam.

James Baldwin

But Anthropology gone mad, which is the right name for Race, means everlastingly looking for your own countrymen in other people's countries.

G.K. Chesterton

We must obey God rather than men.

Acts 5:29

The worst thing about victimhood (embracing the victim role) is that it makes one hateful and revengeful, either of which prevents resolution and confluence. One of the remarkable aspects of Christianity is that it counters the victimhood mentality by a salutary resignation to the struggle with the sufferings of life.

Samuel A. Nigro

If it is not sacramental or potentially sacramental, ignore it.

Name Lost

The community is where the Divine comes to realization between man and man.

Joseph Mauceri

Psychoanalysis is responsible for the fiction, promulgated largely by Freud, that culture is predominately restrictive; the reverse is true, it is predominately directive.

Abram Kardiner

One thing is always certain: The real facts are different than what the news industry has reported. So listen to or read the news. Know that they probably have it wrong and most assuredly have it incomplete. Then forget about it or go find the truth.

Samuel A. Nigro

I curse those sob sisters who moan about the so-called ruination of past "civilizations" wherein those "civilized" had little worthy of sustaining. And a moment's reflection reveals that these are the very same people who unabashedly try to ruin our current Western Civilization. Their's is equivalent to the remarkable feat of someone standing on his head and shooting himself in his foot while it was in his mouth.

Samuel A. Nigro

The one grace is that we are not masters of our own lives. Therefore, something new can be given to us.

James V. Schall

In the temporal order, *force* is that which affects matter particles. Grace is the same for Spirit. Resignedly, take charge.

CHAPTER 11:

PRAYERS

This Chapter contains prayers which should be familiar to anyone calling themselves Roman Catholic. Some prayers are ancient, some are contemporary, some are mere definitions which have a prayerful connotation. All deserve to be put to memory and prayed daily. Prayers make one's chemistry work better.

The Roman Catholic Tradition has many other prayers which should be of interest and can be found elsewhere.

All prayers listed in this book can be reduced, photocopied and then cut and placed in strategic places to be used whenever.

An aside about memorization is pertinent here as drawn from my experience as a psychiatrist and a student of the mind: The mind is greatly invigorated by forced, rote memorization of *meaningful* ideas. Such improves one's mental chemistry. In fact, ideas may not have real meaning for anyone unless they are committed to memory with a capacity to recite them at will. Therefore, the reader is encouraged to memorize prayers and say them. They will bring Loving Truth and better mental functioning. Other less recognized benefits of such memorizing are improved mental capacity, enhanced thought processing, increased perceptibility, and more fluent articulateness. A person who frequently memorizes important messages such as these prayers is truly at no small advantage in dealing with life.

In contrast, mantra mumbling is mental nonsense (even if emotionally comforting), while mantra-like solemn meditation on the mysteries of the Rosary, Gregorian Chant, or prayers among other examples, is to harmonize into the divine energy placing mind, intellect, will and emotions into ascending (Is-ness, Such-ness, and It-is-ness as Buddhists say) unity with God. Fifteen minutes (at least) daily of prayerful harmonizing with the real prayers using real ideas will relax and rejuvenate like nothing else.

The silly humming of phonemes does nothing. But the memorizing and repetitive harmonic recitation of prayers that have meaning are tantamount to mental power. Beware of the do-nothing think-nothing anergia of non-Christian mantra mysticism. It does not free.

Prayer helps to focus on the Other — resulting in a fulfillment which can only occur as a by-product of the intense solo investment in the transcendentals. There is no such thing as *self*-fulfillment, which is an illusion. Fulfillment comes only through prayer as it brings nearer the infinite Trinity by incarnating us into Christ.

Finally, if you know these prayers, you will truly know your faith and be better able to articulate and defend it.

My favorite — easily memorized — and said each day (driving, walking, cooking, shaving, often) — are the following prayers, each worth *thinking* about deeply:

OUR FATHER

Our Father, Who art in Heaven,
Hallowed by Thy Name;
They Kingdom come;
Thy will be done on earth
As it is in Heaven.
Give us this day our daily bread;
And forgive us our trespasses
As we forgive those
Who trespass against us;
And lead us not into temptation,
But deliver us from evil. Amen.

THE HAIL MARY

Hail, Mary! Full of grace,
The Lord is with thee,
Blessed are thou among women,
And blessed is the fruit of thy womb, Jesus.
Holy Mary, Mother of God,
Pray for us sinners,
Now, and at the hour of our death. Amen.

ADORATION

Glory be to the Father, and to the Son, and to the
Holy Spirit; As it was in the beginning is now,
and ever shall be, world without end. Amen.

APOSTLE'S CREED

I believe in God the Father Almighty, Creator of heaven and earth; and in Jesus Christ, His only Son, our Lord, Who was conceived of the Holy Spirit, born of the Virgin Mary, suffered under Pontius Pilate, was crucified, died, and was buried.

He descended into hell; the third day He rose again from the dead.

He ascended into heaven, sits at the right hand of God, the Father Almighty. From thence He shall come to judge the living and the dead.

I believe in the Holy Spirit, the Holy Catholic Church, the communion of Saints, the forgiveness of sins, the resurrection of the body, and life everlasting. Amen.

HAIL, HOLY QUEEN

Hail, Holy Queen, Mother of mercy, our life, our sweetness, and our hope;
To thee do we cry, poor banished children of Eve, to thee do
we send up our sighs, mourning and weeping in this valley of tears.
Turn then, most gracious advocate, thine eyes of mercy towards us, and after this, our exile, show unto the blessed fruit of thy womb, Jesus.
Oh clement, Oh loving, Oh sweet Virgin Mary!

THE MEMORARE

Remember, O most gracious Virgin Mary that never was it known that anyone who fled to your protection, implored your help, or sought your intercession was left unaided.

Inspired with this confidence, I fly to you O Virgin of virgins, my mother. To you I come; before you
I stand, sinful and sorrowful.

O Mother of the world Incarnate, despise not my petitions, but in your mercy, hear and answer me.

Amen.

MORNING OFFERING

O Jesus,
through the Immaculate Heart of Mary, I offer You all my prayers, works, and sufferings of this day. For all the intentions of Your Sacred Heart. In union with the Holy Sacrifice of the Mass throughout the world. In reparation for all my sins. For the intentions of all our associates, and, in particular, for the intention of our Holy Father for this month. Amen.

PRAYER TO ST. MICHAEL

Saint Michael, the Archangel, defend us in battle; be our defense against the wickedness and snares of the devil. May God rebuke him, we humbly pray; and do you, O prince of the heavenly host, by the power of God, thrust into hell Satan and the other evil spirits who prowl about the world seeking the ruin of souls. Amen.

Most Sacred Heart of Jesus, have mercy on us. (Three times)

THE ACT OF CONTRITION

O my God! I am heartily sorry for having offended Thee, and I detest all my sins, because I dread the loss of heaven and the pains of hell, but most of all because they offend Thee, my God, Who art all good and deserving of all my love. I firmly resolve, with the help of Thy grace, to confess my sins, to do penance, and to amend my life.

ADDICTION PRAYER

Unnatural deeds
Do breed unnatural troubles.
Infected minds to their deaf pillows will discharge their secrets.
More need they the Divine than the physician.
Help them conquer their addiction, Oh God.
(Modification of William Shakespeare, MacBeth)

THE SHEMA

Hear, O Israel, the Lord our God is one Lord. Thou shalt love the Lord thy God, with thy whole heart and thy whole soul and with thy whole strength. And these words which I command thee this day shall be in thy heart. And thou shalt tell them to thy children, and thou shalt meditate on them sitting in thy house and walking on thy journey, sleeping and rising. And thou shalt bind them as a sign on thy hand, and they shall be, and shall move between thy eyes. And thou shalt write them in the entry and on the doors of thy house (Deuteronomy 6:4-9).

I WILL NOT SHED INNOCENT BLOOD, NOR HAVE ANY PART OF IT

"Deliver those who are being taken away to death and those who are staggering towards slaughter. Hold them back, oh Lord. Hold them back, oh Lord, and help them out!"

(Proverbs 24:11)

HEAVENLY CONCLUSION

I have had a tremor of bliss,
A wink of heaven, A whisper,
And I would no longer be denied; all things
Proceed to a joyful consummation.

(T.S. Eliott)

PRAYER TO THE HOLY SPIRIT

Breathe into me, Holy Spirit,
  that my thoughts may all be holy.
Move in me, Holy Spirit,
  that my work, too, may be holy.
Attract my heart, Holy Spirit,
  that I may love only what is holy.
Strengthen me, Holy Spirit,
  that I may defend all that is holy.
Protect me, Holy Spirit,
  that I always may be holy.

(St. Augustine)

SELF-DISCIPLINE PRAYER

What business have you reciting my statutes,
standing there mouthing my covenant,
since you detest my discipline?

(Psalm 50:17)

WOMEN

Sing aloud, O daughter of Zion;
shout, O Israel!
The Lord, your God, is in your midst,
he will rejoice over you with gladness,
he will renew you with his love;
he will exult over you with loud singing,
as on a day of festival.

(Zephaniah 3:14-17)

THE FATIHAH

In the name of Allah,
The Beneficent, the Merciful,
Praise be to Allah,
Lord of Creation.
The Beneficent, the Merciful.
King of the Last Judgment!
You alone we worship, and to
You alone we pray for help.
Guide us to the straight path,
The path of those
Whom You have favored, and
Not of those who have incurred
Your wrath
Nor of those who have gone stray.

(The Lord's Prayer of Islam)

GOD IS WITH ME

GOD has created me to do Him some definite service: he has committed some work to me which He has not committed to another. I have my mission — I may never know it in this life but I shall be told it in the next.

I am a link in a chain, a bond or connection between persons. He has not created me for naught. I shall do good, I shall do His work, I shall be an angel of peace, a preacher of truth in my own place while not intending it — if I do but keep His Commandments.

Therefore I will trust Him. Whatever, wherever I am, I can never be thrown away. If I am in sickness, my sickness may serve Him; in perplexity, my perplexity may serve Him; if I am in sorrow, my sorrow may serve Him. He does nothing in vain. He knows what He is about. He may take away my friends. He may throw me among strangers. He may make me feel desolate, make my spirits sink, hide my future from me — still He knows what He is about.

God be with you.

(Cardinal Newman)

LIBERALISM / MODERNISM

Good, we wanted good:
  to set the world right.
We didn't lack integrity:
  we lacked humility.
What we wanted was not
  innocently wanted.
Precepts and concepts,
  the arrogance of theologians,
to beat with a cross,
  to institute with
    blood. . . .

      Some
became secretaries to the
  secretary
to the General Secretary of the
  Inferno.
      Rage
became philosophy,
  its drivel has covered the
planet.

(Octavio Paz)

THE LAST GOSPEL

In the beginning was the Word, and the Word was with God; and the Word was God. He was in the beginning with God. All things were made through Him, and without Him was made nothing that has been made. In Him was life, and the life was the light of all. And the light shines in the darkness; and the darkness grasped it not. There was a man, one sent from God, whose name was John. This man came as a witness, to bear witness concerning the light, that all might believe through him. He was not himself the light, but was to bear witness to the light. It was the true light that enlightens every person who comes into the world. He was in the world, and the world was made through Him, and the world knew Him not. He came unto His own, and His own received Him not. But to as many as received Him He gave the power of becoming sons of God; to those who believe in His name: Who were born not of blood, nor of the will of the flesh, nor of the will of man, but of God. And the Word was made flesh, and dwelt among us. And we saw His glory — glory as of the only-begotten of the Father — full of grace and of truth.

(St. John)

HUMANBEINGNESS PRINCIPLES

1. Since humans have *dignity*, they should always be respected as inviolable ends and never used as means.
2. Since humans have *unity*, they should be honored as whole entireties, and none of their parts should be treated in isolation of their entirety.
3. Since humans have *integrity*, their moral good should be upheld and their morality should never be divorced from their nature.
4. Since humans have *identity*, both as members of the human race and as unique individual persons, these identities should be valued and allowed to develop and no attempt should be made radically to alter or deform them.
5. Since humans have *spirituality*, that quality should be affirmed, and no attempt should be made to reduce humans to their material components or to limit them to what is merely natural.

Without the benefits that humans stand to gain through the application of these moral principles, there exists the imminent danger of humans falling victim to these forms of dissolution: exploitation, fragmentation, disintegration or demoralization, dehumanization, and despiritualization.

(Modification of Principles of Donald DeMarco)

NATURE AS THE LIVING GARMENT OF THE HOLY SPIRIT

I am that supreme and fiery force that sends forth all the sparks of life. Death has no part in me, yet do I allot it, whereforce I am girt about with wisdom as with wings. I am that living and fiery essence of the divine substance that flows in the beauty of the fields. I shine in the water, I burn in the sun and the moon and the stars. Mine is that mysterious force of the invisible wind; I sustain the breath of all living. I breathe in the verdure, and in the flowers, and when the waters flow like living things, it is I. I found those columns that support the whole earth. I am the force that lies hid in the winds, from me they take their source, and as a man may move because he breathes, so doth a fire burn but by my blast. All these live because I am in them and am of their life. I am wisdom. Mine is the blast of the thundered word by which all things were made. I permeate all things that may not die even when they seem to die. I am eternal life.

(St. Hildegard circa 1141)

TEN COMMANDMENTS

Old Testament	*New Testament*
1. I am the Lord thy God; Thou shalt not have strange gods before me	1. You have come from God out of nothing, and to God you shall return with everything.
2. Thou shalt not take the name of the Lord thy God in vain.	2. Clean up your act.
3. Remember thou shalt keep holy the Sabbath Day	3. Stay in touch with God by weekly Mass and monthly Confession.
4. Honor thy father and thy mother.	4. Respect, honor, and listen to those who know more than you do.
5. Thou shalt not kill.	5. Living things are precious and violence is to be avoided.
6. Thou shalt not commit adultery.	6. Extramarital sex is nothing but trouble.
7. Thou shalt not steal.	7. You have a right to your own personal and private property; so does everybody else.
8. Thou shalt not bear false witness against thy neighbor.	8. Loving Truth will set and keep you free.
9. Thou shalt not covet thy neighbor's wife.	9. Keep your relationships holy, uplifting and honorable.
10. Thou shalt not covet thy neighbor's goods.	10. Keep "things" from running your life.

In physics, a *string* is a force which occupies a line in space at each moment of time. The Ten Commandments are strings between people.

PRAYER FOR OPTIMAL FAMILY

A family is a head* of a household, living with one or more related individuals, in a process of mutual growth, reciprocal commitment, shared responsibility, persistent desirability, and self-sacrificing performance on transcendental behalf of themselves, family, neighborhood, and community in the priorities of Life first, Liberty next, and then the peaceful Pursuit of Happiness.

(*May change from day to day, situationally dependent, from one member to another.)

INVOCATION

In the name of Life, Liberty, and Pursuit of Happiness
In the name of Yahweh — the Lord our God is one Lord,
In the name of I-Am-Who-Am,
In the name of Allah, the Beneficent, the Merciful,
In the name of the Trinity,
In the name of the Father, Son, and Holy Ghost,
In nomine Patris, et Filiei, et Spiritus Sancti,
In the name of God:
We even fight over what to call You.
We even fight over Your name.
Mea culpa, mea culpa, mea maxima culpa,
We are an obnoxious and feisty people, oh God, who can only prove our true love by having freedom to hate. And we have hated too much. Because of this hatred, we are not worthy. . . .
We do not deserve. . .
So with deep gratitude, We give thanks for:. . . .
But especially we give thanks for the opportunity to learn, experience, recognize, and promote Loving Truth moving between our eyes in relating in Thy name, bringing us to our true destiny, which is
You from Whom we came.

PEACE PRAYER

Peace is productive tranquility based on *Order* emanating from *Truth* established according to norms of empathic *Justice*, *Temperance*, *Fortitude* and *Prudence*, under the auspices of gentle *Liberty*, and sustained by life-loving, happiness-pursuing *Charity*.

Gentle Liberty

								} Justice
		Productive					Empathic	} Temperance
PEACE	=	Tranquility	=	Order	+	(Truth)		} Fortitude
								} Prudence

Life-Loving Happiness-Pursuing Charity

WHO CARES?

Let nothing disturb you.
Let nothing frighten you.
All things are passing;
GOD only is changeless.
Patience gains all things.
Who has GOD wants nothing.
GOD alone suffices.

(St. Theresa of Avila)

THE BEATITUDES

1. Blessed are the poor in spirit, for theirs is the kingdom of heaven.
2. Blessed are the meek, for they shall possess the land.
3. Blessed are they that mourn, for they shall be comforted.
4. Blessed are they that hunger and thirst after justice, for they shall be filled.
5. Blessed are the merciful, for they shall obtain mercy.
6. Blessed are the pure of heart, for they shall see God.
7. Blessed are the peacemakers, for they shall be called the children of God.
8. Blessed are they that suffer persecution for God's sake, for theirs is the kingdom of heaven.

(Baltimore Catechism)

SPIRITUAL WORKS OF MERCY

The spiritual works of mercy are seven: To admonish the sinner, to instruct the ignorant, to counsel the doubtful, to comfort the sorrowful, to bear wrongs patiently, to forgive all injuries, and to pray for the living and the dead.

(Baltimore Catechism)

CORPORAL WORKS OF MERCY

The corporal works of mercy are seven: To feed the hungry, to give drink to the thirsty, to clothe the naked, to rehabilitate prisoners, to shelter the homeless, to visit the sick, and to bury the dead.

(Baltimore Catechism)

PUBLIC PRAYER

It is the duty of all nations to acknowledge the providence of Almighty God, to obey His will, to be grateful for His benefits, and humbly to implore His protection and favor. . . . That great and glorious Being who is the beneficent author of all the good that was, that is, or that ever will be, that we may then unite in rendering unto Him our sincere and humble thanks for His kind care and protection of the people.

President George Washington's proclamation designating a national day of prayer and thanksgiving (the origin of our current legal holiday) as requested by the House of Representatives the day after the First Amendment was adopted on September 24, 1789

THE ROSARY

The Mysteries Of The Rosary	*Old Testament Link*	*Stage of Development*
Joyful Mysteries—Monday and Thursday		
1. The Annunciation (Humility)	Exodus 3:1-4	In utero conception
2. The Visitation (Charity)	II Samuel 6:9-11	In utero development
3. The Nativity (Poverty)	Isaiah 7:12-14	Birth
4. The Presentation (Obedience)	I Samuel 1:24-28	Baptism
5. The Finding in the Temple (Piety)	Daniel 13:45-68	Adolescence
Sorrowful Mysteries—Tuesday and Friday		
1. Agony in the Garden (Contrition)	Genesis 3:23-24	Penance
2. Scourging at the Pillar (Purity)	Jeremiah 37:13-20	Holy Eucharist
3. Crowning with Thorns (Courage)	IV Kings 24:12-13	Mental work
4. Carrying of the Cross (Patience)	Genesis 22:6-9	Physical work
5. The Crucifixion (Self-Denial)	Exodus 12:1-6	Confirmation
Glorious Mysteries—Sunday, Wednesday, Saturday		
1. The Resurrection (Faith)	Genesis 37	Extreme Unction
2. The Ascension (Hope)	IV Kings 2	Sudden death in grace - Holy Orders
3. Descent of the Holy Spirit (Love)	Exodus 19, 20:1-17	Matrimony
4. The Assumption (Eternal Happiness)	Psalms 131:8	Transition through purgatory
5. Crowning of Mary (Devotion to Mary)	III Kings 2:19	One's own crown of glory

HOW TO SAY THE ROSARY

1 Apostle Creed
1 Our Father
10 Hail Marys
1 Glory Be

The first Mysteries of the Rosary:

In glory, the Resurrection—Yes, we shall rise from the dead.
In joy, the Annunciation—This young woman embraces Life joyfully.
In sorrow, the Agony in the Garden—Reflecting on one's impending death.
Oh Mary and Joseph, intercede to God for us as we reflect on these first mysteries—that we may accept our pending fears, as Mary joyfully accepted a bewildering Life event, that we too may rise to meet God.

1 Our Father
10 Hail Mary
1 Glory Be

The second Mysteries of the Rosary:

In glory, the Ascension of our Lord into heaven—Jesus opened the gates for us, blazed a trail for us, and left tracks for us to follow.
In joy, the Visitation—Not one, but two pregnant women, one very young and one very old, both accepting joyfully their mission from God.
In sorrow, the Scourging at the Pillar.

Oh Mary and Joseph, intercede to God for us as we reflect on these second mysteries—that we may accept life's scourgings, beatings, and physical stresses, as Mary and Elizabeth joyfully accepted and promoted the will of Life, and enable us to follow the trail that Jesus left.

1 Our Father
10 Hail Marys
1 Glory Be

The third Mysteries of the Rosary:

In glory, the Coming of the Holy Spirit—Who speaks to us so that everyone understands in their own language.

In joy, the Birth of our Lord—The birth of true freedom as God becomes human.

In sorrow, the Crowning of Thorns.

Oh Mary and Joseph, intercede to God for us as we reflect on these third mysteries—that we can accept thornlike disappointments and mental anguishes, in the positive spirit of genuine freedom when we live by the universal language of Christ's love which as Pentecost everyone understands.

1 Our Father
10 Hail Marys
1 Glory Be

The fourth Mysteries of the Rosary:

In glory, the Assumption of Mary into heaven—As she follows her Son and leaves another trail for us to follow.

In joy, the Presentation of our Lord at the Temple—

In sorrow, the Carrying of the Cross.

Oh Mary and Joseph, intercede to God for us as we reflect on these fourth mysteries—that we may accept the crosses given to us to carry, by offering all to "the temple" as at our Baptisms, our confessions, our Communions, our Confirmations, and at our vows of marriage and religious life,that we may follow the trails of Mary and Joseph and Jesus, leading us to our heavenly reward.

1 Our Father
10 Hail Marys
1 Glory Be

The fifth Mysteries of the Rosary:

In glory, the Coronation of Mary as Queen of Heaven—And mothers are special,so why not?

In joy, the Finding of our Lord—Who was never lost, but Mary and Joseph lost Him —just as we repeatedly lose Him but take joy in finding Him every time as with the joy of a parent who has found their lost child.

In sorrow, the Crucifixion and Death of Our Lord.

Oh Mary and Joseph, intercede to God for us, as we reflect on these fifth mysteries—that we may understand and live our lives knowing that our own death is a state of transition to the Infinite Eternity if we have found Jesus, enabling us to wear our own crown of glory.

1 Our Father
10 Hail Marys
1 Glory Be
1 Hail Holy Queen
1 St. Michael's Prayer
1 Memorare

SOURCES OF SIN

The chief sources of sin are seven: pride, covetousness, lust, anger, gluttony, envy, and sloth.

(Baltimore Catechism)

GIFTS OF THE HOLY SPIRIT

The gifts of the Holy Ghost are Wisdom, Understanding, Counsel, Fortitude, Knowledge, Piety, and Fear of the Lord.

(Baltimore Catechism)

WHERE ARE YOU?

Too late I loved Thee, oh Thou Beauty of ancient days, yet ever new! Too late I loved Thee! And behold, Thou wert within, and I outside, and outside I searched for Thee; deformed I, plunging amid those fair forms which Thou hast made. Thou wert with me, but I was not with Thee. Things held me far from Thee, which, unless they were in Thee, were not at all. Thou calledst, and shoutedst, and burstest my deafness. . . .Thou touchedst me, and I burned for Thy peace.

(Saint Augustine)

DYING WHEN YOU ARE INNOCENT

I shall now speak of myself, of the reasons for my repentance. . . .For when you ask yourself: "If you must die, what are you dying for?" An absolutely black vacuity suddenly rises before you with startling vividness. There was nothing to die for if one wanted to die unrepentant. . . .This, in the end, disarmed me completely and led me to bend my knees before the Party and the country. And when you ask yourself: "Very well, suppose you do not die; suppose by some miracle you remain alive?" . . .again for what? Isolated from everybody, an enemy of the people, in an inhuman position, completely isolated from everything that constitutes the essence of life. And at once the same reply arises. At such moments, Citizen Judges, everything personal, all personal incrustation, all rancor, pride and a number of other things, fall away, disappear. . . .I am about to finish. I am perhaps speaking for the last time in my life.

The innocent Bukharin's last words to the Soviet Court which condemned him to death—for his uncommitted crime to which he pleaded guilty

DIVORCE PRAYER

Oh, God, marriage is so uncertain it is an uncertainty. Only You know if it was a real marriage. We passionately meant well. We promised sincerely. We suffered it through until we realized it was not so. If we sundered what You made, forgive us; but if we broke free from what we made, thank You. And may we be more in tune with You, oh, God, in all future relationships.

(Prayer for/by the divorced)

SERENITY PRAYER

God, grant me the serenity to accept the things I cannot change, the courage to change the things that I can, and the wisdom to know the difference.

GUARDIAN ANGEL PRAYER

Angel of God, my Guardian dear, to whom God's love commits me here, ever this day be at my side, to light and guard, to rule and guide.

GENUFLECTION PRAYER

We adore Thee, Oh God, and we bless Thee because by thy Holy Cross, Thou hast redeemed the world."

ABORTION PRAYER

Oh my God, seeking relief, millions of men and women have allowed their children to die by abortion. And you, God, allowed your Son, Jesus, to die by crucifixion—a horrible death for our salvation. With compassion, may You see those persons aborted and their parents in similarity of sacrifice rather than as the persecuted and the persecutors. May all involved in abortion come to know and love Life and to savor all moments of Beingness. May healing and forgiveness occur. May the real problems creating the alleged need for any abortion be solved. May Grace empower all that God's will be done.

PRAYER TO ST. DYMPHNA FOR THE MENTALLY AFFLICTED

O GOD, we humbly beseech Thee through Thy servant, St. Dymphna, who sealed with her blood the love she bore Thee, to grant relief to those who suffer from mental afflictions and nervous disorders, especially N. . . .
St. Dymphna, helper of the mentally afflicted, pray for us!

Glory be to the Father (3 times)

ACT OF FAITH

O my God, I firmly believe that You are one God in three divine Persons, Father, Son, and Holy Spirit. I believe that Your divine Son became man, died for our sins, and that He will come to judge the living and the dead. I believe these and all the truths which the holy Catholic Church teaches, because You have revealed them Who can neither deceive nor be deceived.

ACT OF HOPE

O my God, relying on Your almighty power and infinite mercy and promises, I hope to obtain pardon of my sins, the help of Your grace, and life everlasting through the merits of Jesus Christ, my Lord and Redeemer.

ACT OF LOVE

O my God, I love You above all things, with my whole heart and soul, because You are all-good and worthy of all love. I love my neighbor as myself for the love of You. I forgive all who have injured me, and ask pardon of all whom I have injured. Amen.

ANIMA CHRISTI

Soul of Christ sanctify me;
Body of Christ save me;
Blood of Christ inebriate me;
Water from the side of Christ wash me;
Passion of Christ strengthen me;
O good Jesus hear me;
Within Your wounds hide me;
Never let me be separated from You;
From the evil one protect me;
At the hour of my death call me,
And bid me come to You
That with your saints
I may praise You forever. Amen.

PRAYER OF ST. FRANCIS OF ASSISI

Lord, make me an instrument of Your peace.
Where there is hatred, let me sow love;
Where there is heresy, let me sow truth.**(G.K. Chesterton insert)**
Where there is discord, let me sow harmony.**(G.K. Chesterton insert)**
Where there is injury, pardon;
Where there is doubt, faith;
Where there is despair, hope;
Where there is darkness, light;
And where there is sadness, joy.
O Divine Master, grant that I may not so much
seek to be consoled as to console; to be
understood as to understand; to be loved as to love.
For it is in giving that we receive, it is in
pardoning that we are pardoned, and it is in dying
that we are born to eternal life.

SORROW

At last, at even, to my hearth I hark,
  Still faithful to my sorrow. And inside
  Even I and all my old magnanimous pride
Are broken down before her in the dark.

Sorrow's bare arm about my neck doth strain.
  Sorrow doth lift me to her living mouth
  And whispers, fierce and loving like the South.
Saying, "Dear Pilgrim, have you come again?

"Whether you walked by wastes of upland green.
  Whether you walked by wastes of ocean blue.
  Have you not felt me step by step with you.
A thing that was both certain and unseen?

"Or haply is it ended? haply you.
  Conquering and wholly cured of loving me.
  Are but a wavering lover who would be
Off with the old love ere he take the new?"

But, seeing my head did but in silence sink
  Before her ruthless irony and strong.
She gave me then that dreadful kiss to drink
  That is the bitter spring of art and song.

Then with strange gentleness she said. "I choose
  To be thine only, thine in all ways: yes.
Thy daughter and thy sister and thy muse.
  Thy wife and thine immortal ancestress.

"Feed not thy hate against my rule and rod.
  For I am very clean, my son, and sane.
Because I bring all brave hearts back to God.
  In my embraces being born again."

Thus spoke she low and rocked me like a child.
  And as I stared at her, as stunned awhile.
On her stern face there fell more slow and mild
  The splendour of a supernatural smile.

by Charles Guerin
(Translated by G.K. Chesterton)

PRAYER TO ST. JOSEPH

Oh, St. Joseph, whose protection is so great, so strong, so prompt before the throne of God, I place in you all my interest and desires. Oh, St. Joseph, do assist me by your powerful intercession, and obtain for me from your divine Son all spiritual blessings, through Jesus Christ, our Lord. So that, having engaged here below your heavenly power, I may offer my thanksgiving and homage to the most loving of Fathers. Oh, St. Joseph, I never weary contemplating you, and Jesus asleep in your arms; I dare not approach while He reposes near your heart. Press Him in my name and kiss His fine head for me and ask Him to return the Kiss when I draw my dying breath. St. Joseph, Patron of departing souls—Pray for me.

PRAYER TO THE HOLY SPIRIT

Come, Holy Spirit,
fill my heart with Your holy gifts.

Let my weakness be penetrated with Your strength this very day that I may fulfill all the duties of my state conscientiously, that I may do what is right and just.

Let my charity be such as to offend no one, and hurt no one's feelings; so generous as to pardon sincerely any wrong done to me.

Assist me, O Holy Spirit,
in all my trials of life, enlighten me in my ignorance, advise me in my doubts, strengthen me in my weakness, help me in all my needs, protect me in temptations and console me in afflictions.

Graciously hear me, O Holy Spirit,
and pour Your light into my heart, my soul, and my mind.

Assist me to live a holy life and to grow in goodness and grace. Amen.

PRAYER TO SAINT JOSEPH

O Blessed Saint Joseph, faithful guardian and protector of virgins, to whom God entrusted Jesus and Mary, I implore you by the love which you did bear them, to preserve me from every defilement of soul and body, that I may always serve them in holiness and purity of love. Amen.

ALL THAT I AM

All that I am, all that I do,
All that I'll ever have, I offer now to you.
Take and sanctify these gifts for your honor, Lord.
Knowing that I love and serve you is enough reward.
All that I am, all that I do,
All that I'll ever have I offer now to you.

All that I dream, all that I pray,
All that I'll ever make, I give to you today.
Take and sanctify these gifts for your honor, Lord.
Knowing that I love and serve you is enough reward.
All that I dream, all that I pray,
All that I'll ever make, I give to you today.

Sebastian Temple

PRAYER TO CHRIST THE KING

Christ Jesus, I acknowledge You King of the universe. All that has been created has been made for You. Make full use of Your rights over me.

I renew the promises I made in Baptism, when I renounced Satan and all his pomps and works, and I promise to live a good Christian life and to do all in my power to procure the triumph of the rights of God and Your Church.

Divine Heart of Jesus, I offer you my efforts in order to obtain that all hearts may acknowledge your Sacred Royalty, and that thus the Kingdom of Your peace may be established throughout the universe. Amen.

PRAYER OF REPARATION

Eternal Father, I offer Thee the Sacred Heart of Jesus, with all Its love, all Its sufferings and all Its merits;

To expiate all the sins I have committed this day, and during all my life.

Glory be to the Father, etc.

To purify the good I have done in my poor way this day, and during all my life.

Glory be to the Father, etc.

To make up for the good I ought to have done and that I have neglected this day and during all my life.

Glory be to the Father, etc.

DAILY PRAYER TO THE SACRED HEART

Sacred Heart of Jesus today I wish to live in You, in Your grace, in which I desire at all costs to persevere.

Keep me from sin and strengthn my will by helping me to keep watch over my senses, my imagination, and my heart.

Help me to correct my faults which are the source of sin.

I beg You to do this, O Jesus, through Mary, Your Immaculate Mother.

IGNATIUS PRAYER

Dearest Lord, teach me to be generous; teach me to serve You as You deserve: to give and not to count the cost, to fight and not to heed the wounds, to toil and not to seek for rest, to labor and not to ask for reward save that of knowing I am doing Your will.

St. Ignatius Loyola

PRAYER FOR THE HELPLESS UNBORN

Heavenly Father, You create men in Your own image, and You desire that not even the least among us should perish. In Your love for us, You entrusted Your only Son to the holy Virgin Mary. Now, in Your love, protect against the wickedness of the devil, those little ones to whom You have given the gift of life.

PRAYER TO THE HOLY TRINITY

Glory be to the Father,

Who by His almighty power and love created me, making me in the image and likeness of God.

Glory be to the Son,

Who by His Precious Blood delivered me from hell, and opened for me the gates of heaven.

Glory be to the Holy Spirit,

Who has sanctified me in the sacrament of Baptism, and continues to sanctify me by the graces I receive daily from His bounty.

Glory be to the Three adorable Persons of the Holy Trinity, now and forever. Amen.

PRAYER FOR FAITH

Lord, I believe: I wish to believe in Thee.
Lord, let my faith be full and unreserved, and let it penetrate my thought, my way of judging Divine things and human things.
Lord, let my faith be joyful and give peace and gladness to my spirit, and dispose it for prayer with God and conversation with men, so that the inner bliss of its fortunate possession may shine forth in sacred and secular conversation.
Lord, let my faith be humble and not presume to be based on the experience of my thought and of my feeling; but let it surrender to the testimony of the Holy Spirit, and not have any better guarantee than in docility to Tradition and to the authority of the *magisterium* of Holy Church. Amen.

Pope Paul VI

CHRISTIANITY

In the home it is kindness;
In the business it is honesty;
In society it is courtesy;
In work it is fairness;
Toward the unfortunate it is sympathy;
Toward the weak it is help;
Toward the wicked it is resistance;
Toward the strong it is trust;
Toward the penitent it is forgiveness;
Toward the successful it is congratulation;
And toward God it is reverence and obedience.

MARY STEWART'S PRAYER

Keep us, O God, from all pettiness.
Let us be large in thought, in word, in deed.
Let us be done with fault-finding and leave off all self-seeking.
May we put away all pretense and meet each other face to face, without self-pity and without prejudice.
May we never be hasty in judgment, and always be generous.
Let us always take time for all things, and make us to grow calm, serene and gentle.

Teach us to put into action our better impulses,
to be straightforward and unafraid.
Grant that we may realize that it is the little
things of life that create differences, that in
the big things of life, we are as one.
And, O Lord God, let us not forget to be
kind! Amen.

PRAYER FOR A FAMILY

O dear Jesus,
I humbly implore You to grant Your special
graces to our family. May our home be the
shrine of peace, purity, love, labor and faith.
I beg You, dear Jesus, to protect and bless
all of us, absent and present, living and dead.
O Mary,
loving Mother of Jesus, and our Mother,
pray to Jesus for our family, for all the families
of the world, to guard the cradle of the
newborn, the schools of the young and their vocations.
Blessed Saint Joseph,
holy guardian of Jesus and Mary, assist us
by your prayers in all the necessities of life.
Ask of Jesus that special grace which He
granted to you, to watch over our home at
the pillow of the sick and the dying, so that
with Mary and with you, heaven may find
our family unbroken in the Sacred Heart of
Jesus. Amen.

SELF-DEDICATION

(Crossing Forehead): Oh Holy Spirit, Energy of Pursuit of Happiness by relationship, let me interiorize for Thee, Oh God. Infuse into me the moral, intellectual, and theological virtues upon which I may base all my relationships. Let my mental functioning be quick and true, my interactions pleasant, and my research uncover Thy glory.

(Crossing Lips): Oh Jesus, Energy of Liberty, let me exteriorize for Thee, Oh God. Let my freedom imitate You, and may all see Thee in me by my words, actions, and works. Imitating Liberty is difficult: Because Your Presence in me means rejection by others, personal entropy, and perhaps never seeing success. In fact, if I imitate You, I shall mainly feel suffering and see entropy. Regardless, Thy will be done, and I will gladly accept whatever happiness I receive, because true happiness is in knowing that entropy has value through You and the Freedom which You are.

(Crossing Heart): Oh Father, Energy of Life, keep me physically and mentally healthy, Oh God. May my meager energy play a meaningful role in organizing the energy of the earth to greater spirituality and higher synthesis, thereby bringing all to You from whence all came.

Thus by means of my commitment to You, the ultimate Triune Personification(s) of Life (The Father), Liberty (The Son), and Pursuit of Happiness (The Holy Spirit), may the evolutionary continuum on this planet achieve the Absolute Statimuum in which all pervades all, eternal, infinite, from beginning to end, forever in one never ending moment.

12-STEP PRAYER FOR ADDICTION CONTROL

1. We admitted we were powerless over—(alcohol)—that our lives had become unmanageable.
2. Came to believe that a Power greater than ourselves could restore us to sanity.
3. Made a decision to turn our will and our lives over to the care of God as we understood Him.
4. Made a searching and fearless moral inventory of ourselves.
5. Admitted to God, to ourselves, and to another human being the exact nature of our wrongs.
6. Were entirely ready to have God remove all these defects of character.
7. Humbly asked Him to remove our shortcomings.
8. Made a list of all persons we have harmed, and became willing to make amends to them all.
9. Made direct amends to such people wherever possible, except when to do so would injure them or others.
10. Continued to take personal inventory and when we were wrong promptly admitted it.
11. Sought through prayer and meditation to improve our conscious contact with God as we understood Him, praying only for knowledge of His will for us and the power to carry that out.
12. Having had a spiritual awakening as the result of these Steps, we tried to carry this message to others, and to practice these principles in all our affairs.

(Modification of the 12-Steps of Alcoholics Anonymous)

Make Me a Channel of Your Peace

Make me a channel of your peace.
Where there is hatred, let me bring your love.
Where there is injury, your pardon, Lord.
And where there's doubt, true faith in you.
Make me a channel of your peace.
Where there's despair in life,
let me bring hope.
Where there is darkness only light,
and where there's sadness ever joy.
Oh, Master, grant that I may never seek
so much to be consoled as to console,
to be understood as to understand,
to be loved, as to love, with all my soul.
Make me a channel of your peace.
It is in pardoning that we are pardoned,
in giving to all men that we receive,
and in dying that we're born to eternal life.

Sebastian Temple

A SCIENTIST'S NICENE PROFESSION OF FAITH

I believe in one ultimate Triune Personification(s) of
Life, Liberty, and the Pursuit of Happiness,
the Father, the Almighty, the Personification of Life;
the being and maker of heaven and earth,
of all that is seen and unseen.

I believe in one Lord, Jesus Christ, the Personification of Liberty
the unique Freedom of the Triune
the eternal spontaneous part of life,
ultimate Freedom from ultimate Energy, Spontaneity from ascendancy,
an intrinsic identity with Life,
one in being with the Father.
Through him all things were made
through free spontaneous Liberty in the organizing continuum of Life.
For our human energy and for our future synthesis
He came from the ultimate synthesis;
by the power of the Pursuit of Happiness by relationship
the Personification of Liberty was born of the Virgin Mary,
as all genuine liberty is born without entropic sexuality,
and Liberty became human.

For our sake, however, Liberty was crucified under Pontius Pilate,
as all liberty is stifled by intractable authority, entropized by
anti-life actions, or devitalized by neutral non-commitment.
Liberty suffered, died, and disappeared from visible reality,

But, in no time at all, Liberty rose again, as He shall always
rise again as described in prophetic Writings;
He ascended to the highest synthesis and rejoined Life.
He will come again in glory to embrace all creatures,
A Liberating synthesis which will have no end.

I believe in the Holy Spirit, the Personification of the Pursuit
of Happiness by conscious relationship and by aware interaction,
the Lord, the giver and personalizer of Life.
the unique Interational Pattern of the Triune,
who proceeds from paternal Life and filial Liberty.
With the Father and the Son he is worshipped and glorified.
He has spoken through the prophets by their Words which describe
happiness-pursuing relationships.

I believe in one holy Catholic and apostolic church—the Phylum of
Life, Liberty, and the Pursuit of Happiness.
I acknowledge one baptism which establishes my relationship with the
Triune, by which entropy may be converted to higher synthesis.
I look for the transformation of human entropy,
and the Infinite Embracing into the Absolute Statimuum awaiting us.
Amen.

HYMN OF JOY

Joyful, joyful, we adore you, God of glory, Lord of love;
Hearts unfold like flowers before you, Opening to the sun above.
Melt the clouds of sin and sadness; Drive the dark of doubt away;
Giver of immortal gladness, Fill us with the light of day!

All your works with joy surround you, Earth and heav'n reflect your rays,
Stars and angels sing around you, Center of unbroken praise;
Field and forest, vale and mountain, Flowery meadow, flashing sea,
Chanting bird and flowing fountain, Praising you eternally!

Always giving and forgiving, Ever blessing, ever blest,
Well spring of the joy of living, Ocean depth of happy rest!
Loving Father, Christ our brother, Let your light upon us shine;
Teach us how to love each other, Lift us to the joy divine.

Mortals join the mighty chorus, Which the morning stars began;
God's own love is reigning o'er us, Joining people hand in hand.
Ever singing, march we onward, Victors in the midst of strife;
Joyful music leads us sunward In the triumph song of life.

Words to Beethoven's Ninth Symphony by Henry van Dyke
(a chance to *feel* the Incarnation)

If you recite these prayers, you will be able to sustain Faith, promote Loving Truth, and claim your Destiny. Prayer is nourishment. Prayer makes your brain chemistry work better. Prayer puts you with God.

CHAPTER 12:

GIFTS OF THE HOLY SPIRIT, VIRTUES AND SIN

Virtues are offense (power) mechanisms. That is, they are not negations or protective measures of what is going on in a person, but they are efforts of seeking Loving Truth. Virtues are active rather than passive. They are habits — a habit is an acquired or infused quality or disposition which influences a person's actions. Good habits (virtues) are necessary for successful and mentally healthy living.

(Most of these definitions are derived from
The Catholic Encyclopedia by Robert C. Broderick
published by Our Sunday Visitor, Inc., Huntington, Indiana.)

Gifts of the Holy Spirit

"And the Spirit of the Lord shall rest upon Him: the spirit of wisdom and understanding, the spirit of counsel and fortitude, the spirit of knowledge and piety, and the spirit of the fear of the Lord."

Isaiah 11:2,3 (as quoted by St. Bernard)

Before describing the virtues, the seven gifts of the Holy Spirit should be defined. These are considered superior to the intellectual and moral virtues because they help people be influenced by the Holy Spirit. They are habits that can be cultivated to respond to the inspiration of the Holy Spirit. The gifts perfect the exercise of the virtues. They create the means of satisfaction to virtue. They are known as:

1. Wisdom — Truths profounder and beyond the effect of thought. (Sound judgment)
2. Understanding — To discern and grasp more clearly the mysteries of faith. (Comprehending and reasoning)
3. Counsel — Deliberated directing towards good and cautioning against evil. The evangelical counsels are the voluntary obligations of poverty, chastity, and obedience (with these three firmly espoused, genuine trustability occurs). (Trustworthiness)
4. Fortitude — Impulse, will, and joy of acting rightly in face of adversity. (Courage)

5. Knowledge — Familiarizing with the nature, value and utility of created things. (In-depth familiarity)
6. Piety — Applies charity as a loving duty. (Fidelity to duty)
7. Fear of (offending) the Lord — All genuine wisdom begins here. (Consequential Reverence) There are two forms:
   a. Servile fear — mental anxiety and emotions arising from knowledge of God's potential inflicting of punishment.

   b. Filial fear — Dread of offending an all-good God and dread of being separated from God's great Being.

An example will be offered as to how the gifts of the Holy Spirit can be used in practice, i.e. to reflect and apply the seven gifts to any given issue. This is the practice of the seven gifts applying them to you and to any anticipated activity.

While the gifts are *not* an ethical system, they function as "informers of conscience." The end-result will be the influence of the Holy Spirit upon one's actions, whatever they may be. The end-result will be beyond ethical systems but legitimately take into consideration the agent and person performing the act, the activity itself in terms of duty, and the utilitarian consequential results.

Ethical systems are man-made, philosophical predispositions that provide analysis and dialogue but no answers satisfactory to all. In contrast, the gifts of the Holy Spirit are ancient secrets about which the end-results will be acceptable in terms of the ethical analysis to be done; in terms of the freedom and liberty of the individual to respond to life; and in terms of one's image and likeness of God projected to others of similar physiognomy.

Example:

A psychotic patient with AIDS has an aggressive, self-destructive, threatening delusional system which compels him to bang his head, attempt to bite, injure, spit and bleed on others. With great consternation, agitation and fears, he has been brought to the psychiatric unit and is in a secluded room. Two previous physicians have been informed of the nature of his disorder and they have declined to take him as a patient. Similarly, the nurses and aides are also threatened and are very hesitant to get too involved.

Having been so informed and requested to be the attending psychiatrist, the decision is now mine: Will I take this patient? On what grounds can I refuse? On what grounds must I take this patient?

Using the gifts of the Holy Spirit:

1. Wisdom. This is search for the truth beyond the effect of thought. To care for this patient is dangerous and risky. AIDS is an incurable, contagious disease. The patient is delusional and cannot be dealt with. Wisdom is *not* to take the patient.

2. Understanding. "Understanding" is not simple understanding of what is going on. Understanding as a gift of the Holy Spirit is to grasp clearly the mysteries of faith and to comprehend and to reason about one's faith as it applies to the task at hand, as it applies to the impact of this on me, on my duty as a physician, and on the benefits that I can provide this patient. My religious beliefs, my faith gives an understanding that I must take this patient and provide care.

3. Counsel. The core of counsel is *trustworthiness*. In practice, it is advising to do good and avoid evil. In these senses, my trustworthiness in the human relationship in which I have been thrust means that I should positively accept this patient.

Furthermore, the evangelical counsels apply here also. They are poverty, chastity, and obedience. They truly comprise the basis of genuine trustability of anybody, if the evangelical counsels are genuinely held and embraced. These elementary obligations do apply voluntarily in human relationships. I may be impoverished to some extent; chastity is a given; and obedience to "doing what one has to do." All three provide my trustworthiness as congruent with the gift of Counsel. In the final analysis, this gift says to take the patient.

4. Fortitude. Adversity looms large and courage is called for. This one is simple. Perhaps Fortitude is always a "yes."

5. Knowledge. Knowledge means familiarizing myself in depth with what actions are needed. Familiarization reveals many safeguards are possible such as gloves, gowns, medications, transparent coverings and restraints. Knowledge shows the way to minimize risks and maximize treatment. Knowledge of what can be done specifically offers another positive to the question.

6. Piety. Piety has a mundane connotation but the denotation is very deep. Piety impels a charitable fidelity to duty. Thus charity as a loving duty demands I take him as a patient. And fidelity to my duty as a physician demands I take him as a patient also.

7. Fear of the Lord. In reverence I consider the consequences which takes me right back to the first gift of the Holy Spirit, Wisdom, because all genuine Wisdom is said to originate from Fear of the Lord. So, if my patient is in the image of my Lord and I am in the image of my Lord, then I cannot refuse this task for both forms of Fear of the Lord.

With servile fear, I must realize there is a penalty, perhaps a punishment, for not responding to my neighbor's needs.

In filial fear, I lose my own beingness because I am separating myself from God's beingness which He has offered to me.

Thus, the final score is 6 to 1 — six "yes" and one "no." I will take care of this patient. Ethicists can come to their conclusions while I do what I can as a Christian Catholic physician.

The reader might puzzle over the application of the gifts to these problems:

— fetal tissue transplantation techniques,
— in vitro fertilization,
— discontinuing fluid and hydration, and
— abortion.

These seven gifts of the Holy Spirit are predispositions that lead to grace and the insertion of the person into the Body of Christ by follow-through to activities known as virtues.

Virtues

Virtues are active habits which lead to salutary actions. All virtues can be seen to overlap and interrelate. Some of those listed are very old and traditional. Others are proposed (beautification, community, deliberation, materialization, unification, validation and verification) as contemporary habits appropriate to contemporary standards and for transcendental focusing. St. Augustine said it best: "The person who possesses one virtue, possesses them all, and the one who lacks a single virtue, lacks them all." Virtues are interrelated and encompass the panopoly of salutary human behavior. Virtues feed off of one another and lead into one another. Sometimes the distinctions are difficult to make. Whatever it is, if it is salutary and you do it habitually, it can be a virtue however named.

To respiritualize society and the universe, words are needed which "do the will of God" so to speak. Words must be available which gain and direct the attitudes of people more often if not routinely to the "habit of being," i.e. to a transcendental understanding and reinforcement in all aspects of life. In the ultimate sense, all the virtues do exactly this.

1. Beautification — the transcendental virtue of arranging attributes in a manner seeking beauty (*bella*) which pleases one's senses and uplifts the spirit. (Uplifting)
2. Charity — the supernatural and theological virtue of Love of God above all. Charity as love of God is the greatest virtue. It also includes love of neighbor and self with Christ-like conduct. (Christ-like)
3. Chastity — the virtue which checks, controls, modulates, or excludes desire and pleasure of sexual intercourse specifically and of carnal or sexual thoughts or actions in general. It effectively means fidelity if married, virginity if not. (Sexual fidelity)
4. Community — the virtue of individual and collective strivings for salvation by environmental concern, gentle freedom, family support, common interests, and bonding of faith and love. (Neighborliness)
5. Constancy — the virtue of perseverance and fidelity in struggles and sufferings of life. (Persistence)
6. Continence — the virtue derived from charity which preserves the mind from impurity and restrains the will from actions following aroused sexual desire, by voluntary abstinence either partial as in mar-

riage or absolute as in unmarried. (Discrimination)

7. Deliberation — the transcendental virtue of committing one's self to good (*bonum*) in all activities by pursuing the proper end of all things conforming will and being. (Proper Choice)
8. Detachment — the virtue of balanced proportion of attitude about the natural goods of the world. It is an exercise towards perfection from the three theological virtues (faith, hope, and charity) and the three counsels (poverty, chastity, and obedience). (A spiritual separation from the world, i.e., the act of transcending)
9. Faith — the supernatural and theological virtue of adhering by intellect to truths from God because of God's authority rather than needing evidence. (Accepting witness)
10. Fortitude — one of the four cardinal virtues — the virtue of strength of soul to practice all the virtues in pursuit of the good and love of God; unyielding courage in the endurance of pain or adversity. It is the conforming of the irascible appetite (the "difficult good") to reason. (Moral strength)
11. Hope — the supernatural and theological virtue in which the will trusts for eternal happiness in and through God. (Positive and confident expectation)
12. Humility — the virtue of true and just self-estimation whereby excessive self-love, self-will, and self-interest are relinquished. It is the opposite of pride. (Accurate self-awareness)
13. Joy — the virtue of pleasure, delight, and satisfaction. It is related to charity. (Savoring)
14. Justice — one of the four cardinal virtues — the virtue regarding law and duty wherein everyone is given his due because of his dignity. It is the conforming of the will to reason. It implies obedience, truthfulness, gratitude, and religion and is violated by all sin (Fair distribution)
15. Knowledge — the intellectual virtue exercised by the act of knowing through and by striving for information and understanding. It grasps the forms of other beings. (In-depth familiarity)
16. Liberality — the virtue of balanced attitude towards wealth and desires. It is the opposite of covetousness. (Generosity)
17. Longanimity — the virtue of long-suffering and forbearance; waiting with patience anticipating and considering the future good. (Composure under tension)
18. Magnanimity — the virtue of undertaking great things for God and neighbor from noble motivations. It is a combination and free practice of all the virtues. (Altruistic honor)
19. Materialization — the transcendental virtue of accepting and processing matter (*res*) met. (Active Engagement)
20. Meekness — the virtue wherein anger is controlled or moderated by "manly resignation" to adversity. It is related to temperance and it is the opposite of anger. It is not indifference or spinelessness. (Compassionate confrontation)

21. Mercy — the virtue of treating others with forgiving protection. Loving one's undeserving neighbor as oneself, provided you love yourself. (Compassionate aid)
22. Modesty — the virtue of moderation in external manner, dress, deportment, and conversation. It is related to temperance and is an index of positive restraint of thought and feelings. (Decency)
23. Obedience — the virtue which enables one to submit to the will or law of one in authority or representative of authority. (Honorable compliance)
24. Patience — the virtue which moderates inclination to sadness or rebellion. It is related to fortitude and is opposed by impatience and insensibility. (Imperturbability)
25. Penance — the virtue of coming to know and to recognize one's own sins. It turns one towards contrition. (Self-criticism)
26. Piety — the virtue of conscious, sense of duty and willingness to respond. (Fidelity to duty)
27. Prudence — one of the four cardinal virtues — the virtue of judging rightly about acts of virtue. It is the intellect being consistent with itself. It is practical reason and is violated by all sin. (Discerning discretion)
28. Religion — the virtue by which men give due worship and reverence to God and by which men recognize their origin from and future progress to God. (Awareness of a higher power)
29. Temperance — one of the four cardinal virtues — the virtue of moderation and self-control in action and thoughts; mastery over the instincts. It is conforming the concupiscible appetite (the "easy good") to reason. (Self-restraint or self-control facing desirables)
30. Unification — the transcendental virtue of maintaining oneness (*unum*) with all desirables of family, community, world and universe. (Unity)
31. Validation — the transcendental virtue which promotes the identity and essence of one's *aliquid* as an individual and as a member of the human species. (Complete Identity)
32. Verification — the transcendental virtue of committing one's self to truth (*verum*) in all activities by abstracting forms in conformity to being. (Accurate Abstraction)
33. Wisdom — the virtue of truth beyond the effect of thought. It is knowledge arriving at Natural Law. It is applied conscience. (Sound judgment)

PARTICIPATE IN BEING

Incarnating Act (Virtue)	*Transcendental*	*Sin Prevented*
Beautification - uplifting work	Beauty	Gluttony
Charity - Christ-like	Goodness	Hatred
Chastity - sexual fidelity to spouse	Dignity	Lust, Adultery
Community - Neighborliness (democratic cooperation)	Spirituality	Pollution
Constancy - persisting	Unity	Despair
Continence - discrimination	Integrity	Impurity
Deliberation - proper choice	Good	All sin
Detachment - transcending	Spirituality	Blasphemy
Faith - accepting witness	Truth	Ignorance
Fortitude - moral strength	Truth	Pusillanimity
Hope - confident expectation	Beauty	Despair
Humility - accurate self-awareness	Identity	Pride
Joy - savoring	Integrity	Hatred
Justice - fair distribution	Spirituality	Injustice
Knowledge - in depth familiarity	Dignity	Ignorance
Liberality - generosity	Identity	Covetousness
Longanimity - composure under tension	Spirituality	Contumely
Magnanimity - altruistic honor	Unity	Envy
Materialization - active engagement	Matter	Blasphemy
Meekness - compassionate confrontation	Dignity	Anger
Mercy - compassionate aid	Spirituality	Usury
Modesty - "class" (decency)	Dignity	Prostitution
Obedience - honorable compliance	Identity	Contumacy
Patience - time imperturbability	Unity	Rashness
Penance - self-criticism	Unity	Presumption
Piety - fidelity to duty	Integrity	Sloth
Prudence - discerning discretion	Identity	Imprudence
Religion - awareness of a higher power	Identity	Profanity
Temperance - self-control when facing desirables	Beauty	Gluttony
Unification - unity	Oneness	Pollution
Validation - complete identity	Identity	Ignorance
Verification - accurate abstraction	Truth	Pusillanimity
Wisdom - sound judgment	Integrity	Slander, calumny, detraction

HYLOMORPHIC FOCUSING* ON VIRTUE (OR EXAMINING YOUR LIFE)

a is the form of	b in the matter of	c
Beautification	Uplifting	Attributes
Charity	Christ-like	Living
Chastity	Sexual Fidelity	Marriage
Community	Neighborliness (Democratic Cooperation)	Environment
Constancy	Persistence	Activity
Continence	Discrimination	Sexuality
Detachment	Transcending	The World
Deliberation	Properness	Choice
Faith	Acceptance	Witness
Fortitude	Strength	Adversity
Hope	Confidence	The Future
Humility	Accuracy	Self-Awareness
Joy	Savoring	Everything
Justice	Fairness	Distribution
Knowledge	Familiarity	Information
Liberality	Generosity	Things
Longanimity	Composure	Tension
Magnanimity	Altruism	Honor
Materialization	Activeness	Engagement
Meekness	Compassion	Confrontation
Mercy	Compassion	Aid
Modesty	"Class" (Decency)	Appearance
Obedience	Honor	Compliance
Patience	Imperturbability	Time
Penance	Criticism	Self
Piety	Fidelity	Duty
Prudence	Discernment	Discretion
Religion	Awareness	God
Temperance	Control	Desirables
Unification	Oneness	The Universe
Validation	Completeness	Identity
Verification	Accuracy	Abstraction
Wisdom	Soundness	Judgment

* Done by anyone who claims to be good or correct in anything by knowing the "matter and form" ("hylomorphic") of anything.

Sins

No one wants to talk about sin because sin reminds of ancient truths and traditions people wish would go away. Sin is a concept making people stop and think of dire consequences to their being. This being so, no wonder it is attempted to be rejected. But rejection does not dissolve the reality of sin or the consequences. Most assuredly the ignoring of sin as real is an easy replacement for an awareness of one's immortality and that one's actions do have consequences. But to deny sin is like denying garbage. It will have to be dealt with at some time or another. The sin-garbage analogy is a good one, because sin is as much pollution for behavior as garbage is for the environment.

Sins are negations of self because they place one in an entropic (running down, wasteful, descending, non-productive) direction, instead of a direction which would be towards a synthesis and personal evolving into a higher state of being. Make no mistake about it, sins are moral components to relationship and existence. Sin (evil) occurs when virtue is willfully absent. If the transcendental and immanental forms are not in our intellects, we tend to suffer sinfully.

Sin by default destroys form in matter. (Most definitions are from the *Catholic Encyclopedia*)

1. Adultery — Sexual intercourse between a married person and another who is not his or her spouse. (Marital infidelity)
2. Anger — One of the seven capital sins. It is the inordinate inclination to take revenge. As an emotion, it is neutral. When out-of-control, anger is a sin. (Rage)
3. Blasphemy — Explicit words or actions dishonoring God or agent of God. (Verbal irreverence)
4. Calumny — The creation and uttering of false and harmful statements against another. It includes lying with injustice. (Planned slander)
5. Contumacy — Contempt of authority or rebellious stubbornness. (Unwarranted opposition)
6. Contumely — Ridiculing and insulting of others and causing others to lose their dignity by malicious damage to another's honor and character causing that person to suffer. (Scornful rudeness)
7. Covetousness — One of the seven capital sins. It is the inordinate unreasonable love of temporal and earthly things. (Avarice)
8. Despair — The deliberate willful distrust of God's goodness, fidelity, and power; or abandoning of all hope of salvation and the means necessary to obtain it. (Hopelessness)
9. Detraction — unnecessarily revealing true faults about others. (Harsh judging)
10. Envy — One of the seven capital sins, it is willful grieving or sadness because of another's spiritual or temporal good, looked upon as a per-

sonal disadvantage or the lessening of one's own goods. Wanting something of another for one's self unjustly. (Jealousy)

11. Gluttony — One of the seven capital sins, it is inordinate longing for or an indulgence in food, drink, or that which in excess diminishes reason. (Intemperance)
12. Hatred — Human emotion of the mind and will which is the negation of the proper appetite of the person. It is the direct opposite of charity. It is sinful when misdirected, excessive, or leads to direct action against another. (Malevolence)
13. Ignorance — Absence of knowledge when it could be present. (Mental Amorphy)
    a. Invincible — meaning the absent knowledge is uncorrectible and therefore responsibility is not incurred.
    b. Vincible — which is willful avoidance of knowledge or the refusal to accept the forms of things.
14. Impurity — Unnatural (non-gender, non-mating, or non-reproductive) indulgence in sexual pleasures. (Lewdness, uncleanness)
15. Lust — One of the seven capital sins — it is the inordinate desire for a satisfaction of appetite for sexual or carnal pleasure — opposed by chastity, continence and modesty. It is not for a natural purpose or it is an excessive exercising of the desires. (Degrading animality)
16. Pollution — Disrespect for God's creation and beingness. (Defilement)
17. Presumption — Trusting too much in one's own strength or expecting God to do that which He would not will to do. It is the opposite to hope. (Conceit)
18. Pride — One of the seven capital sins — inordinate desire for honor, recognition, and attraction — from self-love. (Selfishness, grandiosity)
19. Profanity — Disrespect of the name of God. (Desecration)
20. Prostitution — The use of one's body to sexually satisfy another in exchange for money or other payment. (Submission)
21. Pusillanimity — "Smallness of soul" — refraining from acting for others out of fear or failure or "not enough in it for me." (Cowardice)
22. Rashness — A rash judgment — the tendency to assent without sufficient reason or basis to the existence of a moral defect in another. (Inconsiderate haste)
23. Slander — The utterance, communication and attribution of falsehoods about another person. (Prevarication)
24. Sloth — One of the seven capital sins — voluntary laziness. (Indolence)
25. Usury — When a lender demands unjust or unlawful interest on a "loan" of value which deserves to be charity. (Greed)

WITHDRAWAL FROM BEING

DECARNATING ACTS (SINS)	*VIRTUE PRIMARILY VIOLATED*
Adultery — marital infidelity	Chastity
*Anger — rage	Meekness
Blasphemy — calculated irreverence, uncaring	Detachment, Materialization
Calumny — planned slander	Wisdom
Contumacy — unwarranted opposition	Obedience
Contumely — scornful rudeness	Longaminity
*Covetousness — avarice	Liberality
Despair — hopelessness	Constancy, Hope
Detraction — harsh judging	Wisdom
*Envy — jealousy	Magnanimity
*Gluttony — intemperance	Temperance, Beautification
Hatred — malevolence	Joy, Charity
Ignorance — mental amorphy (no form)	Knowledge, Faith, Validation
Impurity — lewdness, uncleanness	Continency
*Lust — degrading animality	Chastity
Pollution — defilement	Community, Unification
Presumption — conceit	Penance
*Pride — selfishness or grandiosity	Humility
Profanity — desecration	Religion
Prostitution — submission	Modesty
Pusillanimity — cowardice	Fortitude, Truth, Verification
Rashness — inconsiderate haste	Patience
Slander — prevarication	Wisdom
*Sloth — indolence	Piety
Usury — greed	Mercy

*Seven Capital Sins from which all others derive.

INCARNATING BEHAVIORS			DECARNATING BEHAVIORS		
Humanbeingness (Sacrament)	Major Virtue	Minor Virtue	Coinciding Major Sin	Decarnating Symptoms	Anti-Humanbeingness
Dignity (Baptism)	Faith (Accepting witness)	Chastity (Sexual Fidelity)	Lust, Adultery	Sexual Dyscontrol	Exploitation
		Knowledge (In depth Familiarity)	Ignorance	Accepting of Untruths	
		Meekness (Compassionate Confrontation)	Anger	Violence	
		Modesty ("Class" - Decency)	Prostitution	Moral Corruption	
		Verification (Accurate Abstraction)	Pusillanimity		
Unity (Penance)	Hope (Confidence)	Constancy (Persistence)	Despair	Depression	Fragmentation
		Magnanimity (Altruistic Honor)	Envy	Paranoia	
		Patience (Time Imperturbability)	Rashness	Impulse Dyscontrol	
		Penance (Self-Criticism)	Presumption	Arrogance, Conceit, Disrespect	
		Unification (Unity)	Pollution		
Integrity (Holy Communion)	Charity (Christ-like)	Continence (Sexual Self-Restraint)	Impurity	Obsessiveness, Perversions	Demoralization/ Disintegration
		Joy (Savoring)	Hatred	Destructiveness	
		Piety (Fidelity to Duty)	Sloth	Inadequacy,Inaccuracy,Daydreaming	
		Wisdom (Sound Judgment)	Slander,Calumny,Detraction	Superficiality, Prevarication	
Identity (Confirmation)	Prudence (Discerning Discretion)	Humility (Accurate Self-Awareness)	Pride	Selfishness, Grandiosity	Dehumanization
		Liberality (Generosity)	Covetousness	Stealing, Greed	
		Obedience (Honorable Compliance)	Contumacy	Learning Failure, Opposition	
		Religion (God Awareness)	Profanity	Impaired Vocabulary	
		Validation (Complete Identity)	Ignorance		
Spirituality (Extreme Unction)	Justice (Fairness)	Community (Good Neighboring Democratic Cooperation)	Pollution Imbalance	Environmental Disruption,	Despiritualization
		Detachment (Transcending)	Blasphemy	Uncaring, Usury	
		Longanimity (Composure under tension)	Contumely	Irascibility	
		Deliberation (Proper Choice)			
Life (Holy Orders)	Fortitude (Moral Strength)	Mercy (Compassionate Aid)	Pusillanimity	Whimpery, Cowardice,	Willful Death
		Materialization (Active Engagement)	Blasphemy	Killing of the Innocent	
Liberty (Matrimony)	Temperance (Self-Control)	Beautification (Uplifting Work)	Gluttony	Eating Disorder, Alcoholism, Substance Abuse, All Addictions, Including Perversions	Willful Sterility
Pursuit of Happiness	Holiness	All Virtue	All Sin Separates	Willful Entropy	Gnosticism (excesses

The principles of humanbeingness and their Sacramental representations (first column) are now dissected into subdivisions of activity conceptualized as incarnating behaviors, i.e., the major and minor virtues (second and third columns).

The left half of the chart describes the incarnating behaviors which are those wherein the human being puts on the Body of Christ. The right half of the chart describes the taking off of the Body of Christ by the major sins, the decarnating symptoms, and the principles of anti-humanbeingness all of which oppose the Sacraments and the principles of actual humanbeingness.

There are six columns to understand and each item in each column coincides horizontally with counterparts in the other columns. The major columns under the **INCARNATING BEHAVIORS** are humanbeingness, major virtues and minor virtues. The columns for the **DECARNATING BEHAVIORS** are the major sins, symptoms and the principles of anti-humanbeingness.

The extreme left column and extreme right column respectively demonstrate *humanbeingness* vs. *anti-humanbeingness*. Dignity is opposed to exploitation. Unity to fragmentation. Integrity to demoralization/disintegration. Identity opposed by dehumanization. Spirituality opposed by despiritualization. Life is opposed by willful death. Liberty is opposed by willful sterility. And the Pursuit of Happiness is opposed to Gnosticism or the excesses of feelings and fantasies.

The breakdown of the four inner columns can be arguably different, but as presented basically holds true. The reader is invited to study the permutations and come to their own conclusions about how the virtues and their lack are demonstrable in our lives. By them, you put on the Body of Christ whether you want to or not. Then there is a happy ending.

CHAPTER 13:

RAPPROACHEMENT: LATIN

"The Church uses the Latin language instead of the national language of its children:

1. To avoid the danger of changing any part of its teaching in using different languages;
2. That all its rulers may be perfectly united and understood in their communication;
3. To show that the Church is not an institute of any particular nation, but the guide of all nations. . . ."

(Baltimore Catechism)

Without a doubt, the collapse of religious vocations has temporarily coincided with the abandonment of Latin. This alone warrants the speculation that Latin did have a positive psychological impact on humanity and Church. Seven reasons are proposed:

(1) First, Latin is a discipline, meaning it gives rules and requires the following of rules. There is nothing unusual here, because this is common to all languages. However, Latin is linked to following the rules *of the Church's language*. Associated with this is a recognition that the Church is special and to be followed. Furthermore, the Latin reinforcement of *following the Church* is subtle, frequent, elementary and automatic (each of these qualities being a major psychological engineering feat enviable by motivators everywhere). Discipline towards right reason is praiseworthy. Comparable to this disciplinary dimension of Latin are Hebrew for Jews and Arabic text of the Koran for Muslims. The same logic for or against Latin must, in fairness at least, apply to these examples also.

(2) Second, Latin prompts mental habits of coherence and lucidity. Deeper thinking and precision in conceptualizing are the norms. There is not much room or time available for wishy-washy, feel-good, solipsistic, psychodramatic, emoting, entertaining technobabble. With Latin, the intellect supercedes feelings.

Anyone who pretends to be a scholar or to have "an answer" to any problem, is forced by Latin to think matters through, or at least to "stop and think a moment." Rooted in an intellectual tradition, it requires a focusing that demands stability and ascension. In such regards, it is a unifying and protective barrier permeable to good. And one can rely on its being such. It demands that you take the time *to think.*

(3) Third, Latin is an "elite" communication (language) link for those who are not really an "elite" because *anyone can join* if only they take the time and make the effort to grasp the language. In this "elite" communication, all languages become one, because Latin is the central axis of translation. Interestingly, Latin as a language is unique in that it has little ethnic or historically based animosities. Objections to Latin as "elite" communication (language) are based on resistance to change, laziness, or ignorance rather than threats to identity (as occurs, for example, when "anglo" words are used in France). Latin tends to be *neutral.*

This "elite" communication function is readily recognized to be important when contemporary New Age pseudospiritualities are studied. What is always found in a contemporary wacko religion is a new-language which requires translation and priest or priestess to do the translating. The beginning of these new-languages is not "I think. . ." but "I feel. . . ." Among current examples of pseudolanguage gibberish can be found: transpersonal, People for the Ethical Treatment of Animals, godself, mystical artist, feminist spirituality, Christic Institute, "born-again," creation spirit, level of joy, Great Apostasy, New Age, whole brain, awareness baseline, astrology, covens, Women's Ordination Conference, confluence, channeling, Greenpeace, cosmic dance, women church, "I've been saved," field of Universal C, visionary life secret, enneagrams, and a plethora of other nonscientific, nonrealistic catch-phrases which have the collective purpose of ensnaring the thoughtless ("Don't you FEEL like this too?") and tying them to someone masquerading as a priest. Whatever these listed phrases mean, they replaced Latin.

Like it or not, for some, Latin filled a communication need, except Latin was real and could be genuinely translated into something more than a pseudomessage from an emoting, glib, arrogant, feel-good expert in weird clothes.

A special "elite" language always occurs. People seem to need a second "elite" language of some degree. As Latin is abandoned, the vacuum created is readily filled by New Age and fundamentalist "communications," which are feeling-filled utterances spread contagiously, causing the "Feeling Disease" or contemporary Gnosticism. At least Latin was based on reality.

(4) Fourth, Latin met the undeniable human need for mystery and intrigue present in everyone. This dimension is obviously related to the communication function previously described and easily recognized in New Age nonsense. Re-

gardless, people will be better served if this need was met by a validated "mystery" rather than avant garde ephemeralities or discredited ancient paganisms. Furthermore, Latin is understandable if desired while New Age gibberish cannot be understood because there is nothing there to understand, except "I feel this way!" said in all sorts of entertaining routines.

(5) Fifth, psychological status acrues to those who use Latin—not laudable in itself but nonetheless a psychological fact important to one's unconscious mind. The human element is gratified when made to be or feel "special."

Only those who have never experienced it, who do not know better, or who are lazy naysayers, reject the subjective charismatic sensation one feels when one is a master of something when others are not. This can be no less true for Latin. The implications for the attraction to and fulfillment of the psychological realities associated with the priesthood and religious life cannot be minimized.

(6) Sixth, Latin is tremendously enhancing of Catholicity by its unifying effect. This is tricky, but upon reflecting, can be readily recognized as a realistic and powerful psychological by-product of Latin use.

That is, in a minute but tangible way Latin helps a person extend beyond his individuality. This is because Latin is an impediment to exalting self. No wonder Latin is rejected by the thoughtless or the lazy: It requires intellect over feelings, and it even makes one, however briefly, relinquish one's own language. One goes beyond finite differences to reach out and not be entrenched in concrete traits which, when aggrandized, can be so destructive to humanity coming together as one. Reverend Stallings and his "black Catholic Church," of 1989 origin, is an example of how delimiting the "Catholic Church" with any adjective results in an oxymoron (except "Roman" which marks "leadership" and not "feeling filled identity").

Also, the rich tradition of the Roman Catholic Church as a counterpoise for the people against oppressive governments has always been succored by Latin. That is, Latin helps people identify with something other than their nation or government, the latter in only rare instances worthy of much allegiance.

Latin temporarily separates us from our native language and our nativity itself, enabling a oneness and a Catholicity that is more totally human. At least Latin promotes that trend. The national and linguistic fissures that separate people are briefly shelved. Thusly, Latin renders one less vulnerable to identify *only* with that which could never enhance *all* mankind. Getting caught up in one's own finite characteristics (such as one's blackness, one's Italianness, one's femaleness, one's maleness, etc.) to the point of espousing those traits to the detriment of total humanity, is diminished.

Obviously, with Latin, one's identity is less constricted and more catholic and Catholic. There was a time when familiarity and participation were possible at Mass anywhere in the world. Now this is rare unless the local language is known. The Mass in the vernacular has created "community" which is good, but without some positive use of Latin, there is no "going beyond" a *limited* community. The global unity and total togetherness of some Latin in Mass wherever you are can be important. In this regard, Latin was and is truly the language of civilized humanity. It UNIQUELY *unified* and reduced barriers which separate people! Nothing else has the potential to do that for everyone.

(7) Seventh, an elementary understanding of Latin is essential to being genuinely educated, because Latin is an integral part of 2000 years of Western Civilization (which is irreplaceably and ideally characterized by search for truth, by fair dialogue and balanced discussion, and by tolerance and intellect superseding emotions and force). Even today, one cannot get away from Latin in law, medicine, the arts and more.

To suddenly pretend Latin never existed is foolish—no, I will say it: It is "stupid" to deny Latin, as well as dishonest. Society is, I suppose, "stuck" with it. To the better for sure, in this observer's opinion.

To summarize, even though old, Latin is perennially young. Rationally romantic, it produces an ascendancy of the mental and a supernatural Spirit gluing together humanity and the Church into the Body of Christ. It gives uniformity, commonality, non-nationality, total humanization, and a protective barrier buffering outrage, violence, feelings, and mendacity by commitment to magnanimous freedom, search for truthful ideas, and *agape*.

In the past, when mellifluous ideas genuinely attracted love, truth, thought and virtue, they were in Latin, and it was ours. Its masters were priests. Latin was and is "quality-control" on ideas.

De-Latinization has, to this observer, contributed greatly to the loss of spirit and associated vocations to religious life. Without Latin, the world is a greater babble, more divisible, and obviously less Catholic.

In summary, de-Latinization removes the psychosocial substructure of Catholicity.

WHY THE PRECEDING IS WRONG

Many would object to all of the foregoing. Their reasons are as follows:

(1) First, the diminution of vocations started before the change from Latin to the vernacular in the Liturgy. The vocational collapse coincided more and more with the dissent against *Humanae Vitae* and with development of communication technology as hypnotic distraction. Vocations have thrived in communities and dioceses where strong clerical and religious discipline has been maintained without the emphasis on Latin.

(2) Second, most people following the Church depend not on Latin but on the depth of faith and being properly instructed in the truths of the faith. Latin itself is not instrumental in maintaining the faith.

(3) Latin may create a mysterious atmosphere for some people, but it does not affect or enhance the essential mystery of the Liturgy. The SACRAMENT does with faith and divine charity which inclines us to celebrate the sacrament holily. The mystery consists in what has been and is being revealed about and in the sacrament. "Feeling special" is essentially improper in both the "feeling" part as well as the "special" part. And any specialness is because God chooses us to belong to His Son's mystical body.

(4) The true unity of the Church is interior and based absolutely on faith. Latin is merely an exterior bond and is such only for those who understand it. For those who do not (the majority of people) it is a block to understanding the instruction imparted by the Liturgy to build up faith. Understanding is better.

(5) As for those who travel, they are able to attend Mass being celebrated in a language which gives them an exposure to diversity and an expanded familiarity with the broadness of mankind. The unanimity of Latin is not automatically virtue-producing. In fact, the Catholicity of the Church is shown more clearly when wherever the mass is celebrated, it is the essential Mass in another one of the world's languages. Catholicity stresses the differences within the one unique Church.

(6) While some people may have their minds "lifted" by the use of Latin, a good literary and poetic translation into English will do the same. Most people do not understand. "All Latin" means one may as well be in a foreign city so what is the problem?

(7) It is purely a matter of opinion whether de-Latinization removed the psychosocial substructure of Catholicity. Still, NOTHING, NOT EVEN LATIN, SHOULD BE ALLOWED to stand in the way of ordinary people's assimilation of the faith-instruction that comes with celebration of the Liturgy in a GOOD translation.

(8) It is difficult to keep Latin genuinely spiritual except by Procrustian methods. Latin was not part of the original liturgical language in Rome itself until the end of the fourth century. Before then it was Greek.

A BALANCED APPROACH

While controversy rages, Latin will never go away completely and it can never be denied as part of Church history. And it is also very unlikely that it will ever be as predominate as it once was nor should it be. Therefore, a balanced approach is offered believing that Latin should not dominate nor be excluded completely. These suggestions are offered for history's sake and in the name of peace:

1. Memorize and use frequently the phrases listed at the end of this chapter. Memorize them and add to them. Start your own Latin Phrase Book. An excellent book belonging in every library is: *Amo, Amas, Amat, and More* by Eugen Ehrlich.
2. Promote Latin (and translation) selections to be memorized for reception of the Sacraments:
   The *Confiteor* for First Confession;
   The Gloria in Excelsus Deo for First Communion;
   The Pater Noster, O Salutaris Hostia and *Tantum Ergo* for Confirmation.
3. At Mass, at the Sign of Peace, use "Dominus Vobiscum" and "Et cum spiritu tuo."
4. For Mass, promote selective Latin parts such as the Confiteor, the Gloria, the Pater Noster, the Consecration, and the Final Blessing. (Use *both* Latin and vernacular translation).
   Suggestions are:
   I will go to the altar of God, to God the joy of my youth.
   - Introibo ad alteri Dei, ad deum qua latificat juventutum meam.
   Let us pray.
   - Oremus.
   Kyrie eleison (Okay. It's Greek) - and translation.
   Gloria *or* Confiteor *or* Pater Noster — and translations — do only one at each Mass.
   Consecration in Latin with translation.
   Lord, I am not worthy. . . .
   - Domine non sum dignus. . . .
   Other Latin phrases *with* the vernacular translation might include:
   Dominus vobiscum. . . . The Lord be with you;
   Sanctus, sanctus, sanctus. . . . Holy, holy, holy;
   Agnus Dei. . . . Lamb of God;
   The Final Blessing in Latin, followed by the vernacular;
   "Ite, Missa est" — Go, the Mass is over.
5. Sing "O Salutaris" and "Tantum Ergo" once in awhile.
6. Promote one year of Latin in high school and another year in college. Also, develop one semester of conversational Latin — it is fun, secretive, intriguing and simple — plus it means something special. (Youths love to have their own "piglatin" or equivalent — so give them the real thing but make it fun.)

A FEW SECULAR LATIN PHRASES

A cruce salus — Sacrifice is needed! (Literally: Salvation comes from a cross).

Ad unguem — Perfectly! (Literally: To the fingernail).

Aequo animo — With calm mind, composure, and equanimity.

Age quod agis — Pay attention! (Literally: Do what you are doing).

Alter ego — Bosom pal.

Amantes sunt amentes — Lovers are lunatics!

A maximis ad minima — From the greatest to the least.

Anguis in herba — Hidden danger. (Literally: A snake in the grass).

Animis opibusque parati — Ready for anything. (Literally: Prepared in the mind and resources).

Argumentum ab auctoritate — Proof from authority.

Argumentum baculinum — An appeal to force.

Arrectis auribus — On the alert. (Literally: With ears pricked up).

Caveat emptor — Let the buyer beware.

Coniunctus viribus — With united powers.

Consilio manuque — By strategy and hard work.

Cum grano salis — With grain of salt.

De asini umbra disceptare — Little things affect little minds. (Literally: To argue about the shadow of an ass).

Desipere in loco — To play the fool on occasion.

Fama volat — Rumor travels fast.

Fiat lux — Let there be light.

Fortuna favet fortibus — Fortune favors the brave.

Fuit Ilium — Troy has had it—is no more.

Hoc age — Get with it!

In cauda veneuum — Watch out for that which you cannot see. (Literally: In the tail is the poison).

Labor omnia vincit — Work conquers all things.

Mea culpa — My fault!

Mox nox in rem — Let's get on with it! (Literally: Soon night, to the business).

Mundus vult decipi — There is a sucker born every minute.

Ne cede malis — Do not yield to misfortune.

Ne plus ultra — Perfection.

Nullius filius — Bastard. (Literally: No one's son.

Nunc est bibendum — Break out the champagne.

Pollice verso — Thumbs down!

Populus iamdudum defutatus est — The people have been screwed long enough.

Praemonitus praemunitus — Forewarned, forearmed.

Probitare — Prove it.

Scientia est potentia — Knowledge is power.

Semper paratus — Always ready.

Diem perdidi — Another day wasted.

Dixi — That settles it. (Literally: I have spoken).

Ducit amor patriae — Love of country guides me.

Experto credite — Trust me.

Facile princeps — Number one.

Facta non verba — Actions speak louder than words. (Literally: Deeds, not words).

Pacem habete — Peace be upon you.

Vie victis — Cursed by the defeated.

Peste — A plague on you.

Risum teneatis amici? — Can we restrain our laughter?

Sero venientibus ossa — Sorry, too late. (Literally: For latecomers, the bones).

Stupor mundi — Wonder of the universe.

Summum bonum — Highest good.

Te nosce — Know thyself.

Totis viribus — with all one's powers.

Tua mater — Your mama!

Velis et remis — All-out effort. (Literally: With sails and oars).

Veritas odium parit — Truth breeds hatred.

Vicisti Galilaea — You have conquered, O Galilean! (Last words of Roman Emperor Julian the Apostate, A.D. 331-363).

CHAPTER 14:

RAPPROACHEMENT: JUDAISM

Of crucial importance is why and how did the response to the New Testament go awry? After the occurrence of New Testament events, what went wrong? Knowing of people who had actually encountered God in the Person of Jesus Christ, one must ask: What went wrong?

A first question might be why were early Catholics (all Jews) rejected and estranged from their own people?

Leaders of the Jewish community rejected not only Jesus and His teachings, but to a greater extent, they rejected the early believers by deliberate, violent de-Judaicization (removal of Jewish identity).

Jesus said from the cross, "Forgive them for they know not what they do," and we see in St. Paul how a violent anti-Catholic became a saint. But this account of the rejection of Jesus by some Jews should never be a pretext for anti-Semitism in any form.

New Testament persons were God-fearing, self-sacrificing, peace-loving, and nonviolent people. They were revolutionaries for peace, truth, love, self-sacrifice, and "love, thy enemies" — a "Lovelution."

In the Acts of the Apostles, St. Paul, after his conversion, describes how he was treated and he often survived only because he was a Roman citizen. Additionally, he recommended early Catholics be like sheep led to the slaughter and not resist. Imagine what was done to the thousands of early Catholic converts who were not Roman citizens as was St. Paul. This may be a clue to understanding what went wrong.

The early Jewish people were not without their illiberal and violent practices. When the Hebrews were found to be adoring the golden calf, Moses had 3,000 men killed by the sons of Levi in one day (Exodus XXXII:27,28). Later, Moses directed the slaying of 24,000 worshippers of Belphegor (Numbers XXV). Then after wondering why the women and children were not also killed, Moses had all but female virgins put to death, regardless of age. To say violence was part of the Old Covenant is an understatement. Moses may not have been the first Grand Inquisitor, but he put more to death in the name of religion than Torquemada of the Spanish Inquisition.

Jesus said "NO" to violence in what is the logical, necessary, and desired fulfillment of the violent Old Covenant. The Loving Truth of Jesus can be the only message that really makes sense if one is a believer in the Old Testament. Really, would a Messiah from God bring a message more violent than what was extant at the time?

Initially many Jewish people embraced Jesus and His teachings. There existed no great conflict. One could be a believer in Jesus and still go to Temple. There was no exclusivity but rather a single, peaceful difference in terms of commitment to Judaism wherein some believed the Covenant had been fulfilled by the coming of Jesus while some refused to believe that Jesus was the Messiah and claimed that the Covenant was still unfulfilled.

There was no substantial problem with this originally, but some time in the early years, Jewish leaders demanded that Catholicism be excluded from Judaism and oppressed. And herein began problems. Jewish leadership secretly integrated into Judaism a subtle but vicious anti-Catholicism. Accordingly, to be a Jewish Catholic was to be a traitor and de-Judaicization (removal of Jewish identity) was automatic.

The Gospels provide witness accounts of Jewish leaders' initial violence and attempts to discredit Catholicism. Jewish leaders whipped and imprisoned the apostles out of fear and jealousy. They murdered Stephen when he challenged them about previous Jewish leaders selling Joseph into slavery (Acts 7). The Jewish leaders were so pleased when King Herod put the apostle James the Greater to death by the sword, that Peter was next arrested (Acts 12). The story of Saul, a trained rabbi and vicious persecutor of Catholics was not unique. How many other rabbis did likewise? Bribes were offered to soldiers to spread the story that the body of Jesus was stolen, lest more people convert. Jewish leaders pondered the killing of Lazarus, to discredit his own resurrection.

An excommunication Prayer made it impossible for early Catholics to attend temple services because Catholics were easily identified by their refusing to recite this prayer — wherefore they were promptly thrown out of temple and often abused. A horrendous prejudicial aura, first unilateral, but later of mutual intolerance and rejection was created among Jews who did not accept Jesus and those who did.

A damaging series of events involved Jewish General Bar Cochba who was purported to be the Messiah, in a temporal sense, because he proclaimed to free Jews from the yoke of the Roman Empire. Bar Cochba started a war of liberation with the Romans. In his efforts to enlist soldiers, he tortured and massacred many Catholics who refused to fight because of their pacifist trends and, particularly because Bar Cochba himself was parading as "the Messiah." Bar Cochba, the warmonger, for early Jewish Catholics was an unacceptable alternative to Jesus, the nonviolent peacemaker.

Some time in the Middle A es, the Toledoth Jesu appeared as a Talmudic tract which promoted the idea that the Blessed Virgin Mary was a prostitute and that Jesus was a bastard, not descended from the line of David. That this was a fraud is one fact. That it was promoted and developed is another! Its very existence substantiates the prevaricating, violent abuse and rejection of Catholics by Jewish leadership.

Let us note, however, that Catholics circulated similar fraudulent books accusing Jews of ritual murders of Christians. When we add to this, years of violent persecution of Jews by Christians, we see how much forgiveness is needed on both sides. All sides have wronged each other many more times than reported here.

Genuine early Catholics were peace-loving, love-your-enemy, caring, nonviolent people, willing to sacrifice and suffer much on behalf of their beliefs. These people were rejected and mistreated by the Jewish community to which they belonged under the instigation of Jewish leadership who did not want the establishment of Catholicism as a graft onto the roots of Judaism (as St. Paul put it).

I have personally been asked by Orthodox Jewish children: "Did you know the Blessed Virgin Mary was a prostitute?" (Referring to the Toledoth Jesu already mentioned.) On many other occasions, I have heard prominent Jewish businessmen recite incidents of the mistreatment of Jews by Catholics because Catholics were taught "Jews were Christ killers."

I believe the "Christ killer" accusation must be true, because Jewish converts to Catholicism have reported this. I have never experienced "Jews are Christ killers" from anyone in my entire Catholic upbringing or adult life except from Jews saying that is what Catholics say.

On the other hand, is it not obvious that Jews are taught, in effect, that "Catholics are Jew killers," which is true of false Catholics but leaves out all those who have helped Jews?

An example is the erratic treatment of Pope Pius XII as he faced the Nazi holocaust. Obviously, Pope Pius XII did not do enough to help Jews, but no one did. However, no one did more than Pope Pius XII! But such is not enough for some. Would anything ever be enough? Instead of being identified as the only World War II character worthy of genuine hero status because of the hundreds of thousands of Jews he enabled to escape from Hitler, Pope Pius XII is occasionally scapegoated to maintain the myths of Catholic-based anti-Semitism.

However, if Pope Pius XII was discredited by World War II, then Winston Churchill was discredited by the Blitz of London, Malcolm Muggeridge by the

Starving of Ukraine, MacArthur by the Korean War, Noah by the flood; and Jesus was discredited by the Crucifixion. Baloney! All such scapegoating must stop.

The anti-Semitism by Catholics of the past is overwhelmingly repugnant. It can be understood as the basis for contemporary anti-Catholicism — which must be graciously accepted as a valid phase during which mutual trust can be reestablished.

We must work together to stamp out anti-Semitism and to stop the underlying subtle anti-Catholic forces which contribute (self-fulfilling?) in evoking more anti-Semitism.

This early Jew-on-Jew violence in the first century set the stage for all subsequent Jewish-Catholic relations. The unfair discrediting of Catholicism was present from the beginning and has been present for two millennia. It is present now. . .less overtly violent but of the same genre.

For 2,000 years, the fundamental guiding principle for Jewry has been "do not believe" by means of which perceived anti-Semitism, real and imagined, became the touchstone of Jewish integrity. Today must be different from both the Catholic perspective and the Jewish perspective.

This observer's perception is that Catholics have made the most changes since Vatican II. What is troubling is that these changes are not enough. One suspects what Catholics do will never be enough, since the Jewish perspective has not changed.

One can make the case the Jewish leadership desires no change. Is it possible some Jewish leadership has a vested interest in promoting the victim status for themselves because by this means they can maintain their Jewish integrity and self-bonding? One hopes not, but the idea may be a possibility.

Much that is wrong here must cease. I try not to accuse, but to explain. Whatever understanding or misunderstandings persist must change so that unity may be accomplished.

Terrible events which happened 2,000 years ago included more than the death of Jesus. Jewish leadership oppressed a new-to-the-world Jewish loving-truth sect called "Catholic" in 70 A.D. and presages of Roman Catholics. This was a tragedy of the first magnitude. It prevented a compatibility between Jews of the Old Testament and those of the fulfilled New Covenant. It created an abyss of misunderstanding, a horrendous mistrust, and an absolute rejection, all resulting in an inordinate mutual dysphoria.

One can only fantasize how the world might have been had Jewish leadership merely rejected Jesus and his teachings but not their own people who accepted the fulfillment of the Covenant by joining the Mystical Body of Christ. Had the rejections not occurred, the Vatican might have been in Jerusalem! And the Nazi holocaust would never have happened. One can conjure the possible compatibility of Old and New Covenant people praying together without excommunication prayers assaulting the sensitivities of any party. Old Covenant clingers and New Covenant believers might have lived together in peace.

Such did not happen and one must examine the leaders of those who rejected Jesus and more: They rejected their own people by oppressing new ideas in a hostile illiberal manner, reminiscent of today's intolerant liberals who prohibit the pendulum from swinging any way but their own, just as totalitarians always have.

Later, as Gentiles became converted, the Jewish community forgot (or suppressed) the fact that Christianity was a grafting onto Judaic roots, considered to be a vertical fulfillment of the Covenant called "Catholic" since the first century by St. Ignatius of Antioch. "Catholic" included a horizontal enveloping of all peoples into Christianity, but only after a vertical supraimposition of all converts, Jews and Gentiles, firmly onto original Judaic roots.

Genuine Catholics automatically adopt Judaism — we are of Jewish origin in the eyes of Yahweh, in our hearts and in historical fact.

What's wrong with this? Nothing except that Jewish leadership will have no part of it and does not want anyone to convert — 2,000 years ago — or today. Early anti-Catholicism begot anti-Semitism which begot anti-Catholicism which begot anti-Semitism, and we take turns hurting one another. All because the Old Covenant leaders became hateful and as is now evident: What goes around, comes around, over and over again. The waves of rejection still flow.

As my father would often say: "Some damn fool made it either/or 2,000 years ago, and everybody has been suffering ever since."

Enough already! Let there be peace! Shalom!

CHAPTER 15:

RAPPROACHEMENT: ISLAM

It must first be remembered that Islam is rooted in Catholicism. There is no valid way to deny this. What now constitutes almost the entire Islamic world was once Catholic. It is often forgotten that the ancestors of Muslims were Catholics as historical and archeological evidence proves. But because of the misappropriation of God's Wrath and by abuse of power, faith has been disrupted by the severing of union with one's ancestors.

Islam holds that in the sixth century, the "fulfillment" of The Book (the Torah and the Gospels) was accomplished by Mohammed. This proposal was as controversial to Christianity in the sixth century as Jesus' "fulfillment" of the Old Testament was to Judaism in the first century. Or, is it possible and is it more correct to state that the Islamic sixth century proposal was actually a continuation of the same controversy of the first century: the Old Testament versus the New Testament?

THE KORAN

Islamic scholars state that the "Koran cannot be translated." It is described as "the reading" of *the man who knew not how to read*. And it is believed that the Angel Gabriel instructed Mohammed, who could neither read nor write, to "recite" or "read," which Mohammed did with others recording his verses.

This requires a response. To the assertion that the Koran cannot be translated it must be asked: By whose authority? And by what authority is the assertion made that since Mohammed could not read, his verses apply only to those whose language enables them to understand the original words of the Reading? Is it in the Koran itself that these interpretations must be steadfastly adhered to?

If so, then it must be understood that the Koran is not for the mind and is therefore not for everyone. Is it not unjust to limit believers to only those who do not know how to read or only those who can understand the original language? Actually, these traditional assertions about the untranslatability and unreadability of the Koran create an exclusiveness that is incompatible with it being for everyone. To the contrary, Allah has given me a translation, and I have read it.

The official collection of verses from Mohammed was preserved by the Caliphate of Othman, Comrades of the Prophet, and devout students of the Revelation shortly after the death of Mohammed.

That there was an official collaboration for the original versing is surprising and raises questions about the authority to select, omit, and organize the verses. Who is the official collator and interpreter of the verses? What verses give such authority? What psychosocial circumstances existed that would predispose to conflict and error in the official collection of verses? Have all interpreters come from the spirit of Allah and with the expansiveness of Mohammed? Or did they pick and choose and unwittingly but tendentiously sully the genuine meaning of the divine verses?

One major interpreter of the Koran was Petrus Alphonsi or Peter of Tolado also known as the "Annotator." What qualified him is not in the Koran. Nevertheless, in the 1140's, he developed an interpretation of the Koran extremely hostile to all other Europeans. What was that all about? His interpretation followed the 1066 Muslim massacre of Jews of Grenada which actually was the first pogrom of Jews on European soil. Examples like this make it difficult to deny that the Koran was misused and interpreted for secular purposes to the detriment of all.

A malignant eisegesis of the Koran has rendered it incompatible with the Old Testament and the New Testament even though it relies on, supports, and at times contradicts both. Nevertheless, because the Koran uses biblical characters, Abraham, Jesus and Mary, a presupposition of oneness with the Torah and the Gospels cannot be denied. But this harmony was broken by interpreters.

That Allah has given us minds to question and challenge would seem to be beyond controversy. Allah has also given logic in the mind and language for the people. Allah had words written down. These words are for reading! The mind must have a oneness about words and interpretations of the divine verses or else discontinuity and disturbance will be created among human beings. Did not this happen? Did not themes of power, obviously present in the Koran, become overemphasized for personal aggrandizement and control resulting in headlong plunging into misinterpretation and misuse of power?

The element of temporal power is obvious and it is present in the Koran since initially preserved. But the emphasis on power appears to have occurred with unmeasured disregard for mercy causing error whereby the Koran has become a source of power, conflict and strength misused to force others to accept another's own interpretation in conflict with the very mind Allah has given us.

The tradition of power linked to the interpretation (misinterpretation?) of the Koran is in and of itself inimical to the Koran in the absolute sense, because such misinterpreters omit and ignore what actually are the New Testament components of the Koran. Exegetical study is essential. . . . Up to now, all use (misuse?) of the Koran has, instead, been based on a malignant type of eisegesis from unqualified but powerful men, like Peter of Tolado.

For example, Sura IX, Verse 5 says "When the forbidden months are passed, slay the idolaters wherever you find them and take them captive and beseige for them each ambush." Now this is savagery worthy of Moses. Contrast this with II-109: "Forgive and be indulgent (toward them). . . ."

Thus the history of Islam and Roman Catholicism is confused as well as unpleasant reading. The word "sacrilegious" can at times be applied to both sides' presentations, promotions, and actions. Instead of emphasizing common ground, differences have been accentuated and magnified with the harshest interpretations foisted onto believers of both sides.

After reading the Koran, I was struck by the confusing mixture of Old and New Testament.

To be sure, the Old Testament is there with the wrath of Allah, the severe punishments, the shameful doom. Clearly, some verses appear to fall in with the violence of Moses and others in the Old Testament.

Conversely, the New Testament is also contained in the Koran with "Jesus, son of Mary," well accepted as a genuine messenger from Allah. So the New Covenant is also there with Loving Truth and verses quite imitative of Jesus Christ.

There are enough positive messages in the Koran that, by focusing on them, the New Testament verses may prevail thus reestablishing the commonality of Islam and Roman Catholicism. By incorporating baptism by mutual desire for all, we emphasize the New Testament components and leave the Old Testament violence behind. Loving Truth has fulfilled the Old Testament, even the Old Testament parts of the Koran.

The following quotations from the Koran may help readers to see the basis for one faith, one fold, one shepherd: there is only one God but Allah! — I am Who am — the Trinity — He who can do all things — The Father, Son, and Holy Spirit — Yahweh; and from the Koran: the Beneficent — the Merciful — the Compassionate — the Forgiving — the All-embracing — the All-knowing — the Powerful — the Mighty — the Wise — the Sustainer — Knower of Things Hidden — the Hearer — Lord of the Worlds — Best of Deciders — the Just — the Aware — Cleaver of the Daybreak — the Subtle — Protecting Friend — the Absolute — the Lord of Mercy — Lord of the World — the Knower — Relenting — Loving — the Great — the High Exalted — the One — the Almighty — the Owner of Praise — Full of Pity — the Sublime Similitude — Seerer of His Slaves — the True — Full of Mercy — the Glorious One — the Strong — the Manifest Truth — the Trustee — the All-knowing Judge —

the Forgiver — the Sublime — the Majestic — the Tremendous — the Praise worthy. Do we Christians not know God by most if not all of these titles?

Of interest is that throughout the Koran, Allah consistently refers to Himself as "We," quite consistent with the Christian Trinitarian interpretation although some Muslims persist in saying that the Koran only rejects the Trinity.

EXCERPTS FROM THE KORAN, THE BIBLE OF ISLAM

(The source of these quotations is *The Meaning of the Glorious Koran*, an explanatory translation by Mohammed Marmaduke Pickthall, a Mentor book by New American Library, New York and Scarborough, Ontario.)

The Koran is over 13 centuries old. It is organized into 114 chapters of varying length called "Suras." Each Sura is subdivided into numbered verses, some 6,000 in all. The following quotations from the Koran have the Suras in Roman numerals followed by the verse number.

The proudest boast of the Muslim is to be "a slave of Allah" just as we Catholics are ideally "fools for the Lord" or "prisoners for the sake of Jesus Christ." It is with this goal in mind that I have excerpted what I call the "New Testament" verses, because only by such an emphasis can Loving Truth be the unique, necessary, and logical fulfillment of the Old Testament, as it is for Scripture, for the Torah, and for the Koran.

After the Old Testament verses, verses of violence and then slavery will be listed followed by verses containing the word "love" (pages 495-496).

New Testament Verses

This list of Verses are positive in general and consistent with the New Testament or at least they are a peaceful point of departure for explanatory discussion. (Quotations tend to be subject to interpretation. Readers are asked to "do good and avoid evil" in such processes and to search for Loving Truth,then the reader may want to skip to p. 488 and return to read these verses later.)

I In the name of Allah, the Beneficent, the Merciful.
Praise be to Allah, Lord of Worlds,
The Beneficent, the Merciful.
Owner of the Day of Judgment.
Thee (alone) we Worship; Thee (alone) we ask for help.
Show us the straight path,
The path of those whom Thou hast favored;
Not (the path) of those who earned Thine anger nor of those who go astray.

II-58 Enter the gate prostrate and say "Repentance." We will forgive you your sins.

II-72 And (Remember) when ye slew a man and disagreed concerning it and Allah brought forth that which you were hiding.

II-73 And We said: Smite him with some of it. Thus Allah bringeth the dead to life and showeth you His portents so that ye may understand.

II-74 Then, even after that, your hearts were hardened and became as rocks, were worse than rocks, for hardness. For indeed there are rocks from out which rivers gush, and indeed there are rocks which split asunder so that water floweth from them. And indeed there are rocks which fall down for the fear Allah. Allah is not unaware of what ye do.

II-82 And those who believe and do good works: Such are rightful owners of the Garden. They will abide therein.

II-87 And verily We gave unto Moses the Scripture and We caused a train of messengers to follow after him, and We gave unto Jesus, son of Mary, clear proofs (of Allah's sovereignty), and We supported him with the holy Spirit. Is it ever so, that, when there cometh unto you a messenger (from Allah) with that which ye yourselves desire not, ye grow arrogant, and some ye disbelieve and some ye slay?

II-109 Many of the People of Scripture long to make you disbelievers after your belief, through envy on their own account, after the truth hath become manifest onto them. Forgive and be indulgent (toward them) until Allah give command. Lo! Allah is Able to do all things.

II-112 . . .but whosoever surrendereth his purpose to Allah while doing good, his reward is with his Lord; and there shall no fear come upon them, neither shall they grieve.

II-136 Say (Oh Muslims): We believe in Allah and that which is revealed unto us and that which was revealed unto Abraham, and Ishmael, and Isaac, and Jacob, and the tribes, and that which Moses and Jesus received, and that which the Prophets received from their Lord. We make no distinction between any of them, and unto Him we have surrendered.

II-177 It is not righteousness that ye turn your faces to the East and the West; but righteous is he who believeth in Allah and the Last Day and the angels and the Scripture and the Prophets; and giveth his wealth for love of Him, to kinsfolk and to orphans and the needy and the wayfarer and to those who ask, and to set slaves free; and observeth proper worship and payeth the poor-due. And those who keep their treaty when they make one, and the patient in tribulation and adversity and time of stress. Such are they who are sincere. Such are the God-fearing.

II-190 Fight in the way of Allah against those who fight against you, but begin not hostilities. Lo, Allah loveth not aggressors.

II-253 Of those messengers, some of whom We have caused to excel others, and of whom there are some unto whom Allah spake, while some of them He exalted (above others) in degree; and We gave

Jesus, son of Mary, clear proofs (of Allah's sovereignty) and We supported him with the holy Spirit. . . .

II-279 . . .Wrong not, and ye shall not be wronged.

III-42 And when the angels said: Oh, Mary! Lo! Allah hath chosen thee and made thee pure and hath preferred thee above (all) the women of creation.

III-45 (And remember) when the angels said: Oh Mary! Lo! Allah giveth thee glad tidings of word from Him, whose name is the Messiah, Jesus, son of Mary, illustrious in the world and the Hereafter, and one of those brought near (unto Allah).

III-55 When Allah said: Oh, Jesus! Lo! I am gathering thee and causing thee to ascend unto Me, and am cleansing thee of who disbelieve and am setting those who follow thee above those who disbelieve until the Day of Resurrection. Then unto Me, ye will (all) return, and I shall judge between you as to that wherein ye used to differ.

III-84 Say (Oh, Muhammad): We believe in Allah and that which is revealed unto us and that which was revealed unto Abraham and Ishmael and Isaac and Jacob and the tribes, and that which was vouchsafed unto Moses and Jesus and the Prophets from their Lord. We make no distinction between any of them and unto Him we have surrendered.

III-85 And whoso seeketh as religion other than the Surrender (to Allah), it will not be accepted from him and he will be a loser in the Hereafter.

III-95 Say: Allah speaketh truth. So follow the religion of Abraham, the upright. He was not of the idolaters.

III-144 Muhammad is but a messenger, messengers (the like of whom) have passed away before him. Will it be that, when ye dieth or is slain, ye will turn back on your heels? He who turneth back doth no hurt to Allah, and Allah will reward the thankful.

III-169 Think not of those who are slain in the way of Allah, as dead. Nay, they are living. With their Lord, they have provision.

III-170 Jubilant (are they) because of that which Allah hath bestowed upon them of his Bounty, rejoicing for the sake of those who hath not joined them but are left behind: that there shall no fear come upon them and neither shall they grieve.

III-171 They rejoice because of favor from Allah and kindness and that Allah wasteth not the wage of the believers.

III-180 And let not those who hoard up that which Allah hath bestowed upon them of His bounty think that it is better for them. Nay, it is worse for them. That which they hoard will be on their collar on the Day of Resurrection. Allah's is the heritage of the heavens and the earth, and Allah is informed of what ye do.

III-187 And (remember) when Allah laid a charge on those who had received the Scripture (He said): Ye are to expound it to mankind and not to hide it. . . .

III-195 And their Lord hath heard them (and He saith): Lo! I suffer not the work of any worker, male or female, to be lost. Yet proceed one from another.

IV-50 See, how they invent lies about Allah! That of itself is flagrant sin.

IV-57 And as for those who believe and do good works, We shall make them enter Gardens underneath which rivers flow, to dwell therein forever; there for them are pure companions and We shall make them enter plenteous shade.

IV-94 Oh ye who believe! When ye go forth (to fight) in the way of Allah, be careful to discriminate, and say not unto one who offereth you peace: "Thou are not a believer," seeking the chance profits of this life (that ye may despoil him). With Allah are plenteous spoils. Even thus (as he is now) were ye before; but Allah hath since then been gracious unto you. Therefore take care to discriminate. Allah is ever Informed of what ye do.

IV-96 Degrees of rank from Him, and forgiveness and mercy. Allah is every Forgiving, Merciful.

IV-122 But as for those who believe and do good works We shall bring them into Gardens underneath which rivers flow, wherein they will abide forever. It is a promise from Allah in truth; and who can be more truthful than Allah in utterance?

IV-125 Who is better in religion than he who surrendereth his purpose to Allah while doing good (to men) and followeth the tradition of Abraham, the upright? Allah (Himself) chose Abraham for a friend.

IV-149 If ye do good openly or keep it secret, or forgive evil, lo! Allah is Forgiving, Powerful.

IV-157 And because of their saying: We slew the Messiah, Jesus, son of Mary, Allah's messenger — They slew him not nor crucified, but it appeared so unto them; and lo! Those who disagree concerning it are in doubt thereof; they have no knowledge thereof save pursuit of a conjecture; they slew him not for certain.

IV-158 But Allah took him up unto Himself. Allah was ever Mighty, Wise.

IV-171 Oh People of Scripture! Do not exaggerate in your religion or utter aught concerning Allah save the truth. The Messiah, Jesus son of Mary, was only a messenger of Allah, and His word which He conveyed unto Mary, and a spirit from Him. So believe in Allah and His messengers, and say not "Three" -Cease! (it is) better for you! — Allah is only One God. Far it is removed from His transcendent majesty that he should have a son. His is all that is in the heavens and all that is in the earth. And Allah is sufficient as Defender.

V-2 . . .And let not your hatred of a folk who (once) stopped your going to the Inviolable Place of Worship seduce you to transgress; but help ye one another unto righteous and pious duty.

V-8 Oh ye who believe! Be steadfast witnesses for Allah in equity, and not let hatred of any people seduce you that ye deal not justly. Deal justly, that is nearer to your duty. Observe your duty to Allah. Lo! Allah is Informed of what ye do.

V-9 Allah hath promised those who believe and do good works: Theirs will be forgiveness and immense reward.

V-13 . . .Thou will not cease to discover treachery from all save a few of them. But bear with them and pardon them. Lo! Allah loveth the kindly.

V-17 . . .Allah's is the Sovereignty of the heavens and the earth and all that is between them. He createth what He will. And Allah is Able to do all things.

V-28 Even if thou stretch out thy hand against me to kill me, I shall not stretch out my hand against thee to kill thee, lo! I fear Allah, the Lord of the World.

V-32 For that cause We decreed for the Children of Israel that whosoever killeth a human being for other than manslaughter or corruption in the earth, it shall be if he had killed all mankind, and who so saveth the life of one, it shall be as if he had saved the life of all mankind.

V-46 And We caused Jesus, son of Mary, to follow in their footsteps, confirming that which was (revealed) before him, and We bestowed on him the Gospel wherein is guidance and a light, confirming that which was (revealed) before it in the Torah, a guidance and an admonition unto those who ward off (evil).

V-47 Let the People of the Gospel judge by that which Allah hath revealed therein. Whoso judgeth not by that which Allah hath revealed; such are evil-livers.

V-69 Lo! Those who believe, and those who are Jews, and Sabaeans, and Christians — Whosoever believeth in Allah and the Last Day and doeth right — there shall no fear come upon them, neither shall they grieve.

V-77 Say, O People of the Scripture! Stress not in your religion other than the truth, and follow not the vain desires of folk who erred of old and led many astray, and erred from a plain road.

V-83 When they listen to that which hath been revealed unto the messenger, thou seest their eyes overflow with tears because of the recognition of the Truth. They say: Our Lord, we believe. Inscribe us as among the witnesses.

V-93 There shall be no sin (imputed) unto those who believe and do good works for what they may have eaten (in the past). So be mindful of your duty, (to Allah) and do good works; and again: be mindful of your duty, and believe; and once again: be mindful of your duty, and do right. Allah loveth the good.

V-99 The duty of the messenger is only to convey (the message). Allah knoweth what ye proclaim and what ye hide.

V-105 Oh, ye, who believe! Ye have charge of your own souls. He who erreth cannot injure you if ye are rightly guided. Unto Allah ye will all return; and then He will inform you of what ye used to do.

V-110 When Allah saith: Oh, Jesus son of Mary! Remember My favor unto thee and unto the mother; how I strengthened thee with the holy Spirit, so that thou spakest unto mankind in the cradle as in maturity; and how I taught thee the Scripture and Wisdom and the Torah and the Gospel; and how thou didst shape of clay as it were the likeness of a bird by My permission and didst blow upon it and it was a bird by My permission; and how thou didst raise the dead, by My permission; and how I restrained the Children of Israel from (harming) thee when thou camest unto them with clear proofs, and those of them who disbelieved exclaimed: This is naught else than mere magic.

V-112 When the disciples said: Oh, Jesus, son of Mary! Is thy Lord able to send down for us a table spread with food from heaven? He said: Observe your duty to Allah if ye are true believers.

V-113 (They said:) We wish to eat thereof, that we may satisfy our hears and know that thou hast spoken truth to us, and that thereof we may be witnesses.

V-114 Jesus, son of Mary, said: Oh, Allah, Lord of us! Send down for us a table spread with food from heaven, that it may be a feast for us, for the first of us and for the last of us, and a sign from Thee. Give us sustenance, for Thou art the Best of Sustainers.

V-115 Allah said: Lo! I send it down for you. And whoso disbelieveth of you afterward, him surely will I punish with a punishment wherewith I have not punished any of (My) creatures.

V-116 And when Allah saith: Oh Jesus, son of Mary! Didst thou say unto mankind: Take me and my mother for two gods beside Allah? He saith: Be glorified! It was not mine to utter that to which I had no right. If I used to say it, then Thou knewest it. Thou knowest what kind is in my mind, and I know not what is in Thy mind. Lo! Thou, only Thou art the Knower of Things Hidden.

VI-109 Revile not those unto whom they pray beside Allah lest they wrongfully revile Allah through ignorance. Thus unto every nation have We made their deed seem fair. Then unto their Lord is their return, and He will tell them what they used to do.

VII-28 And when they do some lewdness they say: We found our fathers doing it and Allah hath enjoined it on us. Say: Allah, verily, enjoin us not lewdness. Tell ye concerning Allah that which ye knew not?

VII-37 Who doeth greater wrong than he who inventeth a lie concerning Allah or denieth Our tokens. . . .

VII-42 But (as for) those who believe and do good works — We tax not any soul beyond its scope — Such are rightful owners of the Garden. They abide therein.

VII-43 And We remove whatever rancor may be in their hearts. Rivers flow beneath them. And they say: The praise to Allah, Who hath guided us to this. We could not truly have been led aright if Allah had not guided us. Verily, the messengers of our Lord did bring the Truth. And it is cried unto them: This is the Garden. Ye inherit it for what ye used to do.

VII-55 (O mankind!) Call upon your Lord humbly and in secret. Lo! He loveth not aggressors.

VII-156 . . .and My mercy embraceth all things. . . .

VII-167 And (remember) when thy Lord proclaimed that He would raise against them till the Day of Resurrection those who would lay on them a cruel torment. Lo! Verily thy Lord is swift in prosecution and lo! Verily He is Forgiving, Merciful.

VIII-61 And if they incline to peace, incline thou also to it, and trust in Allah. Lo! He is the Hearer, the Knower.

XI-11 Save those who persevere and do good works. Theirs will be forgiveness and a great reward.

XIII-28 Who have believed and whose hearts have rest in the remembrance of Allah. Verily in the remembrance of Allah do hearts find rest!

XIII-29 Those who believe and do right: Joy is for them, and bliss (their) journey's end.

XIII-43 They who disbelieve say: Thou art no messenger (of Allah). Say: Allah, and whosoever hath true knowledge of the Scripture, is sufficient witness between me and you.

XVI-90 Lo! Allah enjoineth justice and kindness, and giving to kinsfolk, and forbiddeth lewdness and abomination and wickedness. He exhorteth you in order that ye may take heed.

XVI-97 Whosoever doeth right, whether male or female, and is a believer, him verily We shall quicken with good life, and We shall pay them a recompense in portion to the best of what they used to do.

XVI-99 Lo! He (Satan) hath no power over those who believe and put trust in their Lord.

XVI-119 Then Lo! Thy Lord — for those who do evil in ignorance and afterward repent and amend — Lo! (for them) thy Lord is afterward indeed Forgiving, Merciful.

XVI-123 And afterward We inspired (Muhammad, saying): Follow the religion of Abraham, as one by nature upright. He was not of the idolaters.

XVI-124 The Sabbath was appointed only for those who differed concerning it, and lo! thy Lord will judge between them on the Day of Resurrection concerning that wherein they used to differ.

XVI-128 Lo! Allah is with those who keep their duty unto Him and those who are doers of good.

XIX-111 Say: I am only a mortal like you. My Lord inspireth in me that your God is only One God. And whoever hopeth for the meeting with his Lord, let him do righteous work, and make none sharer of the worship due unto his Lord.

XXI-91 And she who was chaste, therefor We breathed into her (something) of Our spirit and made her and her son a token for (all) peoples.

XXV-63 The (faithful) slaves of the Beneficent are they who walk upon the earth modestly, and when the foolish ones address them answer: Peace.

XXIX-7 And as for those who believe and do good works, We shall remit from them their evil deeds and shall repay them the best that they did.

XXXI-19 Be modest in thy bearing and subdue thy voice. Lo! The harshest of all voices is the voice of an ass.

XXXIII-35 Lo! Men who surrender unto Allah, and women who surrender, and men who believe and women who believe, and men who obey and women who obey, and men who speak the truth and women who speak the truth, and men who persevere (in righteousness) and women who persevere, and men who are humble and women who are humble, and men who give alms and women who give alms, and men who fast and women who fast, and men who guard their modesty and women who guard (their modesty), and men who remember Allah much and women who remember — Allah hath prepared for them forgiveness and a vast reward.

XXXIV-37 And it is not your wealth nor your children that will bring you unto Us, but he who believeth and doeth good (he draweth near). As for such, theirs will be twofold reward for that they did, and they will dwell secure in lofty halls.

XXXIX-44 Say: Unto Allah belongeth all intercession. His is the Sovereignty of the heavens and the earth. And afterward unto Him ye will be brought back.

XXXIX-63 His are the keys of the heavens and the earth, and they who disbelieve the revelations of Allah — such are those who are the losers.

XL-3 The Forgiver of sin, the Accepter of repentance, the Stern in punishment, the Bountiful. There is no God save Him. Unto Him is the journeying.

XLI-33 And who is better in speech than him who prayeth unto his Lord and doeth right, and saith: Lo! I am of those who surrender (unto Him).

XLII-13 He hath ordained for you that religion which He commended unto Noah, and that which We inspire in thee (Muhammad), and that which We commended unto Abraham and Moses and Jesus, saying: Establish the religion, and be not divided therein.

XLII-19 Allah is gracious unto His slaves. He provideth for whom He will. And He is the Strong, the Mighty.

XLII-42 The way (of blame) is only against those who oppress mankind, and wrongfully rebel in the earth. For such there is a painful doom.

XLII-43 And verily whoso is patient and forgiveth — lo! that, verily, is (of) the steadfast heart of things.

XLIII-63 When Jesus came with clear proofs (of Allah's sovereignty), he said: I have come unto you with wisdom, and to make plain some of that concerning which ye differ. So keep your duty to Allah and obey me.

XLIII-64 Lo! Allah. He is my Lord and your Lord. So worship Him. This is a right path.

LVII-29 That the People of the Scripture (Jews and Christians) may know that they control naught of the bounty of Allah, but that the bounty is in Allah's hand to give to whom He will. And Allah is of infinite bounty.

LXI-6 And when Jesus son of Mary said: Oh, Children of Israel! Lo! I am the messenger of Allah unto you, confirming that which was (revealed) before me in the Torah, and bringing good tidings of a messenger who cometh after me, whose name is the Praised One.

LXI-12 He will forgive you your sins and bring you into Gardens underneath which rivers flow, and pleasant dwellings in Gardens of Eden. That is the supreme triumph.

LXI-14 Oh he who believe! Be Allah's helpers, even if Jesus son of Mary said unto the disciples: Who are my helpers for Allah? They said: We are Allah's helpers. And a party of the Children of Israel believed while a party disbelieved. Then We strengthened those who believed against their foe, and they became the uppermost.

CIX In the name of Allah, the Beneficent, the Merciful. Say: Oh disbelievers!
I worship not that which ye worship;
nor worship ye that which I worship.
And I shall not worship that which ye worship.
Nor will ye worship that which I worship.
Unto you your religion, and unto me my religion.

CXIV In the name of Allah, the Beneficent, the Merciful.
Say: I seek refuge in the Lord of mankind,
The King of mankind,
The God of mankind
From the evil of the sneaking whisperer,
Who whispereth in the hearts of mankind,
Of the jinn and of mankind.

These one hundred (a strange coincidence) verses use words somewhat consistent with New Testament derivation or allusion such that dialogue to togetherness may be possible.

Verses of Violence

These really are Old Testament verses. . .basically unfulfilled by New Testament messages. These verses contain threats of violence and offer violence as a solution. Therein is a monotonous theme that one can do almost anything after reading, embracing and espousing these verses as ways of living. It is this Old Testament aspect of the verses which lead to abuse.

Whoever can learn to use these verses will be able to manipulate and control people in a way which must be against what Allah wants for his subjects. Whatever individual or family or group can learn to use these verses the loudest will be able to deprive people of choice.

While the resonance of the Koran is exhilarating and uplifting, it has been used to abuse. Notwithstanding its purported divine origin, it has become lethal because real infidels masquerading as Muslims have learned to manipulate people by calculated application of these verses. Allah needs no lethal aid nor blackmail nor enslaving families nor sycophantic interpreters turning divine messages into virulence.

By focusing on these verses, one endorses terror as legitimate and religious. One ends up on a monotonous morality hurdy gurdy, i.e. one is confined, controlled, believing it is fun and good to be going around in circles doing the same things over and over again except if you look the wrong way you will be butchered. In this regard, a call to prayer is not a call to prayer as much as it is a regimented genuflection to the families in power and to those who are controlling the people's understanding of the Koran. The abuse of the Koran is their political and social power by interpreting it for their own ends. Indeed, if one wants to get people to go to war for you, make it a religious experience. These self-proclaimed interpreters are themselves threatened by any deviation from what they proclaim, so they demand their followers to be confined, ignorant, believing and in misery without knowing it. The pedigree is one of power and not enlightened stewardship. A rigid approach is absolutely necessary because there is no capacity for self-renewal or flexibility as in changes of leaders.

In the Ottoman Empire, the death of the sultan meant a sudden grab for power by whichever of his offspring or relatives had enough backing; then the new sultan would promptly exterminate all other pretenders, murdering his brothers, nephews, and uncles to get rid of any competitors. While matters are not so gross today, they are little changed in the final analysis. Such is the impact of misinterpreting the Koran. Such recourse is automatically available to anyone who is the loudest in proclaiming that they are the rightful interpreters of the Koran.

This violence of us versus them is necessary to control, contort and manipulate the people. This is a cynical performance mouthing the Koran and at the same time toying with the people of God to do the biddings of those usurping the power and wrath that does not belong to anyone but Allah. Dissent or differences become so threatening that Muslim leaders can only react with violence. They must prevent an awareness or tolerance of different points of view. It is these verses (and more?) which enable the destruction of whoever offers differences. As interpreted, anything goes — even bombs to kill civilians of all ages. These verses remove guilt. In the final analysis, anyone emphasizing these verses are swindlers because by manipulating violently, they steal the Koran from the people (Not all violent verses are quoted).

II-178 O ye who believe! Retaliation is prescribed for you in the matter of the murdered; the freeman for the freeman, and the slave for the slave, and the female for the female. . . .

II-179 And there is life for you in retaliation, O men of understanding, that ye may ward off (evil).

II-191, 193.

II-216 Warfare is ordained for you, though it is hateful unto you; but it may happen that ye hate a thing which is good for you, and it may happen that ye love a thing which is bad for you. Allah knoweth, ye know not.

II-217, 244, 286.

III-106 On the day when (some) faces will be whitened and (some) faces will be blackened; and as for those whose faces have been blackened, it will be said unto them: Disbelieved ye after your (profession of) belief? Then taste the punishment for that ye disbelieve.

III-107 As for those whose faces have been whitened, lo! in the mercy of Allah they dwell for ever.

III-151, 181. 197.

IV-56, 74, 76, 84.

IV-91 Ye will find others who desire that they should have security from you, and security from their own folk. So often as they are returned to hostility they are plunged therein. If they keep not aloof from you nor offer you peace nor hold their hands, then take them and kill them wherever ye find them. Against such We have given you clear warrant.

IV-95 Those of the believers who sit still, other than those who have a (disabling) hurt, are not on an equality with those who strive in the way of Allah with their wealth and lives. . . .

IV-101 And when ye go forth in the land, it is no sin for you to curtail (your) worship if ye fear that those who disbelieve may attack you. In truth the disbelievers are an open enemy to you.

IV-102, 104.

IV-115 And whoso opposeth the messenger after the guidance (of Allah) hath been manifested unto him, and followeth other than the believer's way, We appoint for him that unto which he himself hath turned, and expose him unto hell — a hapless journey's end.

IV-133, 138, 139, 144, 161, 168.

V-14, 33.

V-38 As for the thief, both male and female, cut off their hands. It is the reward of their own deeds, and exemplary punishment from Allah. Allah is Mighty Wise.

V-45, 51, 57, 64, 72.
VI-17, 42, 47, 48, 49, 70, 94, 96, 125, 132, 136, 160.
VII-4, 5, 16, 39, 97, 164, 165, 168, 179.
VIII-2, 12, 13, 14, 16, 18, 29, 30, 32, 33.

VIII-35 And their worship at the (holy) House is naught but whistling and handclapping. Therefore (it is said unto them): Taste of the doom because ye disbelieve.

VIII-36, 37, 39, 50, 57, 58, 65, 67.
IX-3.

IX-5 Then, when the sacred months have passed, slay the idolaters wherever ye find them, and take them (captive), and beseige them, and prepare for them each ambush. . . . But if they repent and establish worship and pay the poor-due, then leave their way free. Lo! Allah is Forgiving, Merciful.

IX-12, 13, 14, 23, 26, 29.

IX-30 And the Jews say: Ezra is the son of Allah, and the Christians say: The Messiah is the son of Allah. That is their saying with their mouths. They imitate the saying of those who disbelieved of old. Allah (Himself) fighteth against them. How perverse are they!

IX-34, 35.

IX-36 . . .so wrong not yourselves in them. And wage war on all the idolaters as they are waging war on all of you. And know that Allah is with those who keep their duty (unto Him).

IX-41.

IX-49 . . .Lo! hell is all around the disbelievers.

IX-52, 63, 66, 68, 73, 74, 79.

IX-80 Ask forgiveness for them (O Mohammed), or ask not forgiveness for them; though thou ask forgiveness for them seventy times Allah will not forgive them. That is because they disbelieved in Allah and His messenger, and Allah guideth not wrongdoing folk.

IX-82, 83, 84, 85, 93, 101, 113, 123.
X-5, 51, 71, 74, 89, 101, 104, 105, 108.
XI-8, 20.
XIII-18, 25, 31, 32, 34, 42.
XIV-13, 16, 17.
XV-4, 23, 79.
XVI-25, 26, 29, 45, 46, 47, 63, 84, 85, 104.
XVII-7, 10.

XVII-16 And when We would destroy a township We send commandment to its folk who live at ease, and afterward they commit abomination therein, and so the Word (of doom) hath effect for it, and We annihilate it with complete annihilation.

XVII-52, 58.
XVIII-30, 51, 59, 60.
XX-48.
XXII-19, 20, 21.

XXII-22 Whenever, in their anguish, they would go forth from thence they are driven back therein and (it is said unto them): Taste the doom of burning.

XXIII-77.
XXIV-2, 4, 11, 23, 39, 57, 64.
XXV-13, 14, 19, 36, 37, 52.
XXVII-37, 51.
XXVIII-82, 86.
XXIX-23.
XXXI-24.
XXXII-21.
XXXIII-64.
XXXV-7.
XLI-6, 16, 27, 50.
XLII-26, 35, 45, 46.
XLIII-41, 42.
XLIV-11, 12, 15, 16, 47, 48.
XLV-7, 8, 9, 10, 11, 12.
XLVI-24, 25, 26, 27, 35.
XLVII-4, 8, 11, 12.
XLVIII-13, 25, 29.
L-24, 26.
LXV-1, 2, 4.

LXV-6 Lodge them where ye dwell, according to your wealth, and harass them not so as to straiten life for them. And if they are with child, then spend for them till they bring forth their burden. Then, if they give suck for you, give them their due payment and consult together in kindness; but if ye make difficulties for one another, then let some other woman give suck for him (the father of the child).

XCVIII-6.

Those are many of the Old Testament violent verses. There are probably more because I have only read the Koran three times.

Reading them, we see how understandable it was for Marco Polo to write in the twelfth century:

> The Saracens (Muslims) of Tobriz are wicked and treacherous. The law which the prophet Mohammed has given them has laid down that any harm they do to one who does not accept their law and any appropriation of goods is no sin at all, and if they suffer death or injury at the hands of Christians, they are accepted martyrs. For this reason they would be wrongdoers if it were not for the government. And all the other Saracens

> act on the same principle. When they are on the point of their death, up comes one of their priests and asks if Mohammed was the true messenger of God. If they answer "yes" then he tells them they are saved. . . . They are allowed great license to sin, and according to their law, no sin is forbidden. . . .
>
> Such is what happens when love is missing.

In any case, these "Old Testament" violent verses are certainly not part of the Western Civilization mode with a willingness to engage all peoples. The misapplication of these verses has defrauded other people by the creation of legends subjecting people to manipulation and abuse. These verses allow, foster and enable a control. They offer power for oneself and not for salvation when taken out of context and when used for the establishment of political and social empires. Any foe becomes a devil deserving of any doom.

It is highly unlikely that any book called "great" could promote such violence. Indeed, the Koran does not. The interpreters have. Such interpreters basically say: "If you can't stop me, Allah wills it."

Verses of Slavery

"Abd Allah" is a phrase which means "slave of God" and is a powerful designation for Muslims bonding to Allah and liberating themselves from all earthly servitude. To be a slave of Allah is what a Muslim professes to be.

With that comes the denotation that slavery is acceptable. Indeed, one sees throughout the social and political history of Islamic countries that slavery was rampant overtly in the past and covertly present today. The slave mentality is in the psychology of living as interpreters of the Koran have decreed. . . . No surprise since it is to the leaders' and any slaveholders' favor to believe and promote such.

Combining the slavery verses with the violence verses, resultant is a dehumanization of the human person to a non-entity deserving of nothing but being treated as chattel with two options: dead or slave. The themes of control and power usurping people's dignity exist in these interpretations. Indeed, whoever speaks for Allah somehow becomes Allah and with The Reading comes a selective, arbitrary, incomplete, self-serving controlling which goes far beyond The Reading itself. If one could only confine oneself to the Reading, the world would have been a better and different place.

It is this emphasis on "slave" which conveys an attitude which allows that one becomes not a slave to Allah but a slave to a family or a pretender of Allah. One becomes a robot of the Koran — or more precisely a robot of the family or families pretending to speak for the messenger and for the Koran. Slavery makes one to believe everything but the Koran. Slavery enables one to believe anybody but the messenger. In fact, one can become so slavish that one has not the faintest idea of an alternative except an intense objecting to the mere idea of becoming anything other than a mindless robot. . .a freedomless ant in a termitary.

The slavery theme is so inherent that it easily becomes misused by anyone who gets to be the slaver. It becomes misused by anyone who pretends to imitate Allah in Allah's name. Not being able to read, the slavers prohibit others from reading, from analyzing, from discussing. The slavers impose an antithesis of freedom and an outright effort to enslave others under the guise of "conversion." This is enhanced by a mythical espousal of The Reading when what they are really for is power, control and empire-building.

It is difficult to have any other interpretation after reading the Koran in view of what all has been done in its name. The trade-off is clear: A contained, coherent, constricted, simple society superficially satisfying and cultically exuberant for those slavers and their slaves as they war against the world.

The following are verses of slavery:

II-177, 178.
IV-3, 24, 92.
V-89, 118.
VI-18.
VII-194.
VIII-51, 67, 70.
XII-24.
XV-40, 42, 49.
XVI-75.
XVII-3, 5, 7, 17, 30, 96.
XVIII-1, 66.
XIX-93.
XXI-26, 105.
XXIII-6, 109.
XXIV-31, 32, 33, 58.
XXVII-15, 19, 59.
XXVIII-82.
XXXIII-55.
XXXIV-9.
XXXV-45.
XXXVII-40, 74, 81, 111, 128, 160, 169.
XXXVIII-84.
XXXIX-36, 46, 53.
XLI-46.
XLII-19.
XLIII-19, 59, 68.

XLIV-23.
L-30
LIII-11.
LVIII-3.
XCVI-10.

Properly understood in the context of the times, there is nothing too wrong with the slave concept as emphasized in the Koran. In fact, a case can be made that there is emphasis on freeing slaves. However, those who misappropriated the Koran, misinterpreted it to incorporate slavery of non-believers into daily culture mores and activities. History reveals that more people were enslaved (if not believers) than were ever set free. Indeed, almost all commercialized slave trade, even that characterized by Western efficiency, has roots traceable back to the methodical dehumanizing slavery endemic to ancient Islamic communities. In the final analysis, if one was a believer in Islam, you could get your own slaves. . .and that had a great appeal. . .and that is where the problem lay, because any group espousing slavery must be very aggressive against those objecting. Anyone against the slavers will perforce be seen as malevolent and a focus onto which leaders will externalize all blame for whatever goes wrong. This tacit slavery and dehumanizing treatment of others can even be seen in the Black Nation of Islam in the United States. It is obviously still present in many Islamic countries especially as child labor.

It is accurate to divide human slavery into two types: (1) social, individual, stabilizing, contractual, i.e. biblical, and (2) brutal, commercial, dehumanizing, total, i.e. Islamic. When the facts of the origin of barbaric exploitative slavery (in contrast to the civilizing trade off slavery of the Bible for example) are known, no person can well embrace Islam if his family has ever been affected by slavery. Without a doubt, Islam, or rather abusers of Islam, taught the world the worst slavery.

The end result of slavery acceptance in excess by interpreters of the Koran has been the subliminal acceptance of slavery and its gross commercialization with the dedignification and dehumanization of disbelieving peoples because they were to be put under believers' control. Such interpreters basically say: "If I'm a slave of Allah, you are a slave of mine."

To the contrary: "I no longer speak of you as slaves, for a slave does not know what his master is about. Instead, I call you friends, since I have made known to you all that I heard from my Father." — Jesus in St. John's Gospel 15:15.

Verses of Love

As I read the Koran, I attempted to list all the verses which merely mentioned the word "love" regardless of context or meaning.

II-190 Allah loveth not aggressors.

II-216 Warfare is ordained for you, though it is hateful unto you; but it may happen that ye hate a thing which is good for you, and it may happen that ye love a thing that is bad for you. Allah knoweth, ye know not.

II-222 They question thee (Oh Muhammad) concerning menstruation. Say: It is an illness, so let women alone at such times and go not in onto them until they are cleansed. And when they have purified themselves, then go in onto them as Allah hath enjoined upon you. Truly Allah loveth those who turn onto Him, and loveth those who have a care for cleanness.

II-276 Allah hath blighted usury and made alms giving fruitful. Allah loveth not the impious and guilty.

III-119 Lo! Ye are those who love them though they love you not, and ye believe in all the Scripture. When they fall in with you they say: We believe; but when they go apart they bite their fingertips at you, for rage. Say: Perish in your rage!

III-159 . . .Allah loveth those who put their trust (in Him).

IV-73 And if a bounty from Allah befell you, he would surely cry, as if there had been no love between you and him: Oh, would that I had been with them, then should I have achieved a great success!

IV-148 Allah loveth not the utterance of harsh speech save by one who hath been wronged. . . .

V-13 . . .Allah loveth the kindly.

V-18 The Jews and Christians say: We are sons of Allah and His Loved ones. . . .

V-64 And Allah loveth not corrupters.

V-93 . . .Allah loveth the good.

VII-55 (Oh mankind!) Call upon your Lord humbly and in secret. Lo! He loveth not aggressors.

IX-7 . . .Allah loveth those who keep their duty.

XI-90 Ask pardon of your Lord and then turn unto Him (repentant). Lo! My Lord is Merciful, Loving.

XXVIII-76 . . .Allah loveth not the exultant;

LXXXIX-20 And love wealth with abounding love.

Of the over six thousand verses in the Koran, I found seventeen that contained the word "love." I believe I must have missed the word "love" a few times in my three readings of the Koran. I certainly hope so.

As used in the Koran, however, the theme of love seems meager and difficult to stretch into "loving one another." In fact, the distinct sense is that love is a dimension that belongs to God alone and such is not possible for and between humans. The idea of love between humans is given short shrift, and it would hardly be authentic to add to the Koran more love than what little is contained therein.

> If I speak in the tongues of mortals and of angels, but do not have love, I am a noisy gong or a clanging cymbal. And if I have prophetic powers, and understand all mysteries and all knowledge, and if I have all faith, so as to remove mountains, but do not have love, I am nothing. If I give away all my possessions, and if I hand over my body so that I may boast, but do not have love, I gain nothing.
> Love is patient; love is kind; love is not envious or boastful or arrogant or rude. It does not insist on its own way; it is not irritable or resentful; it does not rejoice in wrongdoing, but rejoices in the truth. It bears all things, believes all things, hopes all things, endures all things.
> Love never ends. But as for prophecies, they will come to an end; as for tongues, they will cease; as for knowledge, it will come to an end. For we know only in part, and we prophesy only in part; but when the complete comes, the partial will come to an end. When I was a child, I spoke like a child, I thought like a child, I reasoned like a child; when I became an adult, I put an end to childish ways. For now we see in a mirror, dimly, but then we will see face to face. Now I know only in part; then I will know fully, even as I have been fully known. And now faith, hope, and love abide, these three; and the greatest of these is love.
> (Love nine times)—1 Corinthians 13

FIVE PILLARS OF ISLAM

The most common derivation from the Koran is the "Five Pillars" of Islam: (1) Alms giving, (2) Prayer, (3) Pilgrimage to Mecca, (4) Ramadan Fast, and (5) Profession of God's Unity and Mohammed's Prophethood.

To accept these five "pillars" is not a large problem because they tend to be global to being, in a sense. But to derive them is no small feat. Who was delegated to emphasize them and decree their being absolute and exhaustive in one's duty to Allah? On what basis were these pillars emphasized in contrast to other directions in the Koran?

Interpretations of the Koran have resulted in different Islamic sects, an expected outcome when there is no primary interpreter. Indeed, what happened to the Koran has happened to almost all the great books: Interpreters emphasize their particular needs and beliefs with a self-serving dimension to a self-interpretation of the Koran unless all is subjected to the natural reason given to all mankind and to an authority delegated to help all mankind.

OLD TESTAMENT/NEW TESTAMENT

The Koran Allah gave to me is easily recognizable as a poetic rewriting and dramatic rendition of parts of the Christian Bible (Old and New Testaments) as believed dictated by the Angel Gabriel to Mohammed. In a real sense, the Koran cannot be separated from the Old and New Testaments and as such is the Word of God in a derived sense. Obviously, it can be translated. . .although I have my doubts about if it can be *interpreted*. If read, this poetic rendering is appropriately seen to be a point/counterpoint describing of Old Testament events and themes versus New Testament fulfillments. That social conflict was ongoing at the time between Old Testament clingers and New Testament believers is incontrovertible. Perhaps it is the Old Testament/New Testament conflict and confusion that accounts for Angel Gabriel's message: The Koran is to be a compilation of the then present emotional and historical ferment and was not a replacement for the Book but was a condensed and condensing focus. The yes/no bewilderment therein is a kindling for emotion about the exuberant and violent Old Testament alternating with the Loving Truth messages from the New Testament, but few specific directions are given without contradiction. It denies the Trinity having misinterpreted it as three gods but nevertheless Allah is "We" throughout. And it goes on and on with contradictory messages reasonably interpreted as an Old Testament/New Testament choosing. This explains how *power* appropriates the Koran. Power became the decisive interpreter for the Koran rather than the reasoned, unemotional, love and peace orientation of the New Testament, even though this orientation itself is in the Koran!

The Koran is an amalgam of undefined and undistinguishable Old/New Testament ferment giving a persistent emotional and unreasoned lack of understanding consistent with "a reading by someone who knows not how to read." Such is miraculous. But many can read even though not Arabic. . .and those of us in that category demand too to use reason as Allah gave it to us.

No doubt, the social-political controversies of the day added to the power distortions and frustrated a peaceful New Testament resolution of what the Angel Gabriel was telling Mohammed.

Anyone aware of history realizes how this has been a tragedy of no small significance. The reason is that the vengeful Old Testament emphasis is a distortion of Mohammed by his interpreters and a demeaning misrepresentation of the Koran itself. The wrath-of-God style of the Old Testament with the theocratic tyranny, missionary work by sword, slavery of disbelievers, and the inability to apostatize when one's own reasoning, deformed or correct, forces otherwise, create an extreme degree of unfreedom which is incompatible with the Divine Being.

This is not to say that the Old Testament or the Koran is irrational — but the oneness of mankind based on natural reason points to the New Testament fulfillment. All reason must decree that reason itself should provide the truth and the good. Allah has given it to us. One must use it regardless of emotion, poetry, and power.

MOHAMMED

Emphatically, one should not fault Mohammed whom all Christians can believe was a summarizing prophetic reciter of the ferment as the Old passes to the New Testament. Living some 600 years after Christ, he had access to the Old and New Testaments which is obvious when one reads the Koran. Probably a Christian slave tried to convert him with a fervent recitation of the Torah and Gospels which prepared Mohammed somewhat for his visions. Thus, the mission of Mohammed may have been to marry the old and new, offering people an opportunity to embrace them both emotionally in what should have been an effort resolving the book of the old versus the book of the new, with the house of tears converted to the house of joy.

As the Koran says (III, 144), "And Mohammed is but a messenger, messenger the like of whom hath passed away before him." Hardly someone to adore by the Koran's own recognizing. The Koran itself does not appear to exalt Mohammed beyond that of messenger. It does not proclaim him as prophet.

JESUS

Islamic interpreters of the Koran have clearly identified Jesus as a prophet also.

On the one hand, in the Koran, Jesus is called "the Messiah." On the other hand, he is called "only a messenger of Allah." This is clearly an example of the point/counterpoint presentation of the conflict extant at the time without articulated resolution.

But, there really is no problem in that Jesus has two natures as the New Testament clarifies and an evident conclusion of the mind as it studies the New Testament.

Furthermore, there is a troubling self-contradictory dimension if Jesus is accepted as a prophet but his words are not believed. As a prophet, Jesus must be believed. Truly, right reason demands that as "real prophet," Jesus' actual words which identify him as both God and man are to be taken at face value, providing a marvelous linkage of God to humanity. It confirms the New Testament of God reaching out to humanity in a way which must be beyond our reason. Jesus' words are not point/counterpoint. Neither is the New Testament. The New Testament is the answer. The Koran says so but also the opposite in a point/counterpoint way (perhaps as a catalyst to think-it-through rather than power-it-out — or that is how it should have been had psychosocial power factors not usurped the Koran).

In comparable manner, the remainder of Jesus' words in terms of establishing a Church to interpret all the Word (including all Books), Himself as the Son of God, the Trinity, and other revelations must be accepted. To deny Jesus' words but to accept his prophethood results in an internal self-contradiction to any interpretation (misinterpretation really) of Islam.

What is in the Koran is in the Koran. Who can tell us what it means? What can tell us what it means? Do not vicious historical events due to the Road of

Power make it clear that the Koran has been misinterpreted? Is not a dialogue of love at last indicated?

THE ROMAN CATHOLIC CHURCH

Ambiguous points/counterpoints throughout the Koran emphasize that it is not a "catechism" or a guide at all but a poetic perambulation of mental imagery for the nonreader. It provides the questions that those who do read must themselves sort out consistent with the Jewish-Christian (Old Testament-New Testament) conflict that was ongoing at the time. Speaking for the great mass of unreading humanity, these questions must be asked about what is the meaning of language? The Word? God? The Divine Being? And where, oh where, can one get the answers?

It seems obvious that what happened to the Koran is what happened to the Christian Bible. Most of those who have interpreted it have distorted it giving rise to heresy. Hilaire Belloc has written about "the heresy of Mohammed":

> He (Mohammed) preached and insisted upon a whole group of ideas which were peculiar to the Catholic Church and distinguished it from the paganism it had conquered in the Greek and Roman civilizations. Thus the very foundation of his teaching was that prime Catholic doctrine, the unity and omnipotence of God. The attributes of God he also took over in the main from Catholic doctrine: the personal nature, the all-goodness, the timelessness, the providence of God, His creative power as the origin of all things, and His sustenance of all things by His power alone. The world of good spirits and angels and of evil spirits and rebellion against God was part of the teaching, with a chief evil spirit, such as Christendom had recognized. Mohammed preached with insistence that prime Catholic doctrine, on the human side — the immortality of the soul and its responsibility for actions in this life, coupled with the consequent doctrine of punishment and reward after death.

Nevertheless and in fact, the Christian Bible was obviously referred to in the Mohammed-Angel Gabriel collaboration, and therefore it must not be forgotten that the interpretation of the Christian Bible belongs to the group that gave it to the world: The Bible itself of the New Testament was given to the world by the Roman Catholic Church.

From this fact devolves the understanding that the Roman Catholic Church must be looked to not only for a valid interpretation of Old and New Testaments, but also of the Koran, because the Koran itself is an amalgam of poetic conflict impossible to take literally.

The Koran is to enhance the emotional exuberant energies of the people to struggle with the words of the great books. And these great books, in the final analysis, can be found to have but one interpreter from whom answers must genuinely be sought: The Roman Catholic Church. Jesus said so. In a real sense as THE WORD, all words must be ruled by Him. . .and by the Church He founded.

History shows that whenever any of the great books have been interpreted by others, the end-result has been negative with more hate and vengeful discontent than need be. A deeper use of reason rather than emotion from those who indeed can actually read is needed. The Roman Catholic Church must tell us what the Koran means. The Church must tell us what all books mean. Perhaps the Koran can be translated. . .but it cannot be interpreted. . .except by the proper authority.

THIRD MILLENNIUM

If the third millennium is to be characterized by a new world which includes Islam, then Islam must look hard and fast into itself with an appropriate, wise, rational interpretation of the Koran as Mohammed gave it and not as anyone lesser can co-author except the Church created by one of Islam's prophets and upon which Mohammed himself relied: The Roman Catholic Church.

The Church must communicate in dialogue with Islamic scholars themselves over the interpretations of the Koran as it refers to the Old and New Testaments as given to the world by the Roman Catholic Church some 500 years prior to the birth of Mohammed.

The Qiblah (the place where Muslims face when they pray) changed from Jerusalem to Mecca once. It can and must change again, this time to Rome. When that happens, all Muslims will be in genuine oneness once again with their ancestors. . .the ancient pre-Islamic Catholics who covered the Middle East and environs.

This considered dialogue must begin with the historical fact of these sequences of events and a considered effort not to repeat the mistakes of the past caused by misinterpretations and an intolerance which is countenanced neither in the New Testament itself nor in the New Testament verses of the Koran.

To operate under the Old Testament rules is to emphasize power, violence, confusion and emotion. To operate under New Testament rules is to follow charity, love, and reason. The Old Testament is when God reaches out with love, and humans of course mess it up again but not as badly and with great opportunity for oneness. Allah has given us an interpreter of the Words.

To some extent, a case can be made that the Roman Catholic Church abides by and promotes some verses as well as many Muslims. Perhaps those interested in this New Testament emphasis in the Koran could become followers of Allah as Roman Catholic "slaves of Allah" provided the New Testament verses are embraced with themes of love amplified consistent with a genuine reading of the Gospels. The phrase "Al Islam" is "the Surrender to Allah." This would seem to be a surrender in a non-contradictory way to servitude to God and His themes of transcendental humanity, truth, good, oneness and beauty.

Unfortunately, servitude interpreters won't like it. And their wealthy, controlling families won't like it at all. Guess which verses will get most promoted by them. And we now have a list of the New Testament verses which must be promoted in response!

"Islam" means "submission to the will of Allah," and "Muslim" (derived from "Islam") refers to all those who have submitted which automatically places believers into a common togetherness superseding all other considerations of race or nation. Actually, this sounds pretty "Catholic." So why not "New Testament Muslims?" In the final analysis, the New Testament verses belong to the world and to humanity. They may provide a way to prevent the refighting of old battles, battles which will serve no one's best interest except the ruling families and leaders who have pretended to be owners of the Koran by Old Testament approaches.

As written before: the Loving Truth of Jesus can be the only message that really makes sense if one is a believer in the Old Testament and, I add now, the Koran. Would a Messiah from Allah bring a more violent message than what was existent at the time? Is it not true that Judaism, Islam, Buddhism, and Hinduism are all fulfilled by the New Testament, because the New Testament gives solidarity and civilization unduplicated except by the principles of the Roman Catholic Church?

FINAL COMMENT

Allah has given me a translation. I can read. I can reason. It is obvious that the Reading has been misused for power, by power, seeking power. Power has stolen the Reading from the people. Power is not in the reading without contradiction. Power is the infidel.

Indeed, anything but the Words in the Reading itself is added emotionality.

If the Angel Gabriel gave the Reading to Mohammed, that is all that was given. But the Angel Gabriel also is in the New Testament and the Koran depends heavily on the Gospels and the Old Testament. So there is a linkage. And thus a case can be reasonably that the Reading (the Koran) is as Catholic as the Book (Jewish Old Testament and Catholic New Testament) itself, genuinely Catholic even if not "Roman."

Muslim brothers and sisters must reject those who have distorted the Book and the Reading into instruments of power and vengeance. Christians and Jews too must reject those who have distorted the Word of God into instruments of power and vengeance.

THE FATIHAH *(the Lord's Prayer of Islam)*

In the name of Allah
The Beneficent (Yes!)
The Merciful (Absolutely merciful!)
Praise be to Allah (Yes!)
Lord of Creation (over infidels who would impose power)
The Beneficent (Yes!)
The Merciful (Absolutely merciful!)
King of the Last Judgment (no pretenders and no fake interpreters, please!)
You alone we worship (no problem); and to
You alone we pray for help (no problem).
Guide us to the straight path (yes, with love)
The path you have chosen (not what the powerful have imposed for vengeance)
And not of those who have incurred your wrath (It is *Your* wrath, not the wrath of people or pretenders of the Book and Reading)
Nor of those who have gone astray ("Astray" are those who pretend wrath is theirs, act unmercifully and avoid beneficence).

Once upon a time, many of the ancestors of Islamic people were Catholic. This root was lost by doctrinal innovations and power. The only entity to have been present throughout it all from the beginning is the Roman Catholic Church rendering her to be historically qualified to authenticate the oneness of Words. The Christian roots cannot be denied. The oneness of humanity has been subverted by power. It is time to return to Loving Truth. Whatever does not is not the Church. . .nor is it the Mosque.

> . . .to all other men, the Catholic Church is their Father's house. Where else shall human beings turn if they are to keep the freedom and dignity of human beings? As the world we have known passes away, and kingdoms and empires fall, only this unique Institution continues the same; she only, because Christ lives in her, remains a center and norm of sanity in thought and action. (source lost)

CHAPTER 16:

RAPPROACHEMENT: MILITARY SERVICE

Having spent three years in the U.S. Navy Submarine Service, I have mixed feelings about military service. In my generation, *every qualified male* served. It was a good experience. It was an enriching experience. We were together in wanting to defend one's country.

However, the exaggerated implementation of the "separation of church and state" to the degree of oppression and abuse of the Roman Catholic Church has made me reconsider a blind patriotism and involvement in military service. Indeed, the "separation of church and state" has not been implemented well enough, meaning that it has only been implemented "one way." The state cannot help the church. Obviously, the church must be careful about helping the state. Genuine Catholics, therefore, need to rethink their role in the military and indeed the entire system of nations.

No overstatement this: The nation system is moribund. The term "United Nations" is an oxymoron. National orientation has little planetary value and is basically contra-world, because nationalism is universally contaminated with selfish interests as defined by national boundaries in imaginary spheres of national influence. A critical study would reveal that nationalism has rarely proven more than expedient in providing benefits. The most beneficial aspect of any nation is due to the people involved. Truly, if the people are no good, the U.S. Constitution will not work either. In fact, the U.S. model has been tried many, many times without success because the goodness of the people is the most important element in the worth of a "nation" concept. It is possible that there will never be genuine peace until nationalism is recognized to be a false god.

Comparable to what "atheism" purports to believe about God, I propose "negopatriotism" to be how one should feel about nations.

As Teilhard de Chardin stated: "The age of nations is past. If we are to live, now is the time to build the EARTH."

"Building the earth . . ." such is what Roman Catholicism is all about. It goes beyond mere national hyperbole. Nationalism is essentially irrelevant in today's world except for Olympic sports.

There is no question that it is appropriate and morally correct to defend one's homeland. The Catholic tradition has held since St. Augustine that just wars are possible and, as St. Augustine wrote — "soldiers should perform their military duties in behalf of the peace and safety of the community." But today, one must ask: On behalf of a genuine community? Or a mumbo jumbo spent civilization?

To be duped into serving for leaders whose motives are unjust and immoral or to die in provocative actions elsewhere supposedly protecting an immoral society is absurd. If the people back home are no good, military service is stupid.

Catholic youths should be helped to be more discriminating and suspect of military service as it undertakes efforts far removed from "defending one's homeland."

To "render to Caesar" is not the same as listening to or following corrupt, dishonest, and immoral politicians.

While the first formally established principle of religious liberty in the United States if not the world was by the Catholic Calvert family in Maryland in 1634, Catholics have been the victims more than the beneficiaries of United States' style of religious freedom. In numbers, the U.S. press and media have been worse than Roman Emperor Nero's effects on the Roman Catholic Church.

The way Catholics have been used and the way Catholics have been abused both justify the conclusion that United States "pluralism" does not, if it ever did, fully include Catholics *unless* we subvert ourselves. That subverting should no longer encompass Catholic youth as cannon-fodder for an establishment that will not fairly treat Catholics as pluralistic equals.

In three words: Beware of Caesar! Enough militarism. Enough nationalism except for organizational purposes. Do we belong to God or not? Christ did not die for any country, ideology, or state. He died for you and me and the state of our souls — that we may enter eternity.

True freedom is in Catholicism not militarism. This should also hold true for any country and not merely the United States.

Follow the politics of the Apostles Creed and the Our Father if you really want to do some good. Stay out of the military. Keep a "Serve First List." Go into the priesthood or convent instead or take close care of your family. That way you can really make the world a better place. Reach out to others but hunker down and protect your own. Defend your homeland by defending your home at home and your church at church. Let the abortion promoters serve first. Let the press and media owners' offspring serve first. Let judges', legislators' and politicians' offspring serve and die first before your own.

To these purposes I rewrote the words for "The Star Spangled Banner" into an "American Revolutionary Anthem." Compared to the usual song, these words fit rather well and can be sung unobtrusively and comfortably.

O say can you see, the Revolution in me?
What so proudly we hail against oppression, death, and hate?
Whose proud ideals and broad aims give Life and Liberty
O'er happiness we save the Family's fate?
Not for profits we care,
Nor for violence or despair,
Give proof through any blight that all Rights are still here.
O say does that Revolution still rave
O'er the land of the free and the home of the brave?

About military service, the suggestions are to repudiate it totally with the exception of homeguard:

1. Implement fully the church-state separation which has been used so vigorously by not allowing the state to support the church in any way. In the same way, the state should be removed from all church activities and church grounds. No flags. No pledges of allegiance. No state songs. No national anthems. No recruiters. No military units on college campuses. No entertainment by military grandiosities. The anticlericalism of the state must be exactly mirrored by an anti-militarism of the Church.
2. Teach trans-national values of total Catholicity and the world community. To build the earth is what Roman Catholicism is all about. It goes beyond mere national hyperbole. Nationalism should be taught as essentially irrelevant in today's world except for Olympics and organizational purposes.
3. Help youths understand that *governments oppress their people* — which must have been what Thomas Jefferson was thinking when he said: "Governments that govern least govern best." Help youths keep their distance from the government. "Just consider me already to be a military casualty and get out of my way, I want to do some good!" Teach that the state will always turn into an oppressor of people. The truth is that upon analysis government is routinely, if not always, deserving of contempt. It is usually corrupted and corrupting of all who get involved. This is a near truism applying to governments and politicians everywhere, including judges, legislators, presidents, government employees, etc. Deep, accurate study justifies contempt of government except when clearly proving an exception. Teach that the Church has always been the bulwark for the people against the state. Serving the Church serves the earth and the world much better, more efficiently and more effectively than any service for any state. The Church provides an alternative to government.
4. Educational efforts must create a great caution and wariness of governments. The United States government has not supported its soldiers in military operations such as Vietnam, and the public is unlikely to support fully

any military operation anywhere else (and then one should not believe the news reports either). Youth needs to know that they should not be cannon fodder for a government or for a public which will not support them. The U.S. government has let hostages rot for years. Offspring of those who rule (and this includes those in the press and media) must first serve and first die in any military excursion outside one's homeland.

5. The only acceptable uniforms are other than military, i.e. the Roman collar and those charming, distinctive veils for religious, and more . . . .
6. Catholic youths should be helped to be more discriminating and suspect of military service as it undertakes efforts far removed from "defending one's homeland." This can be brought home graphically to today's youth when they discover that more of their U.S. peers have been killed by abortion in *each year since 1972* than *all* U.S. soldiers in *all* combat since the founding of the United States. In essence, *no place outside your homeland is worth a drop of blood.* Conscientious objection to military service outside of one's homeland should be promoted by any group professing to want world peace instead of whimpering about budgets.

If everyone were to follow this chapter, there would be no wars.

While movies are suspect as sources of information, there are two movies based on historical events which can help Catholic youth keep military service in perspective. First is *The Silence* which reveals the abuse a Catholic Italian-American had to take while a student at West Point. While the movie does not emphasize the student's Catholicity or Italianness, its very failure to do so further underscores the blind bigotry of Hollywood. Second is *The Execution of Private Slovik* which tells the true story of a simple Catholic kid who refused to follow orders with which he could not agree. He was the only American executed by the United States Army in World War II. His Catholicism succored him through. To those of us familiar with the anti-Catholic bigotry of Dwight Eisenhower and much of the military services, the reason for his execution is clearly linked to ulterior motives. Every Catholic youth should be familiar with both movies.

CHAPTER 17:

ANTI-CATHOLICISM — GET USED TO IT

The Roman Catholic Church is not a vehicle for hatred. The Church truly does not promote hatred. To the contrary, the Church attempts to keep trust with Christ and the apostles.

Unfortunately, the human dimension of the Church has erred often, but the main thrust of the Church over and over has been Loving Truth and rejection of hatred.

While not a vehicle for hatred, it has been and still is a target of hatred. Just as Jesus Christ was slandered, persecuted, and crucified, so the Roman Catholic Church as the Body of Christ continues still to be persecuted. Such is what happens to those who promote Loving Truth: Do good and avoid evil, imitate Christ — the joy is insurmountable, but the Cross will be yours. Indeed, to slander the Roman Catholic Church is to crucify Christ. Those leaving it usually are unwittingly offering a tribute to it. To promote the Roman Catholic Church is to promote Loving Truth and at the same time Jesus Christ as personal Lord and Savior. That is what those leaving are leaving whether they believe it or not: Jesus and His apostles. And to believe others not in concert with the apostles is absurd.

To reject Jesus Christ and His Church as originally founded and formed by the apostles requires a mammoth degree of arrogant pride which can only be sustained by incessantly projected hostility. Such proud hostility will be directed to and felt often by Roman Catholics when dealing with non-Catholics. Not that all non-Catholics are of such a nature — but many are.

Whenever any one or group attacks the Roman Catholic Church with hostility, you will find, upon investigation, that what they attack is either a deviant historical distortion repudiated by the Church itself, or the attack is a paranoid projection. A good case can be made that when anti-Catholics talk about the Roman Catholic Church, they are talking about themselves.

Some of the frequent errors of such individuals are the following:

1. They often rewrite history, and they often do not care about or do not adequately research their statements.
2. They often are not interested in Loving Truth.
3. They are really into "sales" of their own group — by a plethora of one-line putdowns of the Catholic Church.
4. They are using the Catholic Church as stomping platform to exalt themselves.
5. They will often flood others with many brief distortions, each requiring extensive rebuttal for which much time would be needed to correct them completely.
6. They appear to luxuriate in suspicion and hatred with ominous enticing excitement, flinging one-liners exalting themselves at the expense of the Catholic Church.
7. They preach hatred of Catholicism but pretend love, which is impossible without truth.
8. Their research is not research at all but a repetition of other anti-Catholic lack of research.
9. They are often unfair, untrue, and unreliable, but overcome all that by a sensationalism of self-importance.
10. They are often loud and smugly confident in their berating of Catholicism.
11. Their own messages are often meaningless in and of themselves, so a victim (Catholicism) is needed as a foil about which to build their reputations.
12. At times they convey neither grace nor truth but a sham, a parody, and a "feel good" chorus of "I'm saved and you are damned — so I can do anything" (except be a Catholic?).
13. They do not convey well the word of God but words of hate, and they often wound people unnecessarily.
14. At times they are held together by anti-Catholic glue — rendering the message of the Bible hateful.
15. Relying on *sola Scriptura* wherein each person has free interpretation of the Bible, they deprive Roman Catholics of that very right which they proclaim for themselves in a major self-contradiction.
16. They generally comprise a school for prevarication, providing courses in Catholic hating. They bail out with the pat statement: "God tells me . . .whatever." Which gives them carte blanche to do what they please and to ignore Loving Truth.
17. They basically are good rhetoricians — who are not interested in truth.

Because of all the above, Roman Catholics are generally at a disadvantage in the debates into which they are forced at times. It is no wonder that many Catholics find themselves overwhelmed or doubting the one true Church. However, for those struggling, partial temporary answers may be in the following statements (unfortunately, often true when dealing with anti-Catholics):

1. The Loving Truth of Jesus Christ is not what you say it is.
2. I wonder what you will believe in when you find that all these wild, outrageous statements are not true. Unfortunately, you have dug yourself into a hole — you have made so many of these statements, you could devote your life to finding out how they all are wrong. I am not asking you to search them all out — but just check out a few in depth, using all the library and resource materials available. Perhaps if you heard what genuine Roman Catholics have to say about this, you may allow Catholics to have their own interpretations — which, to your surprise, may be nearer to what Christ taught than what you are now doing and believing. Just take one or two of your negative statements and check them out with Christian fairness, honesty, and balanced search for truth — and not just with Lorraine Boettner (a popular author of anti-Catholic tracts) either. Believe me, if one or two of these outrageous statements do not hold up, you might want to join us Catholics instead of continuing to believe people whom you yourself have demonstrated to have lied to you. If a teacher tells you one lie, they are unbelievable about almost everything else.
3. It would appear that your brand of religion claims that you can only be "good" when you are attacking imaginary evil. Somehow it is sad that one loud "Hallelujah, I have been saved because I take Jesus Christ as my personal Lord and Redeemer" allows you to do and say anything you want and feel right about it.
4. Why cannot we Catholics accept our Church's own interpretation of Scripture if you claim that free interpretation is the norm? Or does *sola Scriptura* only belong to non-Catholic preachers?
5. Whatever the Church teaches and has taught has been thought out by an incredibly deeply researched process. If you grasp what it takes for a term paper or even a doctoral thesis, those efforts pale in comparison to the agonizing appraisal and study that has gone into what the Catholic Church teaches. These are not just old men coming up with wild ideas. It is ignorant to listen to contemporary holler guys and ignore the early writers of Christianity and those who have studied their writings in depth.
6. If you believe you have been saved by proclaiming "Hallelujah, I take Jesus Christ as my personal Lord and Redeemer," then you could even be a Roman Catholic and still be saved. So stop badgering me because I too take Jesus Christ as my personal Lord and Redeemer, only my personal relationship with the Savior is through the Church He founded as confirmed in the Loving Truth of the apostles and early preachers (Fathers) of the Church.
7. As a Catholic, I have a subdued reverential awe pleading for a continuing relationship (grace) with Jesus and I want to do what He would want me to do by active imitation of Christ. In my personal relationship with the Lord, I am justified and saved in your terms, but in my

own terms, I believe I am only justified and must work to be saved by cleaning myself as Jesus would want through the one True Church He founded. Nothing unclean can get to Heaven, and I cannot believe screaming "I'm saved, et cetera" will force my way to God.

8. To me, proclaiming "I'm saved" sounds like a demand out of abject terror — perhaps you'd feel more comfortable doing good works?
9. You remind me of the story about the person who held his hand up with his pointing finger toward the bright object in the sky and said, "Look at the moon." Another person who saw him do that, went up and looked intently at the pointing finger and said, "My, my — is that really the moon?" It seems you are holding up the Bible and saying, "Here is God" and people are mistaking the Bible for God as the other man mistook the pointing finger for the moon.
10. You don't sound like a disciple of Christ to me, but a disciple of Lorraine Boettner and his fake "Bible" *Roman Catholicism* — a book which might be the biggest collection of lies ever under one cover.
11. To me, here is what you seem to be saying: "Hallelujah — I can hate now — I am forever right now — I am infallible now — I have been saved now — No rules, logic, actions, or honesty are needed." That's what you sound like, and that is no message from Jesus.
12. Nowhere in the Bible does it say that the Bible is literally to be believed alone or that the Bible alone is the only basis for true religion. If you mean what you say, that the Bible is perfect as is, how can you ADD to it (which is what you are doing if you claim it to be literally alone on which all rests — when the Bible itself does not claim such)?

Under the heading of "Anti-Catholicism" also belongs the phenomena of despiritualization caused by the contemporary electronic-celluloid culture.

"Thou Shalt not have false gods before you."

Step back and think about it: Electronic-celluloid experiences (of television and movies) dehumanize and, more so, despiritualize as nothing before in history. There is *nothing* there but photons in a box or on a screen! People are flickering lights relating in *absentia* yet intoxicating the viewer to a numbing style of vicarious living (which is really a form of premature death for the observers), subliminally conveying the message that not much really matters except those exciting, flickering-light, ersatz people. Except for occasional information and rare aesthetics, electronic-celluloid experience in totality is a fraud. Television and movies fool us to disdain real life for voyeurism, passioned counterfeit, degrading fantasy and dirty jokes as life-styles. Television and movies subtly engulf us with an electronic-celluloid culture of disgust which creates human inertia. It embalms us.

These dramatizations apply: Television-movie culture is an intellectual vacuum cleaner. It is an automatic brain drain. It destroys spirit. It is a decerebration mechanism for painless lobotomies, converting *terra firma* into *terra video*. The final fallacy is *argumentum ad pulvinar* (the couch). By the electronic-celluloid mode, we now worship not the Golden Calf, but the Illumined Jackass! or is it the Flickering Flashbulb? And you never have to memorize anything! We are controlled by a perpetual illiteracy machine, i.e. one can neither read nor write when the telly is on or when watching a movie. Electronic-celluloid experiences are an exciting waste of time — an intoxicating vapor — a new "Stoned" Age — a marauding muse — a Lorelei (rarely other than bereft of reality or salutary virtue) enslaving by cheap thrills those unable to assert themselves and paralyzing by stimulus overload those who have an assertive capacity. Amusement has run amock with moral suicide by phosphorescence of sex and violence. Humanity is reduced to the most basic of material components: *the color spectrum photons and shadows* emphasizing the human (in contrast to the "divine") component only and then without refinement and, furthermore, even without confidence in having seen the truth (which also does not seem to matter any longer either). No cerebral dominance is needed. Just a little brain. Provided are a plethora of solipsisms, a brain-bypass, and never is oxygen necessary. Television-movies are a new stupor mundi with profound apologies to Emperor Frederick II, although television/movies really do constitute an imperialistic shadow government.

In these electronic-celluloid presentations is little spirit and less uplifting. Even when ascendant, the passivity (of continually being a spectator to a non-event) renders one stagnant rather than vibrant. Minds are kidnapped without coming to know anything. And all become the "dead" living. No longer death by the sword but by flickering lights. Viewers are kept "busy" doing nothing! Self-determination is replaced by the glitzy sexualized theatrics of some actors. As a whimpering carcass or an inactive drone, "being" becomes nonbeing drooling to be waited upon — no more an ACTIVE BEING savoring the divine substance in which we are engulfed.

Entertainment has become "excitement" easily adapted to, so that the more gross is always needed to achieve and to maintain the quick-feeling-change-of-state known as "excitement." The repetitive compulsive euphoria seeking of pleasure-pain "excitement" IS itself an addiction if not a "disease." Excitement is the name; disgust-illumination is the game. Despiritualization is the reign.

Furthermore, electronic-celluloid culture is not committed to Truth or Love. Its content is, from start to finish, marketing hyperbole. All of it. It is un-(if not anti-)intellectual. Television and movies abandon the intellect for *feelings* which is an old disease known as Gnosticism (the psychological basis for any form of Gnosticism is "the willful replacement of knowledge by feelings" and nothing is more dogmatic than "I feel..______.").

By promoting any and all feelings, television and movies promote the pagan old. The dissent from the intellect and the regression into feelings "bottom out" to Satanism after an exciting, flighty spiral through prevaricating "delights" masquerading as liberty. "I feel this way therefore . . ." is the operative paradigm to the ignoring of knowledge and the intellect. This is the theme which pervades all television and movies (and, to a great extent, print journalism).

Electronic-celluloid experiences are the antithesis of the "true light that enlightens all who come into the world" (from the "Last Gospel"). Indeed, when the world is filtered through television-movies, despiritualization and materialism predominate.

The impact on viewers is immense and coincides with the lessening of not only religious vocations but of genuine spirituality. It is as though reality itself no longer matters . . . .Reality is being coopted by flashing lights and feelings.

The next time you watch television, just ask yourself: "What is really happening to me when I watch this?" Rarely can an honest answer be other than "Nothing — absolutely nothing."

You cannot know *yourself*, examine *yourself*, or even be true to *yourself* watching television or movies because most frequently you are a *nothing* at that time except a non-spiritual absorber of light and feelings.

In summary, the electronic-celluloid culture obliterates being which renders its most common use as fundamentally anti-Spiritual, anti-natural law, and anti-Catholic.

The following suggestions are offered and counter the anti-Catholicism of the electronic-celluloid culture.

1. Gently belittle both television and movies by word and deed. Keep a running commentary: "This is stupid." "This is a waste of time." "This is nothing but a fluorescent light show." "There is nothing real here, just photons" and "Do you enjoy staring at lights?" "Getting embalmed?" "This is not recreation — `recreation' means you are doing something," and so on. Belittle television and movies gently, recognizing that the technology is magnificent, but dependency on and apotheosis of the content, the light source, and the time spent watching are negative and not real. More important activities await completion if one wants to be an active member of the human race.
2. Firmly enjoy activities detached from television-movies. Work actively at anything and bring the kids. Plunge into whatever with everyone helping and positive rewards distributed for participating and completing. Complete tasks together and savor a source of achievement — something never possible as a spectator watching television or a movie. Never get a room with a T.V. set when traveling.

3. Develop alternatives to keep everyone busy — from chores to recreational activities. Savor activity. Prohibit television for those under eight years of age and then very careful selection of programming thereafter.
4. Always diminish the credibility of television and movies by "unperturbed" amusement at it all. Diminish the celebrities — The evening news reporter? He is just an entertainer who can read." (This is not only true, but it also applies to almost all celebrities on television and in movies.) Talk about news and programs as being "staged" and "artificial" and "not real." Emphasize all television and movies as: superficial, unbalanced, inaccurate, and sensational salesmanship. Even with truth present, doubt it until confirmed objectively by something other than television. Believe nothing from Hollywood, from electronic moguls, and even from journalism! Demand confirmation in all that you do with youths to help them understand that television and movies (and most newspapers) rarely deserve believing. "Scorn" is not a bad word to describe the proper attitude to cope with the tyranny of electronic-celluloid-print journalism.
5. Since television and movies are so infused with sexuality, this dimension of human existence as presented in television-movies must also be "mocked" by *unperturbed amusement* at it all. A calm, composed (bored?) attitude is more important than what is said: "What they show, do, and suggest about sexual activity differs only by perfume from what was done 10,000 years ago in caves, and this is neither progress nor civilization. Regardless of what you see and hear, sex is not happiness." These are messages to convey with amused composure about whatever titillating is seen or read about.
6. Reinforce the *intellect* over *feelings*. "This junk on television and movies sure makes you feel different. Aren't you glad that feelings are not facts?" "Aren't you glad that feelings are not knowledge?" "This is just a bunch of feelings unrelated to reality." "I feel, therefore I am? . . .Baloney!" Emphasize that feelings and impulses never mastered anything. Emphasize that feelings and impulses are never mastered by other feelings and impulses but by intellect and virtues.
7. Youth needs to grasp the ridiculousness of the unreality of the electronic-celluloid-print culture. Ninety-five percent of it is utter garbage. Youths must be told this over and over to save them from the disaster of not realizing how unreal is most of what they see and read. Truly: "Television, movies, and newspapers are hazardous to your health, and the only group deeply striving for truth and love is the Roman Catholic Church." In other words, provide intellectual faith messages.

Because of the despiritualization, anti-intellectual and anti-natural law trends of television, movies, and commercial journalism, any discussion of contemporary communication must be in the category of anti-Catholicism.

Index

A

B

C

D

F

G

H

I

J

K

M

O

P

Q

R

S

T

U

V

W

Y

Z

SCRIPTURE PASSAGES QUOTED

John